CN00939904

TEAM PHYSICIAN MANUAL

The FIMS *Team Physician Manual* is the official sports medicine handbook of the International Federation of Sports Medicine (FIMS), the world's oldest sports medicine organization. Now in a fully revised and updated third edition, the book offers a complete guide to the background knowledge, practical techniques and professional skills required to become a successful medical practitioner working in sport.

Well illustrated, with clear step-by-step guidance, plus text boxes and checklists for quick reference, the *Team Physician Manual* covers every key area of activity and intervention, from the pre-participation examination to rehabilitation. The book surveys every classification of sports injury, offering clear advice on fieldside assessment, diagnosis and treatment, as well as examining best practice in general aspects of sports medicine, such as prevention and the psychology of injury. Written by a team of world-leading physicians from North and South America, Europe, Africa and Asia, this book is a 'must have' reference for any doctor, physical therapist, or medical professional working in sport.

Lyle J. Micheli is Clinical Professor of Orthopaedic Surgery, Harvard Medical School, and O'Donnell Family Professor of Orthopaedic Sports Medicine and Director of Division of Sports Medicine, Children's Hospital Boston, USA. He is Secretary General of FIMS.

Fabio Pigozzi is Professor of Internal Medicine and Deputy Rector of the University of Rome. He is the President of FIMS.

Kai-Ming Chan is Chair, Professor and Chief of Service, Department of Orthopaedics and Traumatology, Prince of Wales Hospital, The Chinese University of Hong Kong, and a past President of FIMS, 2002–6.

Walter R. Frontera is Professor of Physical Medicine and Rehabilitation and Professor of Physiology, School of Medicine, University of Puerto Rico. He is a past President of FIMS.

Norbert Bachl is Dean of the Faculty for Sports Science and Professor of Exercise Physiology at the University of Vienna, Austria. He is Vice President of FIMS.

Angela D. Smith is Clinical Associate Professor of Orthopaedic Surgery, University of Pennsylvania School of Medicine, and former President of the American College of Sports Medicine (ACSM). She is a member of FIMS' Education Commission.

S. Talia Alenabi is Secretary General of the Iran Sports Medicine Federation and a member of FIMS' Executive Committee.

TEAM PHYSICIAN MANUAL

International Federation of Sports Medicine (FIMS)

EDITED BY
LYLE J. MICHELI, FABIO PIGOZZI,
KAI-MING CHAN, WALTER R. FRONTERA,
NORBERT BACHL, ANGELA D. SMITH,
and S. TALIA ALENABI

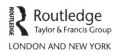 Routledge
Taylor & Francis Group

LONDON AND NEW YORK

First published 2013
by Routledge
2 Park Square, Milton Park, Abingdon, Oxon OX14 4RN

Simultaneously published in the USA and Canada
by Routledge
711 Third Avenue, New York, NY 10017

Routledge is an imprint of the Taylor & Francis Group, an informa business

British Library Cataloguing in Publication Data
A catalogue record for this book is available from the British Library

Library of Congress Cataloging in Publication Data
Team physician manual: FIMS International Federation of Sports Medicine/edited by Lyle Micheli . . . [et al.]. – 3rd ed.
  p. cm.
  Rev. ed. of: FIMS sports medicine manual/senior editor,
  David O'Sullivan McDonagh; editors, Lyle J. Micheli . . . [et al.].
  Includes bibliographical references.
  1. Sports medicine – International cooperation. 2. Sports injuries.
  I. Micheli, Lyle J., 1940– II. International Federation of Sports
  Medicine. III. FIMS sports medicine manual.
  RC1210.F56 2012b
  617.1'027–dc23
  2012016376

ISBN: 978–0–415–50532–1
ISBN: 978–0–415–50533–8
ISBN: 978–0–203–12777–3

Typeset in Zapf Humanist 601 and Eras
by Florence Production Ltd, Stoodeigh, Devon EX16 9PN

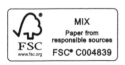

Printed and bound in Great Britain by the MPG Books Group

CONTENTS

V

contents

ILLUSTRATIONS

FIGURES

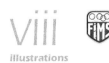

viii

illustrations

xi

illustrations

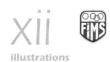

illustrations

illustrations

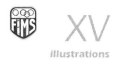

TABLES

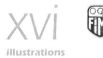

XVi

illustrations

illustrations

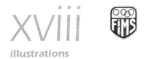

XVIII

illustrations

CONTRIBUTORS

S. Talia Alenabi, MD, MSc (Sports Medicine), is Secretary General of the Iran Sports Medicine Federation and a member of FIMS' Executive Committee.

Julia Alleyne, MD, is Associate Professor, University of Toronto, Department of Family and Community Medicine; Chair, Sport and Exercise Medicine Fellowship; Chair, Education Commission, FIMS 2010–14; CMO, Canadian Olympic Committee, London 2012 Olympic Games.

James R. Andrews, MD, is Medical Director, American Sports Medicine Institute, Medical Director for Intercollegiate Sports at Auburn University, Senior Orthopaedic Consultant at the University of Alabama, Senior Orthopaedic Consultant for the Washington Redskins (NFL).

Norbert Bachl, MD, is Professor, Centre for Sports Science and University Sports, Department of Sports and Physiological Performance, University of Vienna.

Paolo Borrione, MD, Department of Health Sciences, Internal Medicine Unit, University of Rome.

Michelle Burke, MD, is Assistant Professor of Pediatrics, Northeast Ohio Medical University, Sports Medicine Center.

Kai-Ming Chan, is Chair, Professor, and Chief of Service, Department of Orthopaedics and Traumatology, Prince of Wales Hospital, The Chinese University of Hong Kong, President of FIMS, 2002–6.

Eduardo Henrique De Rose, MD, PhD, is Chair, Professor of Sports Medicine, University of Rio Grande do Sul, President of FIMS 1994–2002.

Wayne Derman is Professor of Sport and Exercise Medicine, IOC Research Centre, Cape Town, FIFA Medical Centre of Excellence.

Neil Dilworth, MD, is a 2012 Sport and Exercise Fellow Graduate, University of Toronto.

Sheila A. Dugan, MD, is Associate Professor, Department of Physical Medicine and Rehabilitation, Rush Medical College, Chicago.

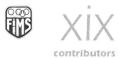

Emin Ergen is Sports Medicine Specialist, Ankara University School of Medicine; Head of Sports Medicine Department, Cebeci, Ankara, Turkey.

Nicholas A. Evans, FRCS(Orth); Consultant Orthopaedic Surgeon

Avery D. Faigenbaum is Professor of Sport and Exercise Medicine, FIMS Executive Committee; Director, IOC Research Centre, Capetown; Director, FIFA Medical Centre of Excellence.

Walter R. Frontera, MD, PhD, is Professor and Chair, Department of Physical Medicine and Rehabilitation, Vanderbilt University School of Medicine; President of FIMS 2006–10.

Peter G. Gerbino, MD, is Chief, Division of Orthopedics, Chairman, Department of Surgery, Community Hospital of the Monterey Peninsula.

Farzin Halabchi, MD, MSc (Sports Medicine), Tehran Medical Sience University, Sports Medicine Research Center, Tehran.

Thomas C. Kim, MD, is Orthopedic Surgeon, Nevada Orthopedic and Spine Center.

Trisha Leahy, PhD, is Chief Executive, Hong Kong Sports Institute.

Keith J. Loud, MDCM, MSc, FAAP, Visiting Associate Professor of Pediatrics, Dartmouth Medical School; Chief, Section of General Academic Pediatrics.

Anthony C. Luke, MD, MPH, is Associate Professor of Clinical Orthopedics, University of California, San Francisco; Director, UCSF Primary Care Sports Medicine; Director, UCSF Human Performance Center.

Oriol Martinez Ferrer is Chairperson, Medical Committee International Paralympic Committee; Facultat Blanquerna, Universitat Ramon Llull, Barcelona, Spain.

Lyle J. Micheli, MD, is Clinical Professor of Orthopaedic Surgery, Harvard Medical School; O'Donnell Familiy Professor of Orthopaedic Sports Medicine; Director of Division of Sports Medicine, Children's Hospital, Boston, Massachusetts.

Marco Michelucci is Sports Physician, Sao Paulo Training and Research Olympic Center 2008–10, Sao Paulo, Brazil, FIFA Medical/Doping Control Officer.

Konstantinos I. Natsis, MD, is Associate Professor, Orthopaedic Surgeon, Director of Anatomy, Medical School, Aristotle University of Thessaloniki; EC member FIMS and EFSMA; Honorary President of Sports Medicine Association of Greece; President of Orthopaedic and Traumatology Association of Macedonia, 2011–12.

Margaret L. Olmedo, MD, is Associate Professor, Department of Orthopaedic Surgery, Louisiana State University Health Science Center, Shreveport.

Dzovig S. Parsehian, ATC, The Children's Hospital of Philadelphia, Department of Orthopedics, Sports Medicine and Performance Center.

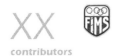

XX

contributors

Fabio Pigozzi, MD, is President, FIMS; Full Professor and Director, Internal Medicine Unit, Department of Health and Sciences of the University of Rome.

Pia Pit-Grosheide is Scientific Study Coordinator, International Paralympic Committee.

Per A.F.H. Renström is Professor Emeritus of Sports Medicine, Karolinska Institutet, Stockholm, Sweden.

Marta Rizzo, MD, Department of Health Sciences, Internal Medicine Unit, University of Rome.

Christer G. Rolf, MD, PhD, is Professor of Sports Medicine, Consultant Orthopaedic Surgeon, Executive Director, Sheffield Centre of Sports Medicine, The University of Sheffield.

Jaspal S. Sandhu, MD, is Dean, Faculty of Sports Medicine, Guru Nanak Dev University, Amritsar, India; Secretary General, Asian Federation of Sports Medicine; Member, Education Commission, FIMS; Immediate Past President, Indian Association of Sports Medicine.

Martin P. Schwellnus, MD, Professor of Sport and Exercise Medicine, FIMS Executive Committee; Director, IOC Research Centre, Capetown; Director, FIFA Medical Centre of Excellence.

Shweta Shenoy, PhD, Associate Professor, Faculty of Sports Medicine and Physiotherapy, Guru Nanak Dev University Amritsar, India; Secretary General, Indian Association of Sports Medicine.

Angela D. Smith, MD, Attending Faculty, Sports Medicine and Performance Center, Children's Hospital of Philadelphia, Past President of the American College of Sports Medicine (ACSM).

William D. Stanish, MD, is Professor of Surgery, Dalhousie University Division of Orthopaedic Surgery; Director of Orthopaedic and Sports Medicine Clinic of Nova Scotia.

Marcus Van Aarsen, Med III, Dalhousie University Division of Orthopaedic Surgery.

Peter Van de Vliet is Medical and Scientific Director, International Paralympic Committee, Bonn, Germany; Professional Affiliate Health, Leisure and Human Performance Research Institute, Faculty of Kinesiology and Recreation Management, University of Manitoba, Canada.

Debra Wein, MS, is President, Wellness Workdays; Assistant Professor/Lecturer, Massachusetts General Hospital.

James A. Whiteside, MD, was Team Physician, Penn State University (retired), Founder, Primary Care Sports Medicine Fellowship, American Sports Medicine Institute (retired), Team Physician, Troy University (retired).

contributors

FOREWORD

I am very pleased to contribute a message to an editorial initiative as important as the third edition of the *Team Physician Manual*.

As President of the International Federation of Sports Medicine (FIMS), and on behalf of the FIMS Executive Committee and all Standing Commissions, my thanks and congratulations go to the editors of this excellent resource: Lyle J. Micheli, Kai-Ming Chan, Walter R. Frontera, Norbert Bachl, Angela D. Smith, and S. Talia Alenabi.

FIMS focuses on educational initiatives with the objective of promoting continuous professional development. In fact, this very book has its origins in the FIMS Team Physician Development Course, which was inaugurated over two decades ago. It is still used as the textbook for these important courses, which are held regularly in different parts of the world. In many instances, FIMS provides the only opportunity for members of the local medical and health community to become qualified to provide care for local sports teams and events.

All of us at FIMS are very proud of this expanded and enhanced iteration of the *Team Physician Manual*, and we trust our vision will continue to be embraced by the broader sports medicine fraternity throughout the world.

Professor Fabio Pigozzi MD
President, FIMS

PREFACE

We are very pleased to introduce this third edition of the FIMS *Team Physician Manual* to our fellow sports medicine practitioners.

Since the first edition was published in 2001, this text has more than doubled in size, which reflects the rapid growth of knowledge in our specialty.

The field of sports and exercise medicine encompasses a wide range of disciplines and interests. Nonetheless, when a physician is in the role of team physician, there is a defined body of knowledge they must master, whatever their background, initial training, or present medical practice, in order to best serve the needs of the athletes under their care. It was the charge of each of our authors to refine information from their particular field of expertise to emphasize the information that would be most useful for team physicians.

This text continues to serve as the primary resource for the FIMS Team Physician Development Course. As such, it is meant to serve as an entry-level curriculum for team physicians and sports medicine providers.

We now know that many sports medicine practitioners also use this text as a resource when they are called upon to serve as team physicians at local, regional, or international competitions.

We have tried to make this third edition as timely and accurate as is possible in this age of electronic medicine. However, we remind our readers that this is an introduction to the subject matter. We recommend that team physicians use this book as a preparation for more advanced training in this subspecialty.

Our primary responsibility as team physicians is the medical welfare of the athletes in our charge. Happily, there is no conflict between sports safety and sports performance. A welcome by-product of the efforts of a qualified, responsible team physician is the enhanced performance of our athletes.

Better health through sports remains the primary goal of all who participate in the Olympic movement.

Lyle J. Micheli, *Secretary General, FIMS*
Fabio Pigozzi, *President, FIMS*
Kai-Ming Chan, *Past President, FIMS*
Walter R. Frontera, *Past and Honorary President, FIMS*
Norbert Bachl, *First Vice President, FIMS*
Angela D. Smith, *Past Chair, Education Commission*
S. Talia Alenabi, *Executive Committee, FIMS*

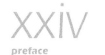

PART I

**SPORTS MEDICINE FOR
THE TEAM PHYSICIAN**

CHAPTER 1

THE MODERN-DAY TEAM PHYSICIAN

Roles, responsibilities, and required qualifications

William D. Stanish, Marcus Van Aarsen, and Nicholas A. Evans

As the international world of sport grows and evolves, so too does the field of sports medicine, and with participation rates in sport on the rise there is an expanding list of countries producing world-class athletes. Modern-day athletes span age groups like never before, and a significant portion of them are recreational athletes who expect that their participation in sport will not adversely affect their day-to-day lives. Consequently, the sports medicine physician continues to play an increasingly important role in the diagnosis and treatment of athletic injuries, injury prevention, and maintenance of general health, as well as optimizing athletic performance through proper training, nutrition, and lifestyle. The health status of an elite athlete is often of such high profile that there is a great onus on the team physician to operate at an elite level by managing the interests of patients, teams, the media, and, unfortunately at times, the legal system.

The modern-day care of athletes requires a broad range of professionals, and as a result the sports medicine physician has an unprecedented level of responsibility to oversee the many aspects of care that an athlete may receive, and must have the ability to communicate effectively in order to ensure optimal outcomes for patients. Moreover, communication skills are essential for properly informing coaches, agents, parents, and other interested parties about the health status of an athlete.

As various sports have dramatically different rules, strategies, cultures, and hazards, there is a tendency for some physicians to become experts in the coverage of a specific sport while maintaining proficiency in all areas of sports medicine. This career path is often fueled by the personal commitment to a team or a sport felt by a physician, and is a testament to the uniqueness and passion that the world of sport provides.

DUTIES OF A TEAM PHYSICIAN

The team physician plays a dynamic role that changes with the time of the season, the location, and the facilities available. Duties in the early season largely consist of health and fitness screening, optimizing of training and nutrition, and other preventative-medicine strategies. The heavy training season requires more management of sports injuries and a mental focus on maintaining motivation, while competition necessitates that the team physician handle many different aspects of athletic care in order to optimize performance and health.

To truly understand their role within each sport, the team physician must possess, not only a strong medical knowledge, but also an understanding of the rules, risks, and culture of the sport. Team physicians must make every effort to ensure that they are available to their athletes pre-, post-, and during competition, as well as after hours. During events that span days or weeks, physicians must keep social and personal commitments to a minimum to ensure that they are available to their team in times of need.

Responsibilities of the team physician include:

- pre-participation health screening and examination;
- assessment and management of athletic injuries both on the field and fieldside;
- triage;
- immediate and long-term management of athletic injuries;
- coordination of athlete's rehabilitation and return-to-play;
- counseling of athletes on proper training and nutrition habits to maintain health;
- ongoing observation of chronic pre-existing medical conditions;
- condemning the use of artificial performance enhancement and counseling athletes on substance abuse;
- staying current with the medical knowledge of the field and upgrading skills as necessary;
- integration of knowledge with other athletic and medical professionals to maximize the quality of care to the team and its athletes.

Having a physician who travels to competitions with a team is a luxury for most amateur sport teams, but a necessity for elite international competition. When traveling with a team and practicing in a foreign venue, there is added responsibility on the team physician to assure the team of safe and fair competition. Additional roles while "on the road" include:

- Preparation for travel: Team members must be aware of the health implications of international travel and be counseled on ways to avoid jet lag as well as other conditions that may be caused by long-term immobility. This education may occur well in advance of travel.

4

- Pre-competition site visit: The team physician should arrive at the competition venue well in advance to look for any potential hazards to athletes during competition, as well as plan and understand the logistics of medical services available at the event and any barriers that may arise. Will the team physician have immediate access to an athlete injured in the field of play? Will there be any barriers to emergency vehicles accessing the venue? Where is the nearest hospital? There may also be other environmental or social hazards in the vicinity that should be considered to keep athletes safe after hours.
- Preparation for medical practice: Many of the resources a team physician will rely on during international competition will come from home, making preparations before travel essential. The team physician should be involved in selecting the medical team, as well as selecting the proper amount of staff to ensure a high standard of care without being overstaffed and causing athletes to be "overdoctored." The medical team should meet prior to travel to delegate foreseen tasks and establish a line of communication between team members. Medical equipment and traveling pharmacy should remain in the care of the team physician, and any substances banned from competitors should be kept to a minimum.
- Event coverage: Effective communication with all medical staff, coaches, athletes, and team officials is paramount during the excitement of competition. Be prepared to treat, educate, advocate for, and listen to the athletes. This is when athletes will experience their highest highs (victory) and lowest lows (defeat or injury). Athletes may also be subject to drug testing at this time. The team physician must be prepared for this by understanding policies and procedures of these tests and being aware of his or her role in the proceedings. Patient confidentiality is to be maintained at all times.
- Finally, the mobile nature of the team physician's practice while traveling should not distract from the necessity of proper documentation of medical occurrences. This will help clarify the status of the athlete during competition and will aid in medical debriefing and continued follow-up of athletes upon their return home.

Considering the amount of time that a physician may spend with a team, it is understandable and invaluable that they feel integrated into the team atmosphere. However, although it is rewarding to feel like part of the team, it is important to keep one's professional role clear. The conduct and dress of a team physician should reflect that of a medical professional rather than a teammate.

CREDENTIALS AND QUALIFICATIONS

The primary concern of the team physician is to provide the best medical care for athletes at all levels of participation. To this end, the following qualifications are necessary for all team physicians:

- have an M.D. or D.O. in good standing, with an unrestricted license to practice medicine;
- possess a fundamental knowledge of emergency care regarding sporting events;
- be trained in CPR;
- have a working knowledge of trauma, musculoskeletal injuries, and medical conditions affecting the athlete.

In addition, it is desirable for team physicians to have clinical training/experience and administrative skills in some or all of the following:

- Specialty Board certification;
- continuing medical education in sports medicine;
- formal training in sports medicine (fellowship training, board-recognized subspecialty in sports medicine (formerly known as a certificate of added qualification in sports medicine));
- additional training in sports medicine;
- 50% or more of practice involving sports medicine;
- membership and participation in a sports medicine society;
- involvement in teaching, research, and publications relating to sports medicine;
- training in advanced cardiac life support;
- knowledge of medical/legal, disability, and workers' compensation issues;
- media-skills training.

There is no single career recipe for becoming an exceptional team physician, as there are many different paths one can take to reach the same level of expertise. Similarly, continuing education will necessarily vary for physicians who cover different sports. The conditions that will be treated most often in weightlifters will be dramatically different from those seen most often in long-distance runners, for example. Consequently, it is good practice to stay current in the sports medicine field as a whole, while maintaining a strong expertise in the sport(s) that will be covered most often.

There are many resources available for physicians to access for continuing education in sports medicine. The FIMS, International Olympic Committee, and the American College of Sports Medicine are excellent resources for accessing ongoing educational programs and meetings.

CODE OF ETHICS

Although the range of duties performed by a team physician is broad, all actions are governed by a core responsibility to "First, do no harm." The team physician must always abide by the regulations of the medical profession and of the sport's governing body.

6

The FIMS and sports medicine physicians throughout the world have embraced the following comprehensive code of ethics. The team physician must:

- always make the health of the athlete a priority;
- understand the medical knowledge in the field being overseen;
- maintain patient confidentiality;
- obtain informed consent;
- not refuse an athlete the right to make their own medical decisions;
- oppose practices that may jeopardize the health of an athlete;
- oppose the use of artificial performance enhancement;
- educate on the health benefits of physical activity;
- not delegate medical decisions to others;
- not allow medical decisions to be influenced by third parties;
- not allow prejudice to bias medical judgment;
- work collaboratively within an interprofessional setting.

The vast majority of team physicians model their careers admirably on this code of ethics, while a minority participate in condemnable practices, such as the promotion or provision of performance-enhancing drugs. There is still ethical debate regarding some practices, notably the administration of local pain masking for the purpose of competition.

LITIGATION

Sports medicine is not detached from the unfortunate trend of lawsuits that has emerged in modern medicine, and the high stakes that are often involved in an elite athlete remaining healthy or being cleared to compete can intensify the litigious element of the profession. Avoiding and combating litigation in this field requires both upstanding practice and an eye for detail.

Although a physician must always ensure that his or her medical liability insurance is in good standing, special consideration must be given to the unique situations in which a sports medicine physician may be involved. Does the insurance policy cover medical practice in a foreign country? Will caring for foreign athletes be covered? Officials? Coaches? Spectators? Special consideration may also be required for coverage of vulnerable populations, such as young or disabled athletes.

A significant strategy for avoiding litigation is inspecting and understanding the medical insurance policies of every individual or group for whom the physician will be providing care. Ensure that the medical insurance of all athletes is in good standing, and be aware of the benefits that may be important for competition at a given venue or country. Beyond standard life and critical-injury insurance, valuable benefits may include coverage of medications or hospitalizations in a foreign country or medical transport within a country or back to the athlete's home country.

There will never be a substitute for the best weapon against litigation: caring for one's patients with skill and compassion. Proper, honest, respectful care leaves little room for the legal system to enter the medical clinic.

MEDIA RELATIONS

Media coverage has become a seemingly ubiquitous component of elite athletics, and with modern technology this coverage has the ability to spread worldwide in a matter of seconds. The pressure from issuing a statement to the media can seem daunting, but with some preparation media interaction can be a positive experience. Training is available and highly recommended for any physician working within elite athletics.

The team physician may be interviewed in positive times (victory) or negative times (serious injury, doping, etc.), but there are guiding principles that must always frame a physician's interaction with the media. Most importantly, an athlete's confidentiality must always be respected. No medical details are to be provided to the media without explicit consent from the athlete, and possibly from the coach or the team. Parental consent is another factor in confidentiality when underage athletes are involved. Even once consent has been obtained, the parties mentioned above have the right to rescind their consent at a later time.

Although the role of the team physician in addressing the media is usually quite clear, this role in amateur athletics tends to be less defined. Before starting with any new team, amateur or professional, a physician should clarify his or her role in media interaction.

Even when the proper medical statements have been issued to the media, there is still the chance of being misquoted or of statements being taken out of context. Although clear, concise communication is the best means of ensuring accurate reporting, there are other strategies that can be employed in order to ensure that the proper message is conveyed. Team physicians will often reserve the right to read a written article before it is published to ensure the proper statement and context are conveyed.

The field of sports medicine is unique and exciting, and sport culture strongly promotes camaraderie and a sense of belonging. Although the commitment may be large and the practice full of unique challenges, devotion to the sport and the well-being of its athletes ensures the team physician of a successful and fulfilling career.

ACKNOWLEDGMENTS

Portions of this manuscript are reprinted with permission of the Project Based Alliance for the Advancement of Clinical Sports Medicine, 2000. The code of ethics contained within this manuscript is an abbreviated reproduction of the code of ethics of the FIMS.

SUGGESTED READING

Brown D.W. Medical issues associated with international competition. *Clin. Sports Med.* 1998; 17:739–54.

Brukner P., Khan K. *Clinical Sports Medicine*. 3rd ed. Sydney: McGraw-Hill; 2007.

The Encyclopedia of Sports Medicine of the International Olympic Committee's Medical Commission. Vol. 6. Oxford, England: Blackwell Science; 1996.

Howe W.B. The Team Physician. *Primary Care* 1991; 18:763–75. *Oxford Textbook of Sports Medicine*. 2nd ed. New York: Oxford University Press; 1996.

Konin J.G. Behind the scenes as a team physician. *Clin. Sports Med.* 2007; 26(2).

Olympic Movement Medical Code. International Olympic Committee Medical Comission; 2009. www.olympic.org/PageFiles/61597/Olympic_Movement_Medical_Code_eng.pdf

Schwellnus M. *The Olympic Textbook of Medicine in Sport*. Chichester, England: Wiley-Blackwell; 2008.

CHAPTER 2

THE PRE-PARTICIPATION EXAMINATION

A cornerstone of sports injury prevention

Lyle J. Micheli

One of the most significant recent developments in sports medicine, especially in the care of young athletes, is that of more comprehensive pre-participation examinations (sometimes called pre-participation screenings), and the increased use of them in preventing sports injuries. Although pre-participation examinations have long been required for school and sometimes community-based sports, such an evaluation was often little more than a "physical," with scant attention paid to the specific or excessive demands that a particular sport places on the athlete. Physicians involved in the care of young athletes now agree that the pre-participation examination is a vital component of sports care. The main goals of pre-participation examination are to assess overall health, detect conditions that may cause injury, detect conditions that may disqualify the athlete from participating in certain sports, assess fitness for the chosen sport, and make recommendations for the exercise program.

In recent years, there has been increased emphasis on using the pre-participation examination for cardiovascular screening to prevent sudden cardiac death (SCD), and so, while this chapter provides an overview of the pre-participation examination, the following chapter will address in depth the importance of cardiac screening as an indispensable tool for preventing SCD in athletes.

TYPES OF PRE-PARTICIPATION EXAMINATION

There are two main types of pre-participation examination – the one-on-one examination of the athlete by an individual doctor, and the station-type, en masse version. Advantages of the personalized examination are that the athlete potentially receives a more detailed assessment, as well as a continuity of care if he/she has been seen by the same doctor. In such circumstances, it is also easier for the physician to take a complete history and discuss sensitive issues with the athlete,

 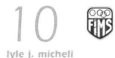

especially when the patient is young, and the examining physician is his/her primary care physician. The most obvious shortcoming of the one-on-one examination is that the examining primary care physician may be relatively unfamiliar with the special demands placed by the sport in question. If the physician has received little, if any, sports medicine training, the examination will probably be little more than a general medical examination.

The station-type examination has the advantage of involving more specialized personnel, including physicians with expertise in a particular sport, athletics trainers, nutritionists, physical therapists, and exercise physiologists. This type of examination is cost-effective and more expeditious for large groups of athletes, and allows performance testing to be offered at the same time.

In a school or community-based sports setting, where local primary care physicians are included in the station-type examination and a private room is set aside for individual consultation, the benefits of both types of pre-participation examination can be achieved.

COMPONENTS OF THE PRE-PARTICIPATION EXAMINATION

In addition to the basal fitness of the athlete, the pre-participation examination should also measure his/her fitness for an individual sport. For instance, when examining a swimmer or tennis player, the physician should check the range of motion in the shoulders – restricted range of motion in the shoulder may predispose swimmers and tennis players to injuries in that area. Runners, on the other hand, need flexibility in the lower back, hip flexors, and hamstrings, or they may sustain injuries in those areas.

When done properly, a pre-participation examination should consist of a medical history, a general medical health evaluation, an anatomical review, a flexibility musculoskeletal examination, and an equipment review. All the components of the examination, including the assessment of body composition, cardiovascular endurance, strength, and flexibility, are important, but the most important components are the medical history and the physical examination.

PRE-PARTICIPATION EXAMINATION GOALS

- Assess overall health.
- Detect conditions that might cause injury.
- Detect conditions that may disqualify the athlete from participating in certain sports.
- Assess fitness for the chosen sport.
- Make recommendations for the exercise program.

Medical history

The medical history is extremely important because it alerts the examining physician to previous illnesses, injuries, and operations that may have a significant bearing on fitness for sports and fitness activities. Well over half the problems athletes encounter can be identified in the history. A common example of a serious or hidden injury that the medical history can reveal is an undiagnosed fracture of the carpal navicular bone in the wrist. Many people dismiss wrist pain, but, in fact, if a carpal navicular bone fracture is undiagnosed, it can have serious arthritic consequences in later life. Because of the importance of the medical history, it is essential to complete the medical history form (Table 2.1) accurately.

The medical history is also extremely important to screen for athletes with a pre-disposing cardiac condition, as described in detail in the following chapter.

It is imperative that the medical history form be available to the athlete for completion well before the actual pre-participation evaluation. Ideally, the coaches or athletic trainer will pass out the forms to the team at least one month before the examination and return the completed forms to the examining physicians at least one week before the examination. One or more physicians involved in the examination process will then have the opportunity to review the medical histories and highlight areas of concern for individual athletes.

Physical examinations

Numerous resources have addressed the cardiovascular component of the physical examination. Without good cardiovascular endurance, fatigue-related injuries such as sprained ankles and twisted knees are more likely to occur. Good cardiovascular endurance is also important for preventing heart and lung disease. The physical examination provides an opportunity to screen for underlying problems that might precipitate cardiac events, as described in the following chapter. Attention should also be given to assessing the strength of muscles and bones, and the flexibility of muscles, ligaments, and joints (Table 2.2).

Most sports injuries result from musculoskeletal problems; the physical examination should therefore include a review of joint function, range of motion, and areas of pain (Figures 2.1 A–N). Restricted range of motion in joints, tight muscles, and lack of muscle strength will create problems for the athlete. The risk of injury increases when there is less flexibility – during dynamic activity, sudden stretching of a tight-ligamented joint, such as a knee or ankle, or the tight muscles crossing that joint may result in injury to the joint or muscle.

Anatomical factors that may predispose the athlete to overuse injury include leg-length discrepancies, bowed legs, knock-knees, hyperextended knees, curvature of the spine, and malalignment of the pelvis.

PHYSICAL EXAMINATION

- Along with medical history, physical examination is the most important component of pre-participation examination.
- Focus not only on cardiovascular endurance, but also on strength and flexibility.
- Lack of strength and flexibility is at the root of many sports injuries.
- Prescribe stretching and strengthening exercises to address deficits.

Table 2.1 Medical history form

■ PREPARTICIPATION PHYSICAL EVALUATION
HISTORY FORM

(Note: This form is to be filled out by the patient and parent prior to seeing the physician. The physician should keep this form in the chart.)

Date of Exam _____

Name _____ Date of birth _____

Sex _____ Age _____ Grade _____ School _____ Sport(s) _____

Medicines and Allergies: Please list all of the prescription and over-the-counter medicines and supplements (herbal and nutritional) that you are currently taking

Do you have any allergies? ☐ Yes ☐ No If yes, please identify specific allergy below.
☐ Medicines ☐ Pollens ☐ Food ☐ Stinging Insects

Explain "Yes" answers below. Circle questions you don't know the answers to.

GENERAL QUESTIONS	Yes	No	MEDICAL QUESTIONS	Yes	No
1. Has a doctor ever denied or restricted your participation in sports for any reason?			26. Do you cough, wheeze, or have difficulty breathing during or after exercise?		
2. Do you have any ongoing medical conditions? If so, please identify below: ☐ Asthma ☐ Anemia ☐ Diabetes ☐ Infections Other: _____			27. Have you ever used an inhaler or taken asthma medicine?		
			28. Is there anyone in your family who has asthma?		
3. Have you ever spent the night in the hospital?			29. Were you born without or are you missing a kidney, an eye, a testicle (males), your spleen, or any other organ?		
4. Have you ever had surgery?			30. Do you have groin pain or a painful bulge or hernia in the groin area?		
HEART HEALTH QUESTIONS ABOUT YOU	**Yes**	**No**	31. Have you had infectious mononucleosis (mono) within the last month?		
5. Have you ever passed out or nearly passed out DURING or AFTER exercise?			32. Do you have any rashes, pressure sores, or other skin problems?		
			33. Have you had a herpes or MRSA skin infection?		
6. Have you ever had discomfort, pain, tightness, or pressure in your chest during exercise?			34. Have you ever had a head injury or concussion?		
7. Does your heart ever race or skip beats (irregular beats) during exercise?			35. Have you ever had a hit or blow to the head that caused confusion, prolonged headache, or memory problems?		
8. Has a doctor ever told you that you have any heart problems? If so, check all that apply: ☐ High blood pressure ☐ A heart murmur ☐ High cholesterol ☐ A heart infection ☐ Kawasaki disease Other: ____			36. Do you have a history of seizure disorder?		
			37. Do you have headaches with exercise?		
			38. Have you ever had numbness, tingling, or weakness in your arms or legs after being hit or falling?		
9. Has a doctor ever ordered a test for your heart? (For example, ECG/EKG, echocardiogram)			39. Have you ever been unable to move your arms or legs after being hit or falling?		
10. Do you get lightheaded or feel more short of breath than expected during exercise?			40. Have you ever become ill while exercising in the heat?		
			41. Do you get frequent muscle cramps when exercising?		
11. Have you ever had an unexplained seizure?			42. Do you or someone in your family have sickle cell trait or disease?		
12. Do you get more tired or short of breath more quickly than your friends during exercise?			43. Have you had any problems with your eyes or vision?		
HEART HEALTH QUESTIONS ABOUT YOUR FAMILY	**Yes**	**No**	44. Have you had any eye injuries?		
13. Has any family member or relative died of heart problems or had an unexpected or unexplained sudden death before age 50 (including drowning, unexplained car accident, or sudden infant death syndrome)?			45. Do you wear glasses or contact lenses?		
			46. Do you wear protective eyewear, such as goggles or a face shield?		
14. Does anyone in your family have hypertrophic cardiomyopathy, Marfan syndrome, arrhythmogenic right ventricular cardiomyopathy, long QT syndrome, short QT syndrome, Brugada syndrome, or catecholaminergic polymorphic ventricular tachycardia?			47. Do you worry about your weight?		
			48. Are you trying to or has anyone recommended that you gain or lose weight?		
			49. Are you on a special diet or do you avoid certain types of foods?		
15. Does anyone in your family have a heart problem, pacemaker, or implanted defibrillator?			50. Have you ever had an eating disorder?		
			51. Do you have any concerns that you would like to discuss with a doctor?		
16. Has anyone in your family had unexplained fainting, unexplained seizures, or near drowning?			**FEMALES ONLY**		
			52. Have you ever had a menstrual period?		
BONE AND JOINT QUESTIONS	**Yes**	**No**	53. How old were you when you had your first menstrual period?		
17. Have you ever had an injury to a bone, muscle, ligament, or tendon that caused you to miss a practice or a game?			54. How many periods have you had in the last 12 months?		
18. Have you ever had any broken or fractured bones or dislocated joints?			**Explain "yes" answers here**		
19. Have you ever had an injury that required x-rays, MRI, CT scan, injections, therapy, a brace, a cast, or crutches?					
20. Have you ever had a stress fracture?					
21. Have you ever been told that you have or have you had an x-ray for neck instability or atlantoaxial instability? (Down syndrome or dwarfism)					
22. Do you regularly use a brace, orthotics, or other assistive device?					
23. Do you have a bone, muscle, or joint injury that bothers you?					
24. Do any of your joints become painful, swollen, feel warm, or look red?					
25. Do you have any history of juvenile arthritis or connective tissue disease?					

I hereby state that, to the best of my knowledge, my answers to the above questions are complete and correct.

Signature of athlete _____ Signature of parent/guardian _____ Date _____

Note: Reprinted with permission from © 1997 American Academy of Family Physicians, American Medical Society for Sports Medicine, American Orthopaedic Society of Sports Medicine, and American Osteopathic Academy of Sports Medicine.

lyle j. micheli

Special emphasis should be given to the ankles and knees because of the high incidence of injury to those areas. If an athlete exhibits a lack of strength or flexibility, which puts them at risk of injury in the chosen sport, he/she should be given a corrective training program before participating. The examining physician should provide exercise programs to help the athlete overcome particular problems.

Although the entire musculoskeletal system of every athlete should be comprehensively assessed, the medical history can direct special focus during the examination. Special attention should be given to an anatomical site that has been previously injured, especially when the chosen sport places special demands on that area.

The musculoskeletal examination should also measure the relative constitutional tightness or looseness of the athlete to address past injuries, as well as provide training recommendations for injury prevention. The relatively "loose" athlete is at increased risk of subluxations of the shoulder, patella, and peroneal tendon, whereas the constitutionally "tighter" athlete is more at risk for muscle tendon strains and apophyseal avulsions.

(A) Inspection, athlete standing, facing toward examiner (symmetry of trunk, upper extremities).
(B) Forward flexion, extension, rotation, lateral flexion of neck (range of motion, cervical spine).
(C) Resisted shoulder shrug (strength, trapezius).
(D) Resisted shoulder abduction (strength, deltoid).
(E) Internal and external rotation of shoulder (range of motion, glenohumeral joint).
(F) Extension and flexion of elbow (range of motion, elbow).
(G) Pronation and supination of elbow (range of motion, elbow and wrist).
(H) Clench fist, then spread fingers (range of motion, hand and fingers).
(I) Inspection, athlete facing away from examiner (symmetry of trunk, upper extremities).
(J) Back extension, knees straight (spondylolysis/spondylolisthesis).
(K) Back flexion with knees straight, facing toward and away from examiner (range of motion, thoracic and lumbosacral spine; spine curvature; hamstring flexibility).
(L) Inspection of lower extremities, contraction of quadriceps muscles (alignment, symmetry).
(M) "Duck walk" four steps (motion of hip, knee, and ankle; strength; balance).
(N) Standing on toes, then on heels (symmetry, calf; strength; balance).

Table 2.2 Physical examination form

PHYSICAL EXAMINATION FORM

Name _____ Date of birth _____

PHYSICIAN REMINDERS
1. Consider additional questions on more sensitive issues
   - Do you feel stressed out or under a lot of pressure?
   - Do you ever feel sad, hopeless, depressed, or anxious?
   - Do you feel safe at your home or residence?
   - Have you ever tried cigarettes, chewing tobacco, snuff, or dip?
   - During the past 30 days, did you use chewing tobacco, snuff, or dip?
   - Do you drink alcohol or use any other drugs?
   - Have you ever taken anabolic steroids or used any other performance supplement?
   - Have you ever taken any supplements to help you gain or lose weight or improve your performance?
   - Do you wear a seat belt, use a helmet, and use condoms?
2. Consider reviewing questions on cardiovascular symptoms (questions 5–14).

EXAMINATION					
Height		Weight	☐ Male ☐ Female		
BP / (/)		Pulse	Vision R 20/	L 20/	Corrected ☐ Y ☐ N

MEDICAL	NORMAL	ABNORMAL FINDINGS
Appearance • Marfan stigmata (kyphoscoliosis, high-arched palate, pectus excavatum, arachnodactyly, arm span > height, hyperlaxity, myopia, MVP, aortic insufficiency)		
Eyes/ears/nose/throat • Pupils equal • Hearing		
Lymph nodes		
Heart ᵃ • Murmurs (auscultation standing, supine, +/- Valsalva) • Location of point of maximal impulse (PMI)		
Pulses • Simultaneous femoral and radial pulses		
Lungs		
Abdomen		
Genitourinary (males only)ᵇ		
Skin • HSV, lesions suggestive of MRSA, tinea corporis		
Neurologic ᶜ		
MUSCULOSKELETAL		
Neck		
Back		
Shoulder/arm		
Elbow/forearm		
Wrist/hand/fingers		
Hip/thigh		
Knee		
Leg/ankle		
Foot/toes		
Functional • Duck-walk, single leg hop		

ᵃConsider ECG, echocardiogram, and referral to cardiology for abnormal cardiac history or exam.
ᵇConsider GU exam if in private setting. Having third party present is recommended.
ᶜConsider cognitive evaluation or baseline neuropsychiatric testing if a history of significant concussion.

☐ Cleared for all sports without restriction

☐ Cleared for all sports without restriction with recommendations for further evaluation or treatment for _____
_____

☐ Not cleared
  ☐ Pending further evaluation
  ☐ For any sports
  ☐ For certain sports _____
    Reason _____

Recommendations _____

I have examined the above-named student and completed the preparticipation physical evaluation. The athlete does not present apparent clinical contraindications to practice and participate in the sport(s) as outlined above. A copy of the physical exam is on record in my office and can be made available to the school at the request of the parents. If conditions arise after the athlete has been cleared for participation, the physician may rescind the clearance until the problem is resolved and the potential consequences are completely explained to the athlete (and parents/guardians).

Name of physician (print/type) _____ Date _____
Address _____ Phone _____
Signature of physician _____, MD or DO

Note: Reprinted with permission from © 1997 American Academy of Family Physicians, American Medical Society for Sport Medicine, American Orthopaedic Society of Sports Medicine, and American Osteopathic Academy of Sports Medicine.

lyle j. micheli

Table 2.2 continued

CLEARANCE FORM

Name _____ Sex ☐ M ☐ F Age _____ Date of birth _____

☐ Cleared for all sports without restriction

☐ Cleared for all sports without restriction with recommendations for further evaluation or treatment for _____

☐ Not cleared

    ☐ Pending further evaluation

    ☐ For any sports

    ☐ For certain sports _____

    Reason _____

Recommendations _____

_____

_____

_____

_____

_____

I have examined the above-named student and completed the preparticipation physical evaluation. The athlete does not present apparent clinical contraindications to practice and participate in the sport(s) as outlined above. A copy of the physical exam is on record in my office and can be made available to the school at the request of the parents. If conditions arise after the athlete has been cleared for participation, the physician may rescind the clearance until the problem is resolved and the potential consequences are completely explained to the athlete (and parents/guardians).

Name of physician (print/type) _____ Date _____

Address _____ Phone _____

Signature of physician _____, MD or DO

EMERGENCY INFORMATION

Allergies _____

_____

_____

_____

_____

Other information _____

_____

_____

_____

_____

_____

_____

_____

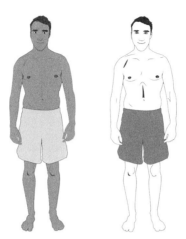

(A) Inspection, athlete standing, facing toward examiner (symmetry of trunk, upper extremities)

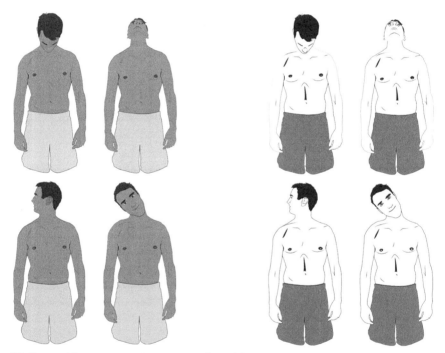

(B) Forward flexion, extension, rotation, lateral flexion of neck (range of motion, cervical spine)

Figure 2.1 The general musculoskeletal screening examination

Source: Reprinted with permission from ©1997 American Academy of Family Physicians, American Medical Society for Sport Medicine, American Orthopaedic Society of Sports Medicine, and American Osteopathic Academy of Sports Medicine

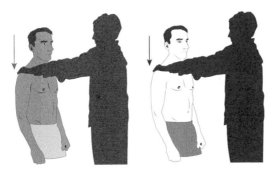

(C) Resisted shoulder shrug (strength, trapezius)

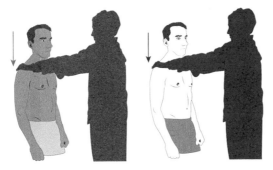

(D) Resisted shoulder abduction (strength, deltoid)

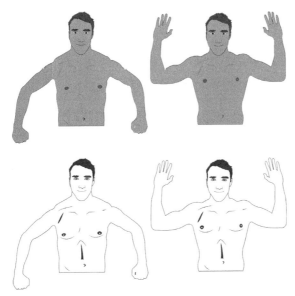

(E) Internal and external rotation of shoulder (range of motion, glenohumeral joint)

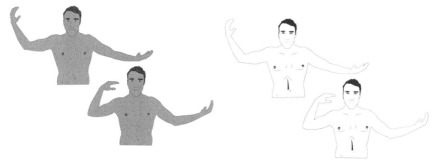

(F) Extension and flexion of elbow (range of motion, elbow)

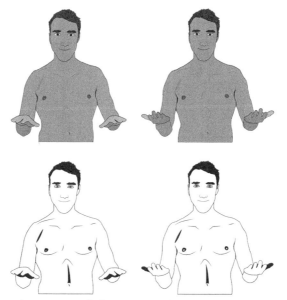

(G) Pronation and supination of elbow (range of motion, elbow and wrist)

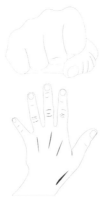

(H) Clench fist, then spread fingers (range of motion, hand and fingers)

Figure 2.1 continued

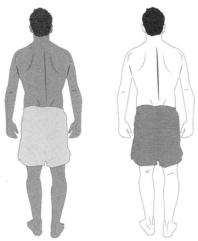

(I) Inspection, athlete facing away from examiner (symmetry of trunk, upper extremities)

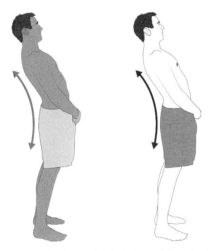

(J) Back extension, knees straight (spondylolysis/spondylolisthesis)

Figure 2.1 continued

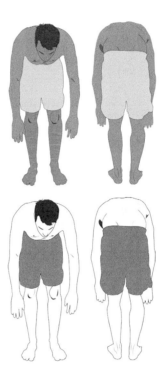

(K) Back flexion with knees straight, facing toward and away from examiner (range of motion, thoracic and lumbosacral spine; spine curvature; hamstring flexibility)

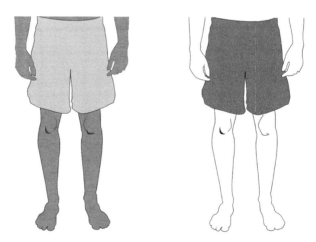

(L) Inspection of lower extremities, contraction of quadriceps muscles (alignment, symmetry)

Figure 2.1 continued

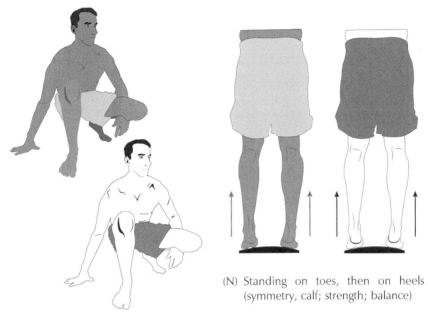

(M) "Duck walk" four steps (motion of hip, knee, and ankle; strength; balance)

(N) Standing on toes, then on heels (symmetry, calf; strength; balance)

Figure 2.1 continued

After the pre-participation examination, the physician should discuss the results with the athlete and focus on conditions that have to be corrected or rehabilitated. After reviewing the history and physical examination result, the physician can choose to:

- recommend full, unlimited participation;
- withhold clearance until a problem is corrected;
- withhold clearance until additional examinations are performed;
- allow participation in certain sports; or
- not allow participation of the athlete.

The physician's decision is often based on guidelines such as the Medical Conditions and Sports Participation of the American Academy of Pediatrics (Table 2.3), which list medical conditions that may disqualify athletes from participating in collision, contact, and non-contact sports. For example, individuals with an enlarged liver should probably not play a contact or collision sport such as football or rugby.

Table 2.3 Medical conditions and sports participation

Condition	May participate
Atlantoaxial instability (instability of the joint between cervical vertebrae 1 and 2) *Explanation*: Athlete (particularly if he or she has Down syndrome or juvenile rheumatoid arthritis with cervical involvement) needs evaluation to assess the risk of spinal cord injury during sports participation, especially when using a trampoline.	Qualified yes
Bleeding disorder *Explanation*: Athlete needs evaluation.	Qualified yes
Cardiovascular disease	
Carditis (inflammation of the heart) *Explanation*: Carditis may result in sudden death with exertion.	No
Hypertension (high blood pressure) *Explanation*: Those with hypertension > 5 mmHg above the 99th percentile for age, gender, and height should avoid heavy weight lifting and power lifting, bodybuilding, and high-static component sports. Those with sustained hypertension (> 95th percentile for age, gender, and height) need evaluation. The National High Blood Pressure Education Program Working Group report defined prehypertension and stage 1 and stage 2 hypertension in children and adolescents younger than 18 years of age.	Qualified yes
Congenital heart disease (structural heart defects present at birth) *Explanation*: Consultation with a cardiologist is recommended. Those who have mild forms may participate fully in most cases; those who have moderate or severe forms or who have undergone surgery need evaluation. The 36th Bethesda Conference defined mild, moderate, and severe disease for common cardiac lesions.	Qualified yes
Dysrhythmia (irregular heart rhythm): – long-QT syndrome – malignant ventricular arrhythmias – symptomatic Wolff–Parkinson–White syndrome – advanced heart block – family history of sudden death or previous sudden cardiac event – implantation of a cardioverter-defibrillator *Explanation*: Consultation with a cardiologist is advised. Those with symptoms (chest pain, syncope, near-syncope, dizziness, shortness of breath, or other symptoms of possible dysrhythmia) or evidence of mitral regurgitation on physical examination need evaluation. All others may participate fully.	Qualified yes

Table 2.3 continued

Condition	May participate
Heart murmur	Qualified yes
Explanation: If the murmur is innocent (does not indicate heart disease), full participation is permitted. Otherwise, athlete needs evaluation (see structural heart disease, especially hypertrophic cardiomyopathy and mitral valve prolapse).	
Structural/acquired heart disease:	
– hypertrophic cardiomyopathy	Qualified no
– coronary artery anomalies	Qualified no
– arrhythmogenic right ventricular cardiomyopathy	Qualified no
– acute rheumatic fever with carditis	Qualified no
– Ehlers–Danlos syndrome, vascular form	Qualified no
– Marfan syndrome	Qualified yes
– mitral valve prolapse	Qualified yes
– anthracycline use	Qualified yes
Explanation: Consultation with a cardiologist is recommended. The 36th Bethesda Conference provided detailed recommendations. Most of these conditions carry a significant risk of sudden cardiac death associated with intense physical exercise. Hypertrophic cardiomyopathy requires thorough and repeated evaluations, because disease may change manifestations during later adolescence. Marfan syndrome with an aortic aneurysm also can cause sudden death during intense physical exercise. Athlete who has ever received chemotherapy with anthracyclines may be at increased risk of cardiac problems because of the cardiotoxic effects of the medications, and resistance training in this population should be approached with caution; strength training that avoids isometric contractions may be permitted. Athlete needs evaluation.	
Vasculitis/vascular disease:	Qualified yes
– Kawasaki disease (coronary artery vasculitis)	
– pulmonary hypertension	
Explanation: Consultation with a cardiologist is recommended. Athlete needs individual evaluation to assess risk on the basis of disease activity, pathologic changes, and medical regimen.	
Cerebral palsy	Qualified yes
Explanation: Athlete needs evaluation to assess functional capacity to perform sport-specific activity.	
Diabetes mellitus	Yes
Explanation: All sports can be played with proper attention and appropriate adjustments to diet (particularly carbohydrate intake), blood glucose concentrations, hydration, and insulin therapy. Blood glucose concentrations should be monitored before exercise, every 30 min during continuous exercise, 15 min after completion of exercise, and at bedtime.	

Table 2.3 continued

Condition	May participate
Diarrhea, infectious *Explanation*: Unless symptoms are mild and athlete is fully hydrated, no participation is permitted, because diarrhea may increase risk of dehydration and heat illness (see fever).	Qualified no
Eating disorders *Explanation*: Athlete with an eating disorder needs medical and psychiatric assessment before participation.	Qualified yes
Eyes:	Qualified yes

– functionally 1-eyed athlete

– loss of an eye

– detached retina or family history of retinal detachment at young age

– high myopia

– connective tissue disorder, such as Marfan or Stickler syndrome

– previous intraocular eye surgery or serious eye injury

   Explanation: A functionally 1-eyed athlete is defined as having best-corrected visual acuity worse than 20/40 in the poorer-seeing eye. Such an athlete would suffer significant disability if the better eye were seriously injured, as would an athlete with loss of an eye. Specifically, boxing and full-contact martial arts are not recommended for functionally 1-eyed athletes, because eye protection is impractical and/or not permitted. Some athletes who previously underwent intraocular eye surgery or had a serious eye injury may have increased risk of injury because of weakened eye tissue. Availability of eye guards approved by the American Society for Testing and Materials and other protective equipment may allow participation in most sports, but this must be judged on an individual basis.

Condition	May participate
Conjunctivitis, infectious *Explanation*: Athlete with active infectious conjunctivitis should be excluded from swimming.	Qualified no
Fever *Explanation*: Elevated core temperature may be indicative of a pathologic medical condition (infection or disease) that is often manifest by increased resting metabolism and heart rate. Accordingly, during athlete's usual exercise regimen, the presence of fever can result in greater heat storage, decreased heat tolerance, increased risk of heat illness, increased cardiopulmonary effort, reduced maximal exercise capacity, and increased risk of hypotension because of altered vascular tone and dehydration. On rare occasions, fever may accompany myocarditis or other conditions that may make usual exercise dangerous.	No
Gastrointestinal:	Qualified yes

– malabsorption syndromes (celiac disease or cystic fibrosis)

   Explanation: Athlete needs individual assessment for general malnutrition or specific deficits resulting in coagulation or other defects; with appropriate

Table 2.3 continued

Condition	May participate
treatment, these deficits can be treated adequately to permit normal activities.	
– short-bowel syndrome or other disorders requiring specialized nutritional support, including parenteral or enteral nutrition *Explanation*: Athlete needs individual assessment for collision, contact, or limited-contact sports. Presence of central or peripheral, indwelling, venous catheter may require special considerations for activities and emergency preparedness for unexpected trauma to the device(s).	
Heat illness, history of *Explanation*: Because of the likelihood of recurrence, athlete needs individual assessment to determine the presence of predisposing conditions and behaviors and to develop a prevention strategy that includes sufficient acclimatization (to the environment and to exercise intensity and duration), conditioning, hydration, and salt intake, as well as other effective measures to improve heat tolerance and to reduce heat injury risk (such as protective equipment and uniform configurations).	Qualified yes
Hepatitis, infectious (primarily hepatitis C) *Explanation*: All athletes should receive hepatitis B vaccination before participation. Because of the apparent minimal risk to others, all sports may be played as athlete's state of health allows. For all athletes, skin lesions should be covered properly, and athletic personnel should use universal precautions when handling blood or body fluids with visible blood.	Yes
HIV infection *Explanation*: Because of the apparent minimal risk to others, all sports may be played as athlete's state of health allows (especially if viral load is undetectable or very low). For all athletes, skin lesions should be covered properly, and athletic personnel should use universal precautions when handling blood or body fluids with visible blood. However, certain sports (such as wrestling and boxing) may create a situation that favors viral transmission (likely bleeding plus skin breaks). If viral load is detectable, then athletes should be advised to avoid such high-contact sports.	Yes
Kidney, absence of one *Explanation*: Athlete needs individual assessment for contact, collision, and limited-contact sports. Protective equipment may reduce risk of injury to the remaining kidney sufficiently to allow participation in most sports, providing such equipment remains in place during activity.	Qualified yes
Liver, enlarged *Explanation*: If the liver is acutely enlarged, then participation should be avoided because of risk of rupture. If the liver is chronically enlarged, then individual assessment is needed before collision, contact, or limited-contact sports are played. Patients with chronic liver disease may have changes in liver function that affect stamina, mental status, coagulation, or nutritional status.	Qualified yes
Malignant neoplasm *Explanation*: Athlete needs individual assessment.	Qualified yes

Table 2.3 continued

Condition	May participate
Musculoskeletal disorders	Qualified yes
Explanation: Athlete needs individual assessment.	
Neurologic disorders:	
– history of serious head or spine trauma or abnormality, including craniotomy, epidural bleeding, subdural hematoma, intracerebral hemorrhage, second-impact syndrome, vascular malformation, and neck fracture.	Qualified yes
Explanation: Athlete needs individual assessment for collision, contact, or limited-contact sports.	
– history of simple concussion (mild traumatic brain multiple simple concussions, and/or complex injury), concussion	Qualified yes
Explanation: Athlete needs individual assessment. Research supports a conservative approach to concussion management, including no athletic participation while symptomatic or when deficits in judgment or cognition are detected, followed by graduated return to full activity.	
– myopathies	Qualified yes
Explanation: Athlete needs individual assessment.	
– recurrent headaches	Yes
Explanation: Athlete needs individual assessment.	
– recurrent plexopathy (burner or stinger) and cervical cord neuropraxia with persistent defects	Qualified yes
Explanation: Athlete needs individual assessment for collision, contact, or limited-contact sports; regaining normal strength is important benchmark for return to play.	
– seizure disorder, well controlled	Yes
Explanation: Risk of seizure during participation is minimal.	
– seizure disorder, poorly controlled	Qualified yes
Explanation: Athlete needs individual assessment for collision, contact, or limited-contact sports. The following non-contact sports should be avoided: archery, riflery, swimming, weight lifting, power lifting, strength training, and sports involving heights. In these sports, occurrence of a seizure during activity may pose a risk to self or others.	
Obesity	Yes
Explanation: Because of the increased risk of heat illness and cardiovascular strain, obese athlete particularly needs careful acclimatization (to the environment and to exercise intensity and duration), sufficient hydration, and potential activity and recovery modifications during competition and training.	
Organ transplant recipient (and those taking immunosuppressive medications)	Qualified yes
Explanation: Athlete needs individual assessment for contact, collision, and limited-contact sports. In addition to potential risk of infections, some medications (e.g., prednisone) may increase tendency for bruising.	

Table 2.3 continued

Condition	May participate
Ovary, absence of one	Yes
Explanation: Risk of severe injury to remaining ovary is minimal.	
Pregnancy/postpartum	Qualified yes
Explanation: Athlete needs individual assessment. As pregnancy progresses, modifications to usual exercise routines will become necessary. Activities with high risk of falling or abdominal trauma should be avoided. Scuba diving and activities posing risk of altitude sickness should also be avoided during pregnancy. After the birth, physiological and morphologic changes of pregnancy take 4–6 weeks to return to baseline.	
Respiratory conditions:	
– pulmonary compromise, including cystic fibrosis	Qualified yes
Explanation: Athlete needs individual assessment but, generally, all sports may be played if oxygenation remains satisfactory during graded exercise test. Athletes with cystic fibrosis need acclimatization and good hydration to reduce risk of heat illness.	
– asthma	Yes
Explanation: With proper medication and education, only athletes with severe asthma need to modify their participation. For those using inhalers, recommend having a written action plan and using a peak flowmeter daily. Athletes with asthma may encounter risks when scuba diving.	
– acute upper respiratory infection	Qualified yes
Explanation: Upper respiratory obstruction may affect pulmonary function. Athlete needs individual assessment for all except mild disease (see fever).	
Rheumatologic diseases:	Qualified yes
– juvenile rheumatoid arthritis	
Explanation: Athletes with systemic or polyarticular juvenile rheumatoid arthritis and history of cervical spine involvement need radiographs of vertebrae C1 and C2 to assess risk of spinal cord injury. Athletes with systemic or HLA-B27-associated arthritis require cardiovascular assessment for possible cardiac complications during exercise. For those with micrognathia (open bite and exposed teeth), mouth guards are helpful. If uveitis is present, risk of eye damage from trauma is increased; ophthalmologic assessment is recommended. If visually impaired, guidelines for functionally 1-eyed athletes should be followed.	
– juvenile dermatomyositis, idiopathic myositis	
– systemic lupus erythematosis	
– Raynaud phenomenon	
Explanation: Athlete with juvenile dermatomyositis or systemic lupus erythematosis with cardiac involvement requires cardiology assessment before participation. Athletes receiving systemic corticosteroid therapy are at higher risk of osteoporotic fractures and avascular necrosis, which should be assessed before clearance; those receiving immunosuppressive	

Table 2.3 continued

Condition	May participate
medications are at higher risk of serious infection. Sports activities should be avoided when myositis is active. Rhabdomyolysis during intensive exercise may cause renal injury in athletes with idiopathic myositis and other myopathies. Because of photosensitivity with juvenile dermatomyositis and systemic lupus erythematosis, sun protection is necessary during outdoor activities. With Raynaud phenomenon, exposure to the cold presents risk to hands and feet.	
Sickle cell disease	Qualified yes
Explanation: Athlete needs individual assessment. In general, if illness status permits, all sports may be played; however, any sport or activity that entails overexertion, overheating, dehydration, or chilling should be avoided. Participation at high altitude, especially when not acclimatized, also poses risk of sickle cell crisis.	
Sickle cell trait	Yes
Explanation: Athletes with sickle cell trait generally do not have increased risk of sudden death or other medical problems during athletic participation under normal environmental conditions. However, when high exertional activity is performed under extreme conditions of heat and humidity or increased altitude, such catastrophic complications have occurred rarely. Athletes with sickle cell trait, like all athletes, should be progressively acclimatized to the environment and to the intensity and duration of activities and should be sufficiently hydrated to reduce the risk of exertional heat illness and/or rhabdomyolysis. According to National Institutes of Health management guidelines, sickle cell trait is not a contraindication to participation in competitive athletics, and there is no requirement for screening before participation. More research is needed to assess fully potential risks and benefits of screening athletes for sickle cell trait.	
Skin infections, including herpes simplex, molluscum contagiosum, verrucae (warts), staphylococcal and streptococcal infections (furuncles (boils), carbuncles, impetigo, methicillin-resistant *Staphylococcus aureus* (cellulitis and/or abscesses)), scabies, and tinea	Qualified yes
Explanation: During contagious periods, participation in gymnastics or cheerleading with mats, martial arts, wrestling, or other collision, contact, or limited-contact sports is not allowed.	
Spleen, enlarged	Qualified yes
Explanation: If the spleen is acutely enlarged, then participation should be avoided because of risk of rupture. If the spleen is chronically enlarged, then individual assessment is needed before collision, contact, or limited-contact sports are played.	
Testicle, undescended or absence of one	Yes
Explanation: Certain sports may require a protective cup.	

Notes: This table is designed for use by medical and non-medical personnel. "Needs evaluation" means that a physician with appropriate knowledge and experience should assess the safety of a given sport for an athlete with the listed medical condition. Unless otherwise noted, this need for special consideration is because of variability in the severity of the disease, the risk of injury for the specific sports listed, or both.

Pediatrics April 2008 vol. 121 no. 4 841–848 doi: 10.1542/peds.2008–0080

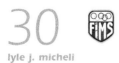

WHEN TO SCHEDULE THE PRE-PARTICIPATION EXAMINATION

The pre-participation examination must be scheduled to allow sufficient time for any necessary corrective measures to be taken before the athletic season starts. Such measures may include strengthening or flexibility exercises or drills to improve agility and skill. These interventions can be as simple as teaching a young athlete with tight hamstrings the proper techniques of hamstring stretching, or as complex as teaching a basketball player the technique of cutting on the basketball court to decrease the chance of injuring the anterior cruciate ligaments.

The minimum interval between the pre-participation evaluation and the start of the athletic season is one month. The ideal interval is 10–12 weeks before the beginning of the athletic season, because time is needed to effectively implement, in a systematic fashion, interventions such as stretching and strengthening. Apart from allowing adequate time to teach specific exercises, or to fit and manufacture specific protective devices, this 10–12-week interval allows sufficient time for re-evaluation and/or reassessment to ensure that the intervention has been effective in addressing the risk factor for injury.

A pre-participation evaluation not only detects risk factors for sports injury, but can also ascertain therapeutic interventions that may prevent or decrease the risk of sports injury. Personnel with a sound understanding of both the intrinsic and extrinsic risk factors for sports injury are better prepared to make recommendations that will correct or compensate for detected risk factors in the athlete.

The pre-participation examination is also an opportunity to screen for pre-existing and often silent cardiac abnormalities that may predispose the athlete to SCD, as we see in the following chapter.

SUGGESTED READING

American Academy of Family Physicians, American Academy of Pediatrics, American College of Sports Medicine, American Medical Society for Sports Medicine, American Orthopaedic Society for Sports Medicine, and American Osteopathic Academy of Sports Medicine. *Pre-participation Physical Evaluation*, 3rd ed. McGraw-Hill, Minneapolis, MN, 2005.

American Academy of Family Physicians, American Academy of Pediatrics, American College of Sports Medicine, American Medical Society for Sports Medicine, American Orthopaedic Society for Sports Medicine, and American Osteopathic Academy of Sports Medicine. *Pre-participation Physical Evaluation*, 4th ed. D. Bernhardt and W. Roberts (Eds.), American Academy of Pediatrics, Elk Grove, IL, 2010.

Barrett, J.R., Kuhlman, G.S., Stanitski, C.L., et al. The pre-participation physical examination. In: *Care of the Young Athlete*. American Academy of Orthopedic Surgeons and American Academy of Pediatrics, Elk Grove Village, IL, 2000.

Glover D.W., Maron B.J., Matheson G.O. The pre-participation physical examination: Steps toward consensus and uniformity. *Phys. Sportsmed*. 1999 (Aug); 27(8):29–34.

Koester M.C., Amundson C.L. Pre-participation screening of high school athletes: Are recommendations enough? *Phys. Sportsmed*. 2003 (Aug); 31(8):35–8.

Lively M.W. Pre-participation physical examinations: A collegiate experience. *Clin. J. Sport Med*. 1999; 9:3–8.

Peterson A.R., Bernhardt D.T. The pre-participation sports evaluation. *Pediatr. Rev*. 2011; 32:53–65.

Rice S.G., American Academy of Pediatrics Council on Sports Medicine and Fitness. Medical conditions affecting sports participation. *Pediatrics*. 2008; 121:841.

CHAPTER 3

THE CARDIOVASCULAR PRE-PARTICIPATION SCREENING OF ATHLETES

A cornerstone of sport-related sudden cardiac death prevention

Fabio Pigozzi, Marta Rizzo, and Paolo Borrione

As described in the previous chapter, the main goals of pre-participation examination are the assessment of the athlete's overall health; the detection of conditions that may cause injury; the identification of underlying disease that may disqualify the athlete from participating in certain sports; and assessing fitness for the chosen sport.

Another of the main goals of the athlete's pre-participation examination should also be to identify subjects at risk for sport-related illness, with particular regard to sudden death. It is significant to note that, while non-traumatic athletic-field deaths are often considered "tragic fatalities," in most instances they are preventable. And, although they may be attributed to non-cardiac causes (cerebral aneurysm, heat stroke, bronchial asthma, drug abuse), more than 90% of these tragic events occur in subjects who have pre-existing and usually clinically silent cardiac abnormalities, most of which are congenital and identifiable with an accurate cardiologic evaluation (see Figures 3.1 and 3.2).

Fortunately, the majority of cardiac abnormalities with the potential to cause SCD can be identified by cardiovascular screening, although this depends on the specific abnormality and the content of the cardiovascular screening applied.

Although with some important differences, cardiovascular screening for competitive athletes is currently universally recommended by the cardiac societies (European Society of Cardiology (ESC) and American Heart Association (AHA)), required by the major sporting bodies (e.g. Fédération Internationale de Football Association (FIFA), and Union of European Football Associations (UEFA)), and applied in most countries.

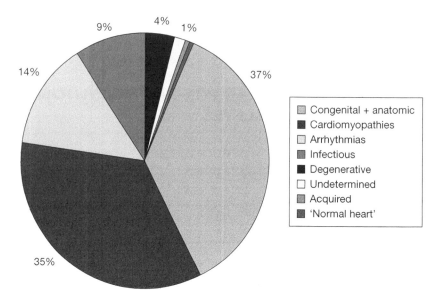

Figure 3.1 Global causes of SCD in young athletes

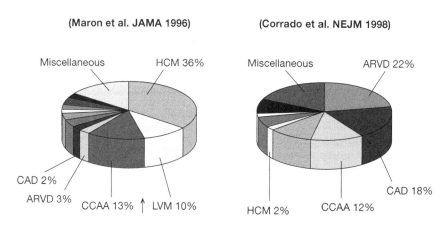

Figure 3.2 Specific causes of SCD in young American and Italian athletes. Note that in the United States, hypertrophic cardiomyopathy (HCM) is the leading cause, whereas in Italy the most frequent cause is arrhythmogenic right ventricular dysplasia (ARVD). This difference is mainly due to the Italian national pre-participation screening program based on ECG that allows the identification of athletes affected by HCM by the characteristic ECG abnormalities of this disease. (CAD: coronary atherosclerotic disease; CCAA: congenital coronary artery anomalies)

The cardiovascular screening of competitive athletes is composed of three main elements:

- the medical (familial and personal) and athletic history;
- the physical examination;
- the 12-lead ECG.

Although the medical history and physical examination are universally applied, a 12-lead ECG is applied only in some countries.

MEDICAL AND ATHLETIC HISTORY

A careful medical history of the athlete and his/her family, as well as a careful physical examination, represent the basis of the screening. In particular, the familial medical history must be guided to the identification of a "genetic predisposition" to cardiovascular disease. To attain this goal, major cardiovascular risk factors that are known to have a multifactorial (genetic and environmental) genesis (i.e., hypertension, diabetes, hypercholesterolemia), as well as symptomatic coronary artery disease, must be investigated in first-degree relatives. Great attention must be paid to cases of sudden death in relatives under 50 years of age that may suggest the presence of inherited cardiac disorders.

The personal medical history must investigate:

- the presence of major cardiovascular risk factors (smoking, hypertension, hypercholesterolemia) and substance abuse (alcohol, drugs, doping);
- a past clinical history, mainly focusing on cardiovascular problems;
- a recent clinical history, with the purpose of identifying the presence of exercise-related cardiovascular symptoms, with particular regard for:
  - chest pain or discomfort;
  - dyspnea or breathlessness;
  - palpitations;
  - syncope or pre-syncope;
  - unexplained worsening in physical performance.

Athletes are likely to underestimate their symptoms, even when they are of some importance, hence the need for careful questioning.

To obtain a complete and informative history, the use of a checklist, as reported in Tables 3.1 and 3.2, could be suggested.

Table 3.1 Checklist for familial medical history

Questions	Answers
1. Did someone of your first-degree relatives die suddenly before 50 years of age for cardiac causes or for unexplainable causes?	NO/YES
2. Do any of your first-degree relatives suffer from:	
– unexplainable syncope or unexplainable convulsions?	NO/YES
– any disabling cardiac problem (pacemaker, implantable defibrillator, heart transplant, cardiac surgery, antiarrhythmic teraphy)?	NO/YES
– HCM, DCM, Marfan syndrome, ARVD, long-QT syndrome, CPTV, premature CAD (M < 55 years; W < 65 years)	NO/YES
– diabetes, arterial hypertension, hypercholesterolemia	NO/YES

Criteria for positive medical history

Family history:

- family history of premature heart attack or sudden death (< 50 years);
- family history of cardiomyopathy, Marfan syndrome, long-QT syndrome, Brugada syndrome, severe arrhythmias, coronary artery disease or other disabling cardiovascular disease.

Personal history:

- exertional chest pain or discomfort;
- syncope or near syncope;
- irregular heartbeat or palpitations;
- shortness of breath or fatigue out of proportion to the degree of exertion.

Finally, investigating the type, duration, and intensity of training allows correlation of these data with the further clinical and instrumental findings. A checklist, as reported in Table 3.3, is suggested.

PHYSICAL EXAMINATION

The main elements of the cardiovascular physical examination are:

- evaluation of the presence and features of heart murmurs; cardiac auscultation should be performed in a noiseless room, both in supine and standing positions;
- evaluation of the presence of femoral pulses to exclude aortic coarctation;
- examination for physical stigmata of Marfan's syndrome;
- measurement of brachial artery blood pressure (preferably at both arms, in sitting position).

36

Table 3.2 Checklist for personal medical history

Questions	Answers
Have you ever experienced syncope or pre-syncope?	
– during physical effort	NO/YES
– after physical effort	NO/YES
– out of physical effort	NO/YES
Have you ever experienced chest pain?	
– during physical effort	NO/YES
– after physical effort	NO/YES
– out of physical effort	NO/YES
Have you ever experienced dizziness?	
– during physical effort	NO/YES
– after physical effort	NO/YES
– out of physical effort	NO/YES
Have you ever experienced breathlessness or breathing trouble?	
– during physical effort	NO/YES
– after physical effort	NO/YES
– out of physical effort	NO/YES
Have you ever experienced palpitation?	
– during physical effort	NO/YES
– after physical effort	NO/YES
– out of physical effort	NO/YES
Are you taking any drugs or other substances?	NO/YES
Do you smoke?	NO/YES
Have you ever been recommended to undergo cardiac tests (Holter ECG, echo, exercise test)?	NO/YES
Have you had any cardiovascular problem in the past?	NO/YES

Criteria for positive physical examination:

- musculoskeletal and ocular features suggestive of Marfan syndrome;
- diminished and delayed femoral artery pulses;
- mid- or end-systolic clicks;
- second heart sound single or widely split and fixed with respiration;
- marked heart murmurs (any diastolic and systolic grade ≥ 2/6);
- irregular heart rhythm;
- brachial blood pressure > 140/90 mmHg (on > 1 reading).

Table 3.3 Checklist for athletic history

1. Type of sport	....
2. Years of practice	....
3. Number of training sessions/week	....
4. Duration of a single training session (minutes)	....
5. Number of competitions/month	....

A cardiac screening based only on medical history and physical examination is currently applied in the United States, where the exceptionally large number of athletes required to be evaluated, compared with the relative rarity of SCD, is considered the major obstacle for the implementation of pre-participation examination with instrumental tests. However, such screening fails to recognize most athletes at increased cardiac risk.

THE 12-LEAD ECG

On the other hand, implementing the screening with 12-lead ECG appears to significantly increase the diagnostic power (in particular, specificity) of the screening itself. Indeed, ECG abnormalities are commonly found in patients who have potentially lethal congenital cardiac diseases.

Unfortunately, the increase in specificity and sensibility of the screening due to ECG implementation is associated with an increase in the rate of false-positive results. Actually, in healthy, highly trained athletes, abnormal ECG patterns are frequently observed, and the correct interpretation of these patterns represents a crucial point of the athlete's evaluation.

ECG abnormalities that may be found in athletes are of two types, listed in Table 3.4:

- physiologic ECG variants, related to athletic training and extremely common (up to 80% of the athletes);
- non-physiologic variants, not related to athletic training.

Athletes trained in sports with high cardiovascular involvement frequently present with physiologic ECG alterations that reflect the adaptation of the autonomic cardiac nervous system and, specifically, the increased vagal tone and/or reduction of sympathetic tone. These alterations include sinus bradycardia, first-degree AV block, and early repolarization. Moreover, the increased QRS voltages and the incomplete right-branch block reflect the physiologic cardiac hypertrophy of the

38

Table 3.4 Classification of ECG alteration that could be found in competitive athletes

Physiologic and common ECG alterations	Non-physiologic and uncommon ECG alterations
Sinus bradycardia	Inverted T waves
First-degree AV block	Pathologic Q waves
Incomplete right-branch block	Left atrial hypertrophy
Early repolarization	Left axis deviation
Increased isolated QRS voltages	Right axis deviation
	Left ventricular hypetrophy
	Wolf–Parkinsons–White
	Complete left or right branch block
	Long or short QT interval
	Brugada-like early repolarization
	Ventricular or supraventricular premature beats
	Second-degree AV block
	Third-degree AV block

athlete's heart. These ECG alterations are not alarming and do not require further diagnostic tests.

On the other hand, the non-physiologic ECG alterations, listed in Table 3.4, are generally expressive of a structural or electrical cardiac alteration, including those with the potential to cause SCD. Therefore when found, these alterations must be considered expressions of disease until proved otherwise and dictate second-level (echocardiogram, maximal exercise test, 24-hour Holter ECG), and eventually third-level, diagnostic tests (cardiac MRN, T-wave voltages, late potentials, electrophysiologic studies), in order to evaluate concretely the athlete's risk and evaluate his/her qualification for training and competition (Figure 3.1).

Criteria for a positive 12-lead ECG

The 12-lead ECG was introduced as a part of Italian mandatory pre-participation examinations for competitive athletes in 1982. Analysis of data from long-term Italian experience indicates that ECG screening has provided adequate sensitivity and specificity for the detection of potentially lethal cardiomyopathy or arrhythmias and has led to a substantial reduction of mortality in young competitive athletes by approximately 90%.

Despite the reported evidence in favor of ECG, the debate about its actual effectiveness in screening competitive athletes remains open. The main, recognized limitation of ECG is the demonstrated occurrence of false-positive results. In its

CRITERIA FOR A POSITIVE 12-LEAD ECG

- P wave.
- Left atrial enlargement: negative portion of the P wave in lead V1 ≥ 0.1 mV in depth and ≥ 0.04 s in duration.
- Right atrial enlargement: peaked P wave in leads II and III or V1 ≥ 0.25 mV in amplitude.
- QRS complex.
- Frontal plane axis deviation: right ≥ + 120° or left 30° to -90°.
- Increased voltage: amplitude or R or S wave in a standard lead ≥ 2 mV, S wave in lead V1 or V2 ≥ 3 mV, or R wave in lead V5 or V6 ≥ 3 mV.
- Abnormal Q waves ≥ 0.04 s in duration or ≥ 25% of the height of the ensuing R wave or QS pattern in two or more leads.
- Right or left bundle branch block with QRS duration ≥ 0.12 s.
- R or R' wave in lead V1 ≥ 0.5 mV in amplitude and R/S ratio ≥ 1.
- ST-segment, T waves and QT interval.
- ST-segment depression or T-wave flattening or inversion in two or more leads.
- Prolongation of heart rate corrected QT interval > 0.44 s in males and > 0.46 s in females.
- Rhythm and conduction abnormalities.
- Premature ventricular beats or more severe ventricular arrhythmias.
- Supraventricular tachycardias, atrial flutter, or atrial fibrillation.
- Short PR interval (0.12 s) with or without "delta" wave.
- Sinus bradycardia with resting heart rate ≤ 40 beats/min.
- First- (PR ≥ 0.21 s), second-, or third-degree atrioventricular block.

recent document, the AHA stated that ECG could also be potentially deleterious to the athletes with false-positive results, as it would lead to further, unnecessary evaluations and testing, anxiety, and possibly to disqualification without merit. Evidence from the Italian experience does not agree with this consideration. A correct ECG interpretation, that is, distinguishing the physiological from the non-physiological patterns, is the first step. Moreover, in the vast majority of cases, echocardiography allows clarification of whether the ECG abnormalities are the consequence of structural alterations or just the expression of the physiological cardiac hypertrophy of the athlete's heart. However, when the ECG alterations are marked, even in the absence of echocardiographic evidence of disease, continuing surveillance is requested, especially in adolescent athletes in whom ECG abnormalities may precede the development of structural alterations in adulthood. In fact, long-term follow-up studies demonstrated that markedly abnormal ECGs

f. pigozzi, m. rizzo, and p. borrione

in young, apparently healthy athletes may represent the initial expression of underlying cardiomyopathies that may not be evident until many years later and that may ultimately be associated with adverse outcomes, thus requiring continued clinical surveillance.

THE ROLE OF ECHOCARDIOGRAM IN THE SCREENING OF COMPETITIVE ATHLETES

Echocardiography is a non-invasive, readily available, and relatively inexpensive diagnostic tool with the ability to detect subclinical abnormalities early in their natural history. Currently, it is considered a second-level test to perform in the presence of clinical and/or instrumental abnormalities. Actually, pre-participation examination with ECG allows identification of most of the cardiac disease responsible for SCD, and routine echocardiogram is considered not to increase the sensitivity of this screening. However, over the last decade, a new debate concerning the possible role of echocardiography in the routine screening of competitive athletes has been growing in Europe. Actually, many congenital cardiac abnormalities may not be revealed even by accurate physical examination and may be not associated with ECG alterations. These anomalies, which include mild and innocent to severe and potentially threatening conditions, are likely to be common in the athletic population, with particular regard to mitral valve prolapse, myocarditis, and aortic valve diseases.

It is likely that implementing athletes' pre-participation examinations based on history, physical examination, and ECG with a limited two-dimensional echo-cardiographic study would not significantly increase the cost-effectiveness of the screening itself, but it would significantly increase its diagnostic power and, perhaps, its effectiveness in terms of SCD prevention. However, because the cardiac abnormalities that are detected by echocardiography are mostly congenital defects, it could be suggested that echocardiography should be performed at the first cardiovascular clearance, at the beginning of the competitive career.

Figure 3.3 summarizes the progressive steps of an athlete's cardiovascular evaluation. The screening (first-level evaluation) includes medical history, physical examination, and 12-lead ECG. If no abnormalities were found, the athlete would be qualified for training and competitions. On the other hand, if any abnormalities (clinical or instrumental) arose, second-level tests would be performed, including echocardiography, maximal exercise test (on cycloergometer or treadmill), and 24-hour Holter monitoring. If no evidence of cardiac disease were found, the athlete would be qualified for training and competitions. Finally, if any abnormalities were detected, third-level tests would be performed, depending on the specific findings, including cardiac MNR, the search for the presence of ventricular late potentials by signal averaging, T-wave alternans, transesophageal electrophysiologic study, or endocavitary electrophysiologic study.

Athletes with any cardiovascular conditions would be managed according to established cardiovascular protocols, such as the Italian Cardiological Guidelines for Competitive Sports Eligibility (COCIS) or the recommendations of the European Society of Cardiology (Bethesda Conference).

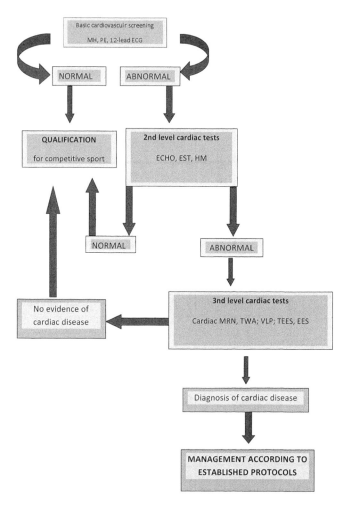

Figure 3.3 Flowchart of cardiovascular pre-participation examination for competitive athletes. MH: medical history; PE: physical examination, ECHO: echocardiography; EST: maximal exercise stress testing; HM: 24-hour Holter monitoring; TWA: T-wave alternans; VLP: ventricular late potentials; TEES: transesophageal electrophysiologic study; EES: endocavitary electrophysiologic study

SUGGESTED READING

Bille K., Schamasch P., et al. Sudden deaths in athletes: the basic of the "Lausanne Recommendations" of the International Olympic Committee. *Circulation* 2005; 112 (suppl. II): II-830.

Corrado D., Basso C., et al. Trends in sudden cardiovascular death in young competitive athletes after implementation of a pre-participation screening program. *JAMA* 2006; 291:1593–1601.

Corrado D., Pelliccia A., Bjornstad H.H., et al. Cardiovascular pre-participation screening of young competitive athletes for prevention of sudden death: proposal for a common European protocol. Consensus Statement of the Study Group of Sport Cardiology of the Working Group of Cardiac Rehabilitation and Exercise Physiology and the Working Group of Myocardial and Pericardial Diseases of the European Society of Cardiology. Eur Heart J 2005; 26:516–24.

Pelliccia A., Di Paolo F., et al. Evidence for efficacy of the Italian national pre-participation screening programme for identification of hypertrophic cardiomyopathy in competitive athletes. *Heart J* 2006; 27(18):2196–200.

Pelliccia A., Zipes D.P., Maron B.J. Bethesda Conference #36 and the European Society of Cardiology Consensus Recommendations revisited a comparison of U.S. and European criteria for eligibility and disqualification of competitive athletes with cardiovascular abnormalities. *J. Am. Coll. Cardiol.* 2008 Dec 9; 52(24):1990–6.

Pigozzi F., Rizzo M. Sudden death in competitive athletes. *Clin. Sports Med.* 2008; 27:153–81.

CHAPTER 4

PRINCIPLES OF EXERCISE PHYSIOLOGY

Norbert Bachl and Avery D. Faigenbaum

The principles of sports science are based on an understanding of the production and use of energy in biological systems. With an awareness of the contributions of the different energy systems across a variety of activities, effective training programs can be designed. Activities such as marathon rely almost exclusively on aerobic energy systems, whereas others, such as the 50-m swim, are quite anaerobic; the predominant energy systems in team sports such as basketball and soccer, on the other hand, are constantly changing. To improve an athlete's ability to perform a certain task, a training program must be designed and implemented to specifically develop the muscles, organs (e.g. heart, lungs), and energy systems involved in the sport or activity. This means training the involved muscles, organs, and energy systems at an increased level, so that they adapt and achieve a greater maximal energy potential. The end result is faster, stronger, and more powerful movements that will likely enhance sports performance and increase resistance to injury. Although a training program is designed with the specific goals, needs, and medical concerns of the athlete carefully evaluated by the team physician, its quality is defined by the ability to apply scientific principles efficiently and effectively in its design. Extensive amounts of literature have been published on aerobic training; more recently, the acute and chronic responses to anaerobic training have received increasing public and medical attention. Because of the potential influence of exercise training on sports performance and injury prevention, the team physician needs to understand the principles of sports science and their implications for the design and evaluation of sports training programs.

FUELS FOR EXERCISE

The body uses carbohydrates, fats, and proteins (Figure 4.1) consumed daily to provide the necessary energy to maintain cellular functions at rest and during exercise. The energy generated in the breakdown of food macronutrients serves to phosphorylate adenosine diphosphate (ADP) and reform the energy-rich compound adenosine triphosphate (ATP). This energy is used to pull the actin

44

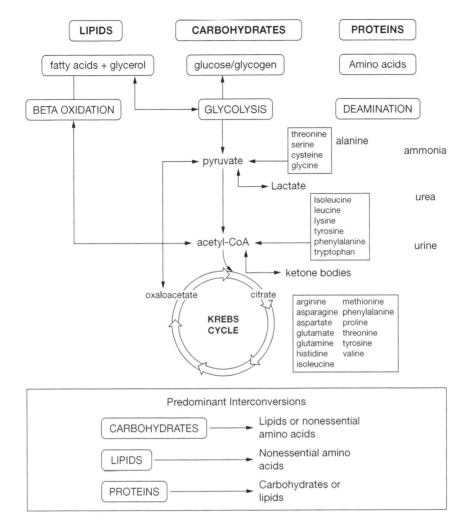

Figure 4.1 Lipids, carbohydrates, proteins

filaments across the myosin filaments and cause shortening of the muscle. Without adequate amounts of ATP, muscular contraction, and thus human movement, would not be possible. Adenosine triphosphate is stored in limited amounts in muscle cells, and its production processes occur in the cell.

The primary nutrients used for energy during exercise are carbohydrates and fats (Table 4.1), with proteins contributing a small amount.

Table 4.1 Body stores for fuels and energy

	Untrained, kcal	Untrained, kJoule	Trained, kcal	Trained, kJoule	Untrained, grams	Trained, grams
Carbohydrates						
Liver glycogen	328	1,373.2	492	2,059.9	80	120
Muscle glycogen	1,025	4,291.4	1,640	6,866.6	250	400
Glucose in body fluids	62	259.5	74	309.8	15	18
Total	1,415	5,924.1	2,206	9,236.3	345	538
Fats						
Subcutaneous	74,000	309,838	55,880	233,970	8,000	6,000
Intramuscular	465	1,946.9	2,790	11,681.2	50	300
Total	74,465	311,784.9	58,670	245,651.2	8,050	6,300
Amino acids	410	1,716.6	451	1,888.3	100	110
Proteins					6,000	7,000

Estimates based on body size of 70kg and 12% body fat (male)

55 kg = 121.254 lb
58 kg = 127.868 lb
70 kg = 154.324 lb
74 kg = 163.142 lb

Carbohydrates

Stored carbohydrates provide the body with a rapidly available form of energy, with 1 g of carbohydrate yielding approximately 4 kcal (16.74 kJ) of energy. Carbohydrates exist as monosaccharides (e.g. glucose and fructose), disaccharides (e.g. sucrose and maltose), and polysaccharides (cellulose and starch). Under resting conditions, muscle and liver take up glucose and convert it into a storage form of carbohydrate called glycogen. Cells store glycogen in their cytoplasm until it is needed as an energy source. During exercise, muscle cells break down glycogen into glucose (a process called glycogenolysis), which is used as a source of energy for muscle contraction. Glycogenolysis also occurs in the liver, with free glucose released into the bloodstream and then transported to the active tissues where it is metabolized. Liver and muscle glycogen stores, however, are limited and can become depleted within a few hours of exercise. High-carbohydrate diets tend to enhance glycogen synthesis, whereas low-carbohydrate diets can hamper glycogen synthesis. Unlike fats and proteins, carbohydrates are the only macronutrients whose stored energy can be used to generate ATP aerobically and anaerobically. In general, carbohydrates are used preferentially as an energy fuel at the beginning of exercise and during high-intensity exercise (> 80% maximum oxygen uptake (VO_2 max)).

The complete oxidation of one glucose molecule muscle results in a net yield of about 36 or 38 ATPs, depending on which shuttle system is used to transport nicotinamide adenine dinucleotide (NADH) to the mitochondria.

Fats

Stored fat represents the most plentiful source of potential energy in the body for prolonged exercise – fat molecules contain relatively large quantities of energy per unit weight. One gram of fat contains about 9 kcal (37.66 kJ) of energy, more than double the energy content of carbohydrates and proteins. The quantity of lipid stores available for energy is essentially almost unlimited (between 70,000 and 110,000 kcal, or 292,880–460,240 kJ), depending on the body weight and percentage of body fat. Comparing the lipid stores with carbohydrate (glycogen) stores, the latter are about 2% of the lipid stores. Fatty acids, which are the primary type of fat used by muscle cells for energy, are stored in the body as triglycerides. When needed for energy, triglycerides can be broken down through a process called lipolysis into free fatty acids and glycerol to be used as energy substrates. The free fatty acids will enter the mitochondria and then undergo a series of reactions in which they are converted to acetyl-coenzyme A, a process called beta-oxidation. From this point, the fat metabolism follows the same path as the carbohydrate metabolism when acetyl-coenzyme A enters the Krebs cycle and the electron transport chain (Figures 4.1 and 4.6). Although glycerol is not a direct energy source for muscle, it can be used by the liver to synthesize glucose. Fat is the primary source of energy during lower-intensity, prolonged periods of exercise (> 30 minutes).

Proteins

Proteins are composed of a chain of subunits called amino acids. As a potential energy source, each gram of proteins contains about 4 kcal of energy. In the case of severe energy depletion, starvation, and events of unusual endurance (e.g., triathlons), proteins can supply up to 5–10% of the energy needed. When used as substrates to form high-energy compounds, proteins are broken down into their constituent amino acids. Many amino acids (primarily the branched chain amino acids leucine, isoleucine, alanine, and valine) can be converted into metabolic intermediates, which can enter the pathways for energy release. Some amino acids

---

ENERGY SOURCES

- Carbohydrates stored as liver and muscle glycogen.
- Fatty acids stored as triglycerides.
- Proteins.

can also be converted to glucose in the liver, through a process called gluco-neogenesis, which can be used to synthesize glycogen.

BIOLOGICAL ENERGY SYSTEMS

There are three energy-yielding processes for the production of ATP. Each system differs in its ability to supply energy for activities of various intensities and durations (Figure 4.2). Quick, explosive events such as the 100-m sprint require a rapid rate of energy, whereas longer duration, lower power events such as a marathon rely on energy from other sources. The primary source of energy for activities and sports between these two extremes depends primarily on the exercise intensity and secondarily on the duration. The three metabolic pathways for generating energy are the ATP–phosphocreatine (PCr) system or phosphagen system, the glycolytic system, and the oxidative system.

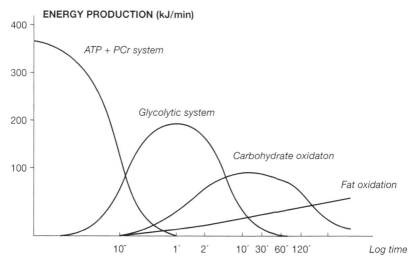

Figure 4.2 Biological energy systems and their interaction with power and time

Formation of ATP via the ATP–phosphocreatine (PCr) and glycolytic systems does not require the use of oxygen, and the systems are called anaerobic (i.e., energy produced without oxygen) pathways. Oxidative formation of ATP is an aerobic process and requires oxygen. Although each energy system has unique charac-teristics, at no time does any single energy system provide the complete supply of energy.

Adenosine triphosphate–phosphocreatine system

Because the energy released from the breakdown of ATP powers all forms of biologic activity, ATP is considered the "energy currency" of the cells. The splitting of ATP to ADP and an inorganic phosphate, Pi, enables the cells to generate energy for immediate use during short-term, high-intensity activities (e.g., sprinting and jumping) – see Figure 4.2.

ATP + H_2O ADP + P_i + energy

During the first few seconds of muscular activity, the ATP–PCr system maintains ATP in the cell at a relatively constant level because cells contain another high-energy phosphagen, PCr, in a concentration three times that of ATP. Because of the small quantity of ATP in the muscle cells, the break down to ADP immediately stimulates the breakdown of PCr to provide energy for ATP resynthesis. This ATP can then be used to generate energy for muscle contraction. This reaction is catalyzed by the enzyme creatinkinase (CK).

ADP + PCr + H + ATP + creatine

When PCr is broken down to creatine and P_i, the energy released is used to combine ADP and P_i back into ATP. The ATP can then be used to generate energy for muscle action. The energy from PCr is not used directly for muscle action because PCr does not have a receptor on the muscle crossbridges.

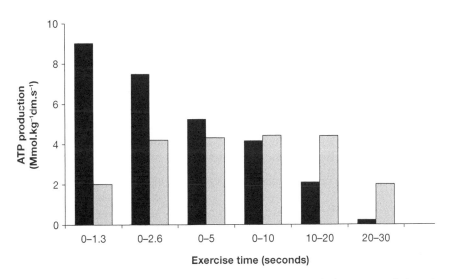

Figure 4.3 Rates of anaerobic ATP resynthesis form PCr hydrolysis (■) and glycosis (□) during maximal isometric contraction in human skeletal muscle. Rates were calculated from measurements of biopsy samples of muscle obtained during intermittent electrically evoked contractions over a period of 30 s
Source: R. J. Maughan et al., 2000, *Nutrition in Sport*

Although the ATP–PCr system provides the highest rate of energy liberation, its capacity is limited to only 3–7 seconds. Thus, during anaerobic, short-term, high-intensity activities, such as the shot put, long jump, and sprinting events, the quantity of intramuscular high-energy phosphagens is of significant importance. For example, during a 100-m dash, high-energy phosphates provide immediate energy for the initial acceleration to maximum speed. During the second phase of the race, when maintaining the desired speed is the goal, other energy sources (i.e., glycolysis) may take a more important role in the energy supply (Figure 4.3).

Glycolytic system

The glycolytic system (also called glycolysis) provides the anaerobic liberation of energy by the breakdown of glucose or glycogen via multiple enzymatically catalyzed reactions. When glycogen stored in the liver or in the muscle is used for energy liberation, it must first be broken down to glucose-1-phosphate in a process called glycogenolysis. Glucose-1-phosphate must then be converted to glucose-6-phosphate before it can be used to generate energy. The process of glycolysis begins once glucose-6-phosphate is formed. Glycolysis is essentially a series of enzymatically controlled chemical reactions that are used to transfer bond energy from glucose to rejoin ADP to P_i (Figures 4.1 and 4.6).

$$3ADP + 3P_i + glucolsyl\ unit\ 3ATP + 2lactate + 2H^+$$

Glycolytic enzymes are located in the cytoplasm of the cells, or the sarcoplasm in muscle cells. Because of its high concentration of glycolytic enzymes and the speed of these reactions, glycolysis can provide significant amounts of energy for muscle action rapidly. However, glycolysis cannot supply as much energy per second as the ATP–PCr system. The highest energy liberation from glycolysis occurs during the first 10–15 seconds of muscle action, because acidification of muscle fibers reduces the rate of glucose and glycogen breakdown (Figure 4.3). In addition, the acidification of the muscle cells decreases the calcium-binding capacity of fiber, which may further impede muscle contraction.

The capacity of the cell for anaerobic glycolysis during "all-out" physical activity is about 1–3 minutes. Activities such as the 200-m free-style swim, 400-m sprint, and strength-training activities with short rest periods between sets (e.g. 30 seconds) rely primarily on glycolysis for energy liberation. Anaerobic energy systems contribute also to energy production at the beginning of less intense exercise, when oxygen uptake kinetics lag behind the total energy demand placed on the system.

Glycolysis produces a net gain of two molecules of ATP (three molecules if glycogen is the substrate) and two molecules of pyruvic acid or lactic acid per glucose molecule. If oxygen is not available, pyruvic acid is converted to lactic acid. This reaction is catalyzed by the enzyme lactate dehydrogenase. Lactic acid quickly dissociates, and the salt known as lactate is formed. The major limitation of anaerobic glycolysis is the accumulation of lactic acid in the muscles and body fluids. If oxygen is present in the mitochondria, pyruvate can participate in the aerobic production of ATP. Thus, glycolysis can be considered a first step in the oxidation of carbohydrates.

Onset of blood lactate

As a result of these theoretical considerations, the concentration of lactic acid in the muscles and in the blood can be used as a reference point for the interaction of the aerobic–anaerobic metabolism during physical load and to optimize the training processes. From resting values of about 1 mmol/l^{-1}, blood lactic acid may increase during maximal physical activity to more than 25 mmol/l^{-1}. In an exercise test with increasing workload, the blood lactate concentration (as an indirect measure of the lactic acid produced in the working muscles) remains fairly stable during the first few minutes of the test, because the energy demand is met adequately by reactions that consume oxygen. Then, at a certain point, the blood lactate concentration will increase exponentially. This can be recognized easily by plotting the blood lactate concentration versus VO$_2$ (litre ml^{-1}; ml.kg.min^{-1}). Although arguments exist over terminology, this point, which is called the aerobic threshold or the first lactate turn point, is the beginning of a so-called "mixed aerobic–anaerobic metabolism." With increasing intensity, a second deflection point will occur, when more lactate in the working muscle will be produced than can be buffered or even removed. This point – as the last balance between lactate

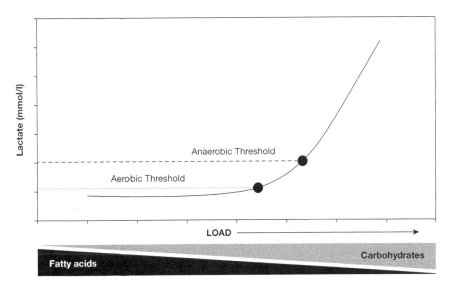

Figure 4.4 Model of the lactate performance curve and energy supply during increasing workload

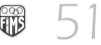

principles of exercise physiology

production and removal – is also called the anaerobic threshold or the respiratoric compensation point or the second lactate turn point. From this point, the lactate production will increase rapidly and then lead to the end of the exercise, because lactate will be accumulated in the muscle cells (Figure 4.4). Although arguments exist over terminology, this point of deflection is also often called the onset of blood lactate accumulation (OBLA). Untrained individuals reach this second deflection point at around 50–65% VO_2 max, whereas endurance athletes reach it at around 80–90% VO_2 max.

Factors related to this lactate accumulation include low tissue O_2, reliance on glycolysis, activation of fast-twitch muscle fibers, and reduced lactate removal. Following endurance training near or above the anaerobic threshold level, lactate accumulation occurs later and at higher exercise intensity. This adaptation training will allow athletes to train at a higher percentage of VO_2 max with less lactate in the blood. Although the VO_2 max or heart rate response of an athlete can be used to gauge the exercise intensity at which the aforementioned adaptations may occur, it must be emphasized that the capacity to maintain the desired exercise intensity cannot be evaluated precisely by these procedures. The accumulated lactate is removed faster if light activity (e.g., slow jogging) instead of rest is taken after the exercise session.

Figure 4.5 contrasts the lactate-performance and the heart rate-performance curves of an untrained person, a marathon runner, and a 400-m runner. The

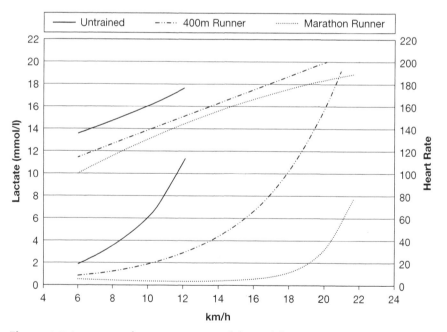

Figure 4.5 Lactate-performance curves of three different trained individuals

untrained person shows a very rapid increase in blood lactate concentration from the resting value, with increasing workload associated with rapid lactate accumulation. The lactate behavior of the marathon runner is characterized by a very distinct plateau with increasing load, which is a result of the aerobic adaptations brought about by endurance training. The anaerobic threshold occurs at a higher percentage of the athlete's aerobic power. This favorable aerobic response may be caused by a decrease in the production of lactic acid and/or a more rapid removal rate of it at any particular level of exercise intensity. In addition, athletes who have undergone endurance training are able to generate ATP to a greater extent through the breakdown of fatty acids, thus conserving glycogen stores. The 400-m runner shows an earlier increase in lactate accumulation than the marathon runner, because of their specific metabolic adaptations resulted from anaerobic training. Anaerobic training also causes a unique adaptation, which is expressed as a long and flatter increase in blood lactate concentration over the anaerobic threshold of about 4 mmol/l), allowing the muscle cells to better tolerate the acidification resulting from increasing levels of blood lactate.

Oxidative (aerobic) system

The anaerobic energy system provides energy at a high liberation rate but with limited supply. Muscles, however, need a continuous and steady supply of energy at rest and during lower-intensity, long-duration activities. Unlike anaerobic ATP production, which has a high liberation rate but low capacity, the oxidative system has lower energy-liberation rates but a tremendous energy-yielding capacity. Thus, aerobic metabolism is the primary method of energy production during endurance events such as the 5,000-m run.

Although the oxidative system cannot produce enough ATP per second to allow the performance of maximal anaerobic activities, at the end of the activity aerobic energy sources are used to replenish anaerobic sources. For example, heavy breathing at the end of an 800-m run is used to replenish the anaerobic energy stores. Aerobic production of ATP occurs in the mitochondria and involves the interaction of the Krebs cycle (also called the citric-acid cycle) and the electron transport chain. Oxygen does not participate in the Krebs-cycle reactions, but it is the final hydrogen acceptor at the end of the electron transport chain.

BASIC ENERGY SYSTEMS

- *ATP–PCr system*: Primarily for high-intensity activities lasting a few seconds.
- *Glycolysis system*: Primarily for "all-out" activities lasting 1–3 minutes.
- *Oxidative system*: Primarily at rest and during low-intensity endurance events.

The maximal amount of oxygen the body can produce aerobically depends on how much oxygen it can obtain and utilize. The term maximal aerobic power, or VO_2 max, reflects the rate at which oxygen can be transported by the cardiorespiratory system to the active muscles. The oxidative system uses primarily carbohydrates and fats as energy substrates.

Oxidation of carbohydrate

The anaerobic breakdown of blood glucose and muscle glycogen is the first step in the metabolism of carbohydrates. In the presence of oxygen, pyruvate – the end product of glycolysis – is converted into acetyl-coenzyme A (Acetyl-CoA), which enters the Krebs cycle. Two ATPs are produced from guanine triphosphate for each molecule of glucose. Six molecules of reduced NADH and two molecules of reduced flavin adenine dinucleotide (FADH2) are also produced from the glucose molecule. The molecules of NADH and FADH2 carry the hydrogen atoms to the electron transport chain, where they are used to rephosphorylate ADP to ATP, a process called oxidative phosphorylation. The complete oxidation of one glucose molecule in skeletal muscle through glycolysis, the Krebs cycle, and the electron transport chain results in a net yield of about 38 ATPs (note that this number may also be reported as 36 ATPs, depending on which shuttle system is used to transport NADH to the mitochondria).

Oxidation of fat

In contrast to carbohydrates, the fat stored inside muscle fibers and fat cells can supply more than 100,000 kcal (418,400 kJ) of energy. However, fat can only be metabolized in the presence of oxygen. Triglycerides, a major energy source of fat oxidation, are stored in fat cells and within skeletal muscles. To be used for energy, the triglycerides are broken down by enzymes known as lipases to their basic units of one molecule of glycerol and three molecules of free fatty acids. After entering mitochondria, free fatty acids undergo a series of reactions in which they are converted to acetyl-CoA and hydrogen atoms, a process called beta oxidation (Figure 4.6).

The fat metabolism then follows the same path as carbohydrate metabolism when acetyl-CoA enters the Krebs cycle and electron transport system. The by-products of the oxidation of free fatty acids are ATP, H_2O, and CO_2. Although different fatty acids result in varying amounts of resynthesized ATP, the complete oxidation of one (18-carbon) triglyceride molecule results in a total energy yield of about 460 ATPs. Although fats provide more kilocalories of energy per gram than carbohydrates, the oxidation of fat requires more oxygen compared with that of carbohydrate. During mild to moderate exercise, such as walking and in-line skating, in which oxygen delivery is not limited by the oxygen transport system, fat is the major energy substrate oxidized. At rest, for example, 70% of the ATP is produced from fat and 30% from carbohydrate, whereas, during high-intensity exercise, a majority of the energy is from carbohydrate, provided an adequate supply is available (Figures 4.7 and 4.8).

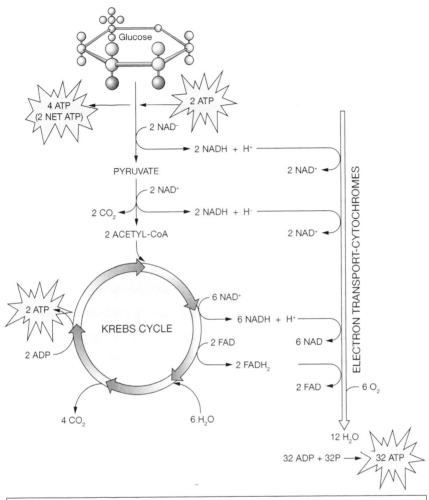

SOURCE	REACTION	NET ATP
Substrate phosphorylation	Glycolysis	2
2 H_2 (4H)	Glycolysis	4
2 H_2 (4H)	Pyruvate → Acetyl-CoA	6
Substrate phosphorylation	Krebs cycle	2
8 H_2 (16H)	Krebs cycle	22
		TOTAL: 36 ATP

Figure 4.6 Complete oxidation of glucose

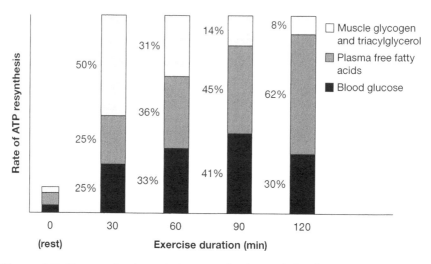

Figure 4.7 Changes in the relative contributions of the basic energy system, prolonged submaximal exercise at an intensity equivalent to about 70% VO_2 max

Source: R.J. Maughan et al., 2000, *Nutrition in Exercise*

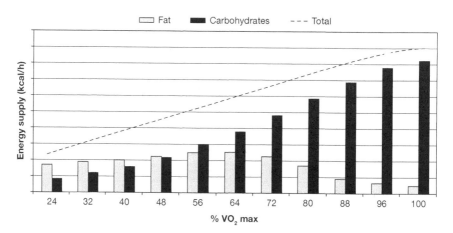

Figure 4.8 Total energy supply and relation of fat and carbohydrates during incremental work load

Source: Estimated from data by J. Achten, Z.E. Jeukendrup, 2003

TRAINING FOR PERFORMANCE AND INJURY PREVENTION

The overall objective of a sports conditioning program is to enhance sports performance by increasing the energy output during a particular activity. Although the specific needs of athletes involved in different sports may vary, the two basic tenets of any training program are to identify the major energy system used in performing a specific sport and to develop a training program that "overloads" that system. To perform well, athletes must train at a level that typically exceeds the amount required for health enhancement. An appropriate sports conditioning program, which includes exercise training and adequate recovery, can improve sports performance, increase resistance to sports-related injuries, and enhance motivation for training. Although total elimination of sports-related injuries is an unrealistic goal, regular participation in a conditioning program, particularly during off- and pre-seasons, will likely enhance a healthy athlete's resistance to injury, and lessen the risk of overuse and severity of injury. This recommendation is particularly important for aspiring young female athletes, who are at greater risk for knee injuries.

An athlete's response to training is variable and depends on many factors, including age, health status, diet, genetics, and initial fitness level. One of the most influential factors is the initial fitness status of the athlete. In general, athletes who are less conditioned make greater gains than those who begin the training program at a higher level of fitness. For example, after several months of training, sedentary adults may improve their aerobic fitness by more than 50%, whereas conditioned athletes may improve by only 3% over the same period of time. However, that 3% improvement may be the difference between getting first place and failing to make it to the final round.

FUNDAMENTAL TRAINING PRINCIPLES

- Specificity.
- Overload.
- Progression.
- Supercompensation.
- Reversibility.
- Tapering.
- Periodization.

Fundamental training principles

The development of effective training programs requires an understanding of fundamental training principles, specific types of training, and individual goals. Physicians and coaches must also be cognizant of the physical and psychological uniqueness of the young athlete. The intensity and volume of most training programs for adults are inappropriate and potentially injurious for children and teenagers, who are still undergoing changes associated with growth and development. The principles of training include specificity, overload, progression, supercompensation, reversibility, tapering, and periodization.

Specificity

Specificity implies that the body's acute and chronic responses and adaptations to exercise training are metabolically and biomechanically specific to the type of exercise performed and the muscle groups involved. When a muscle performs endurance exercise, the number of capillaries and mitochondria increases, which enhances the capacity of the muscle to produce energy aerobically; but, when a muscle performs heavy strength exercise, the primary adaptation is an increase in the number of contractile proteins. This is referred to as the specific adaptation to imposed demand (SAID) principle. Knowing the specific metabolic profile of a sport or activity is important, because, for example, increasing the aerobic power of a sprinter or weightlifter, while neglecting the training of anaerobic power, is of little benefit to the athletes. Aerobic training may in fact reduce speed and power-related performance capabilities in athletes training for anaerobic sports.

In addition, the principle of specificity refers also to the concept that individuals respond differently to the same training stimulus. This variability of the training response, known as high or low responder – respectively, fast or slow responder – maybe influenced by such factors as pretraining status, fitness level, genetic predisposition, and gender.

Overload

The overload principle is based on the need to train the body at a level beyond that to which it is normally accustomed. Overload refers to a level of training above which there is a sufficient training stimulus for chronic adaptations to occur. The amount of overload necessary to elicit a training adaptation depends on the training state of an individual, meaning that an untrained individual needs a very little overload stimulus to improve the performance, whereas an athlete needs to be stimulated with a mix of higher impacts. Overload can be achieved by increasing the frequency, intensity, or duration of exercise.

Adaptations occur when the muscles and physiological systems are no longer overloaded, at which point an otherwise well-designed training program becomes less effective.

Progression

As an athlete adapts to a training stimulus, the exercise load (i.e., intensity, duration, and/or frequency) must be increased so that improvements will continue. The training program can be progressed by increasing the load lifted, training frequency, quality and quantity of drills, or exercise stimulus. However, too great an overload may overstress the physiological systems and increase the risk of sports-related overuse injuries and exercise burnout. The training program that provides an adequate overload stimulus without overstressing the body is optimal. This is important for non-athletes as well as athletes, and the importance of training the muscles and physiological systems while providing adequate time for recovery and adaptation must be stressed.

Supercompensation

The principle of supercompensation is also called stimulus–fatigue–recovery–adaption (SFRA). That means that an appropriate stimulus will cause some level of fatigue, recovery, and then an adaption in a way that performance can be improved. The amount of recovery required after a training session is directly related to the magnitude and duration of the exercise stress. During the recovery period, the restoration process is not stopped once the pre-work-out level is reached, but will progress to an even higher level, which is often called over-compensation or supercompensation. To achieve the most effective improvement in performance capacity, the next training session should commence during this phase. One of the challenges of prescribing training programs is properly balancing the overload and the regeneration period.

Reversibility

Adaptations to regular exercise training begin to return to pre-exercise values when the exercise stimulus is removed. After several weeks of detraining, negative changes in strength and aerobic endurance may be noticed. However, training-induced gains in strength and power seem to diminish at a slower pace compared with gains in aerobic endurance. Under conditions of forced inactivity (e.g., bed-rest), decreases in performance are rapid and significant under these conditions, e.g. VO_2 max can be decreased by 25–30% after three weeks. It is evident that, after a detraining period, both low-, moderately, and highly trained individuals have a more rapid rate of gain after returning to training. However, it is widely accepted that muscle atrophy caused by injury or after an operation will recover in a proportion of 3:1, meaning that an athlete who misses one week of training requires three weeks to return to the same level.

Tapering

Peak performance requires maximal physical and psychological stress tolerance. After periods of intensive training, the athlete's exercise tolerance and performance capacity may start to decrease. Coaches may therefore reduce the training load during a variable period of time, in a progressive, non-linear way, before the next training cycle or a major competition. This practice is referred to as tapering, which may increase muscle power, enhance athletic performance, and decrease the risk of overtraining. The length of a tapering period and the training programs depends on the specific sport, the purpose of the taper, the specific period in a training year, and individual needs. Tapering is an effective training method, and athletes should not be worried about reducing their training volume for several days before an athletic competition.

Periodization

Periodization is a planned variation in the training program. The underlying concept of periodization relates to Selye's general adaptation syndrome, which proposes that, when confronted with a stressor (e.g., exercise), the body will go through the following three stages: shock, adaptation, and staleness. In the latter phase, performance may reach a plateau or decrease. Without a planned variation in the training program, which includes periods of adequate rest, athletes may lose motivation or be overtrained. Periodization allows the training stimulus to remain fresh and therefore can be used to combat staleness, overreaching, and overtraining. The classic model of periodization divides the training program into specific periods of time. In general, a macrocycle is about one year, a mesocycle about three or four months, and a microcycle about one to four weeks. Depending on the number of athletic competitions within a given year, the phases have to be matched with the needs and goals of individual athletes.

A yearlong periodization model generally comprises several mesocycles, which begin with high-volume, low-intensity exercise and gradually progress to lower-volume, higher-intensity training during each of the following mesocycles. Although the names of each phase may differ, the traditional cycle includes the following four mesocycles: (1) preparatory phase; (2) first transition phase; (3) competition phase; and (4) second transition phase or recuperation phase. The last phase consists of low-volume, low-intensity training, or some other types of light physical activity. The goal of the second transition phase is to allow for physical and psychological recovery. In short, periodization involves variations in the training stimulus to optimize gains in performance and reduce the risk of staleness and overtraining. Although this does not mean that new exercises should be performed every training session, noticeable changes in the volume and intensity of training should be made every few weeks.

Exercise guidelines

The design of a training program should be based on many factors, including age, initial fitness level, health status, and individual goals. The amount of gain in strength and aerobic endurance is related to the genetic potential of an individual. A deconditioned person who starts training will make great gains in fitness because of the large adaptational potential that exists. It is therefore not surprising that many different types of training program can enhance the fitness of untrained individuals. However, as training progresses and the individual approaches his/her genetic potential, fitness gains decrease, and it becomes more challenging to continually enhance performance. Thus, expected training outcomes must be kept in perspective when working with different populations. Clearly, training for peak performance is quite different from training for optimal health.

Most endurance events rely heavily on oxidative metabolism for energy production, whereas other activities, such as the 400-m swim, require important contributions from anaerobic glycolysis, and sports such as weight lifting rely primarily on energy from the ATP–PCr system. However, even in events such as the marathon, runners may need to rely on anaerobic metabolism during the final "kick" to the finish line. When designing a training program, it is important to consider the relative contributions of the aerobic and anaerobic energy pathways to sports performance. For example, the overall design of a training program may need to be re-evaluated if prolonged periods of aerobic training diminish gains in muscular power (e.g., jumping height of basketball players). In addition, the importance of training in sport technique, adequate warm-up, cool-down activities, and recovery strategies should not be overlooked. When designing a training program, every coach must use exercise prescriptions based on the four primary program design variables:

- *Training frequency*: the number of training sessions per day or per week, depending on the sport discipline, the training status, and the specific sport season. The training frequency will depend on the interaction of training intensity and duration.
- *Training intensity*: should be calculated from an exercise test (e.g., heart rate or intensity from a stress test in the lab or a field test). There is always an interaction of training intensity and training duration, meaning, in general, the higher the exercise intensity, the shorter the exercise duration.
- *Training duration*: time of a training session.
- *Training mode*: type of a specific physical activity performed by the athlete. That means that all the other three program design variables must be accommodated to the specific type of exercise, e.g., cycling, running, rowing, skiing, cross-country running, etc.

Aerobic training

Aerobic training programs generally involve activities of the large muscle groups, such as in running, swimming, rowing, and cycling. Successful endurance performance depends on several factors, including a high level of VO_2 max, a high lactate threshold, a high percentage of Type 1 (slow-twitch) muscle fibers, effective use of fat as a fuel source, and good exercise economy. When appropriate principles of aerobic training are followed, physiological adaptations in the cardiorespiratory and musculoskeletal systems will result. These adaptations include enhanced oxygen exchange in the lungs, increased cardiac output, enhanced blood flow to skeletal muscles, increased arteriovenous oxygen difference, and increased concentrations of capillaries, mitochondria, myoglobin, and oxidative enzymes in the trained skeletal muscles. In general, to improve aerobic endurance capabilities, an individual should exercise 20–60 minutes for three to five days per week, at an intensity corresponding to between 55/65 and 90% maximum heart rate, and between 40/50 and 85% of oxygen uptake reserve (i.e., the

 61

difference between VO$_2$ max and resting VO$_2$) or heart rate reserve. The range of exercise intensities for enhancing aerobic fitness is broad, reflecting the wide range of intensities that may be used to enhance aerobic fitness in deconditioned individuals and highly trained athletes. Sedentary individuals tend to enjoy continuous aerobic activities, such as walking, at a relatively low intensity (e.g. 20 minutes at 55–65% maximum heart rate), and it is suggested that a more realistic goal for these individuals is a target range of 150–400 kcal (627.6–1673.6 kJ) energy expenditure per day in exercise activities. Highly trained athletes need to exercise at intensities at the high end of the continuum to further enhance their aerobic endurance. To maximize gains in performance, athletes should engage in activities that mimic the movement pattern of the targeted sport. A limitation of continuous training is that the intensity level may be lower than that during competition.

Other types of aerobic endurance training program, including pace/tempo training, interval training, and fartlek training, can be used for specific outcomes. Pace/tempo training involves training at an intensity at, or slightly higher than, the race pace. Pace/tempo training can be performed at a steady pace or using tempo intervals. This type of training allows the athlete to develop a sense of race pace and enhances the body's ability to sustain this exercise intensity. Interval training refers to a type of exercise that involves intense work-out bouts of between 30 seconds and 5 minutes, which are followed by predetermined rest intervals.

SUMMARY OF AEROBIC TRAINING GUIDELINES

- 3–5 days per week.
- 20–60 minutes.
- 60–90% maximum heart rate.

The proposed work-to-rest interval is about 1:1 for the oxidative system, and about 1:2 or 1:4 for anaerobic glycolysis. Interval training allows athletes to train at intensities close to their VO$_2$ max for prolonged periods of time. Fartlek training literally means "speed play." This type of aerobic conditioning involves training at different exercise intensities (e.g., a run at a comfortable pace combined with hill work or short sprints). Although not as systematic or quantifiable as continuous training or interval training, fartlek training can be used to develop a good basis for more intense conditioning, and it also helps to reduce boredom and provides a certain "freedom" during long training sessions.

Fundamentals of fitness training

Despite the training recommendations for athletes, there is a strong consensus about the importance of the relationship between physical activity, health, and well-being. This is based on an accumulation of epidemiological research over the past several decades. Based on that, the Centers for Diseases Control and Prevention and the American College of Sports Medicine recommend a level of at least 30 minutes of moderate-intensity physical activity each day. In addition, as a basis for individual fitness training, the President's Council of Physical Fitness and Sports published the following "Fitness Fundamental Guidelines for Personal Exercise Programs":

- *Cardiorespiratory endurance training*: at least five 30-minute bouts of continuous aerobic exercise each week, e.g., walking, Nordic walking, jogging, cycling, cross-country skiing, swimming, etc.
- *Muscular strength training*: a minimum of two 20-minute sessions per week, including exercises for all the major muscle groups.
- *Muscular endurance training*: at least three 30-minute sessions each week, including exercises such as push-ups, sit-ups, pull-ups, and weight training for all the major muscle-groups.
- *Flexibility training*: 10–12 minutes per day stretching exercises, which can also be included partly in a warm-up or cool-down period. Each work-out should begin with a warm-up, e.g., 5–10 minutes of exercise such as walking, slow jogging, knee lifts, arm circles, or trunk rotations, and should end with a cool-down, e.g., 5–10 minutes of slow walking, low-level exercise combined with stretching.

Anaerobic training

Anaerobic training refers to many different types of conditioning, including sprint work-outs, stair running, plyometrics (stretch–shortening cycle activities), and strength training or resistance training. This type of training enhances speed, strength, and power and relies primarily on the two anaerobic energy sources, namely the ATP-PCr and the glycolytic systems. Anaerobic training that focuses on the ATP–PCr system typically involves relatively intense work intervals of under 10 seconds and adequate recovery between sets, so that lactate does not significantly accumulate. Glycolytic conditioning is characterized by less-intense work intervals and shorter rest periods. For example, strength training with a heavy weight (three repetitions at 90% of the 1 repetition maximum (RM)) and resting 3 minutes between sets relies more on the ATP–PCr system, compared with strength training with moderate loads (12 repetitions at 60% of 1 RM) and resting 1 minute between sets, which relies more on the glycolytic system. Although aerobic metabolism is not typically involved in sustaining these training activities, this energy system is important for recovering energy stores. Physiological adaptations to regular anaerobic training include increases in myofibrillar protein content, anaerobic enzyme activity, metabolic energy stores (e.g. glycogen and phosphagens), and connective-tissue strength. Important adaptations occur within the central and peripheral nervous systems, which further aid in the specific activation of motor units to enhance force and power production.

63

Among the various types of anaerobic training, most athletes include strength training as part of their training program. For the purpose of this chapter, strength training is defined as a specialized type of conditioning that involves the progressive use of resistance to increase one's ability to exert resisting force. This term should be distinguished from the sports of weight lifting and power lifting, in which athletes attempt to lift as much weight as possible in competition. The design of a strength-training program can be complex and requires the manipulation of the following five acute program variables: choice of exercise, order of exercise, number of sets, resistance used, and rest periods between sets and work-outs. By manipulating these variables, an almost infinite number of strength training protocols can be created. Depending on the needs and abilities of athletes, different strength-training programs can be used to optimize gains in strength and power. The use of only one training system over prolonged periods of time will inevitably lead to less than optimal gains, plateaus in progress, or overtraining. Manipulating the acute program variables over time will help optimize gains in performance, reduce the likelihood of injury, and enhance motivation. Basic recommendations for strength training include:

- a training frequency of at least two or three times per week, with adequate rest between training sessions;
- warm-up activities before strength training;
- multijoint and Olympic-style lifts with free weights (barbells and dumbbells), and isolated movements on weight machines;
- multiset training protocols to enhance muscle performance and training adaptations;
- functional exercises for the "core" musculature (i.e., hips, abdomen, and lower back);
- periodized training to enhance performance and decrease risk of overtraining; and
- a safe training environment and qualified instruction.

Four major types of strength training system – isometrics, isokinetics, dynamic constant external resistance, and plyometrics – are discussed below.

Isometric training

Isometric or static training refers to exercises that involve muscle actions without changing the muscle length. Isometric training, which can be performed anywhere with little or no equipment, became popular in the 1950s. Isometrics can be performed by pushing against an immovable object, or by having a weak muscle contract against a stronger muscle; these can be incorporated into rehabilitation programs to counteract strength loss and muscle atrophy. A major limitation of isometric training is that strength gains are specific to the joint angle used during training. Strength gains can be carried over to a small degree of up to about 20° on either side of the trained joint angle, and isometric training at several

64

different joint angles can increase strength throughout the entire range of motion (ROM).

Athletes can use isometric training to increase muscle strength within the ROM where the mechanical advantage is the lowest (i.e., the "sticking point"). Isometric training at a specific joint angle, however, will not enhance motor performance ability.

Isokinetic training

Isokinetics refers to dynamic muscle actions performed at a constant angular velocity. Unlike other types of strength training, the velocity of movement during an isokinetic exercise is controlled mechanically with the aid of an isokinetic machine, which matches the force produced by the muscle group throughout the entire ROM. It is theoretically possible to exert a continual, maximal force throughout a full ROM. Isokinetic training is relatively safe and results in little or no muscle soreness; this may be owing to the fact that most isokinetic devices do not require eccentric muscle actions. Isokinetic training can increase muscle strength and improve motor performance skills such as sprinting and jumping; the optimal training speed, nevertheless, is controversial.

Dynamic constant external resistance training

Dynamic constant external resistance (DCER) training refers to muscle actions performed concentrically and eccentrically with a constant external load. Although the term isotonic has been used to describe free-weight (i.e., barbells and dumbbells) and weight-machine exercises, this term is technically incorrect, because the force exerted by the muscle during these exercises varies with the mechanical advantage of the joint. The term DCER better describes the type of training in which the weight being lifted is constant. DCER training has been proven to enhance muscle strength and power and can result in significant positive changes in motor performance skills. The fact that traditional DCER training with a concentric and eccentric muscle action is more effective than concentric-only training suggests that the eccentric component of DCER is particularly important. Because eccentric force output is greater than concentric force output, in an attempt to optimize strength gains, some athletes may perform eccentric training (also called negative training) with loads up to 120% of their concentric 1 RM. A disadvantage of eccentric training is the development of post-exercise muscle soreness. A spotter is also required to assist with eccentric training.

Compared with training on weight machines, more time is required to learn proper exercise techniques in DCER training, such as the squat and bench press. Also, appropriate spotting procedures need to be followed in DCER training. Common DCER strength training protocols are circuit training, pyramid training, forced repetition training, and super set training.

- *Circuit training*: Circuit training consists of a series of strength exercises performed with minimal rest (about 30 seconds or less) between each set of exercises. This type of training is time efficient, and, in addition to increasing muscle strength, circuit training may also enhance cardiovascular fitness in sedentary individuals. A circuit-training program usually consists of at least 10 exercises performed for 10–15 repetitions, with loads of approximately 40–60% of 1 RM.

- *Pyramid training*: Pyramid training is one of the more effective methods of increasing muscle strength. The design is typically a light-to-heavy (ascending pyramid) mode of training, in which the athlete progresses from a light load to a heavier load while decreasing the number of repetitions performed for each set, continued until only one to three repetitions are performed. Other variations of pyramid training (e.g., heavy-to-light, or descending pyramid) have also proven to be effective.
- *Forced repetition training*: This type of training is an extension of the pyramid training system and is popular among strength athletes. After a set is performed to exhaustion, a spotter assists the lifter by providing just enough assistance for the performance of two to three additional repetitions. Forced repetition training forces the muscle to continue working when it is fatigued. This method of training may result in muscle soreness and is not recommended for beginners.
- *Super set training*: The super set system involves several sets of two exercises for the agonist and antagonist muscle groups, with minimal rest between sets. One example of this type of training is knee extensions immediately followed by knee curls. Another method of super-setting involves performing one set of different exercises for the same muscle group (e.g., bench press and dumbbell fly for the chest). This type of training results in significant gains in strength, local muscular endurance, and muscle hypertrophy.

SUMMARY OF STRENGTH TRAINING GUIDELINES

- At least two or three days per week.
- Perform multiset training protocols.
- Include functional, multijoint exercises.

Plyometric training

Plyometric training, also known as stretch–shortening cycle exercise, refers to activities that allow the muscle to reach maximal force in the shortest possible time. This type of training is often used by track and field athletes to develop explosive strength and power. Plyometric training involves a quick, powerful movement using a pre-stretch or countermovement that involves the stretch–shortening cycle. The slight stretch before the action of concentric muscle stores elastic energy and results in a more forcible action of the concentric muscle.

norbert bachl and avery d. faigenbaum

This type of training may also facilitate the recruitment of additional muscle fibers involved in the movement. Traditional heavy strength training characterized by slow-velocity movements does not necessarily improve the force development at rapid movement, which is required in events such as the discus and high jump.

The potential effects of plyometric training are noticeable in jumping ability. If the jumper bends at the knees and the hips immediately before jumping (countermovement), he/she will jump higher than if the jump were performed from the bent knee position held for 3–5 seconds (no countermovement). Plyometric exercises can be performed for the upper and lower body using medicine balls and jumping drills and are often categorized as low intensity (e.g., squat jump), medium intensity (e.g., double leg tuck jump), or high intensity (e.g., depth jump). Because of the stress placed on the muscles involved, connective tissue, and joints, plyometric exercises need to be carefully prescribed and progressed. Athletes must understand proper plyometric exercise technique and have a sufficient base of muscular strength, speed, and balance to avoid the risk of injury.

Flexibility training

Flexibility refers to the ROM of a joint or combination of joints. Flexibility training can enhance athletic performance, improve posture, and decrease muscle tension and body stiffness. Exercises designed to enhance flexibility should be preceded by at least 5–10 minutes of general warm-up (e.g., slow jogging) to increase heart rate, blood flow, deep muscle temperature, viscosity of joint fluids, and perspiration. In flexibility training, athletes typically perform 8–12 sport-specific stretches or movements. After practice and competition, flexibility exercises may help to decrease muscle stiffness. Four different types of flexibility training are static stretching, dynamic stretching, ballistic stretching, and proprioceptive neuromuscular facilitation (PNF):

Static stretching
This type of stretching involves relaxation and elongation of the stretched muscle. Static stretching is performed slowly, and the end position of each stretch is held for about 20–30 seconds. This type of stretching is easy to learn, and, because it is performed slowly, the likelihood of injury is reduced. Static stretching following practice and competition may be preferable for strength and power athletes. A sitting toe-touch is an example of a static stretch.

Dynamic stretching
Dynamic flexibility refers to the available ROM during active movements. Dynamic stretching involves movements that are specific to a sport or movement pattern. A soccer player performing long walking strides to stretch the hip flexors to enhance flexibility of the hip joints is an example of a dynamic stretch. This type of pre-event activity may augment subsequent performance. Although these stretches utilize speed of movement, they do not involve bouncing.

Ballistic stretching

This type of stretching involves bouncing-type movements and is sometimes used in the pre-exercise warm-up. However, because of the nature of these exercises (i.e., high force and quick movements), ballistic stretching may injure muscles and connective tissue. For example, if an athlete sits on the floor with legs extended and repeatedly bounces while reaching toward both ankles, the high force and quick movements may injure the lower back and hamstrings. Ballistic stretching is not a preferred method of flexibility training.

Proprioceptive neuromuscular facilitation

PNF training is usually performed with a partner and involves both passive movements and active (concentric and isometric) muscle actions. There are different types of PNF stretching, but it typically involves a passive pre-stretch of the involved muscle, a contraction against opposition, and, finally, relaxation and further stretching. Common PNF stretches with a partner are used to enhance hamstring, quadriceps, and chest flexibility. Because it facilitates muscular inhibition, PNF stretching is a very effective method of enhancing flexibility.

SUMMARY OF FLEXIBILITY TRAINING GUIDELINES

- Warm up before stretching with submaximal aerobic activity.
- Perform flexibility exercises for all the major muscle groups.
- Perform 8–12 stretches or dynamic movements.
- Hold static stretches for 20–30 seconds.

Overtraining and overreaching

In an attempt to induce training adaptations and improve performance, athletes expose themselves to planned periods of intensive training. However, if intensive training is not followed by adequate rest and recovery, overtraining or overreaching may result. Burnout, staleness, over-fatigue, and unexplained underperformance syndrome (UPS) are some other terms used to describe a plateau or decrease in performance because of excessive training. Overtraining is caused by training errors (e.g., inappropriate rate of training progression, prolonged monotonous training, inadequate periods of rest and recovery, or failure to taper training before competition). When the effects are short term, overtraining is called overreaching. Overtraining syndrome refers to the conditioning results from overtraining. Whereas recovery from overreaching can be achieved with a few days of rest, overtraining syndrome can last as long as 6 months. Two distinct types of overtraining are sympathetic overtraining syndrome, which includes increased sympathetic activity at rest, and parasympathetic overtraining syndrome, which includes increased parasympathetic activity at rest.

Susceptibility to overtraining may increase when an athlete is highly motivated but has failed to plan long-term training schedules to achieve specific goals. Manifestations of overtraining include increased or decreased resting heart rate, decrease in body mass, muscle tenderness, increased risk for infection, loss of appetite, sleep disturbances, chronic fatigue, psychological staleness, persistent flu-like symptoms, and a decrease in performance. An overtrained athlete may exhibit one or more of these symptoms, and markers of overtraining in endurance athletes may be different from those in athletes involved in anaerobic sports (e.g., weight lifting). Unfortunately, performance decrements typically occur too late to be a good marker of overtraining, and an inexpensive, sensitive gauge of over-training applicable to all athletes is not yet available. Although many parameters of overtraining have been evaluated (e.g., the ratio of total testosterone to cortisol, creatine kinase levels, nocturnal urinary atecholamine excretion, blood lactate profiling, and abnormal T-wave patterns in the electrocardiogram), none of these factors is able to confirm the diagnosis of overtraining syndrome. By the time a coach realizes that an athlete has been pushed too far, it may already be too late.

The best "treatment" for overtraining syndrome is prevention. Training programs need to be carefully prescribed, and athletes should be provided with ample opportunity for rest and recovery. As a general rule, a hard training session should be followed by one or two days of less-intense training and adequate recovery. One of the advantages of a periodized training program is that time for physical and mental recovery is incorporated into the training plan. Too much training for too long a duration is a key factor in the development of overtraining syndrome. Periods of reduced training can provide time for the cardiovascular and neuromuscular systems to recover from the stresses of regular training.

Overtrained athletes usually recover faster from complete rest than from a reduced training level. However, if the rest period lasts several weeks, training-induced adaptations will decline, and performance expectations may therefore need to be modified. Medical examinations, nutritional guidance, and psychological

MARKERS OF OVERTRAINING

- Increase or decrease in resting heart rate.
- Decreased body mass.
- Muscle tenderness.
- Loss of appetite.
- Disturbances.
- Chronic fatigue.
- Psychological staleness.
- Flu-like symptoms.
- Decreased performance.

counseling should also be part of the recovery process. Physicians should get to know their athletes and their individual tolerance for sports training. Training programs for athletes need to be based on knowledge of exercise science and consideration of individual needs and goals. Athletic training programs should be designed to improve athletic performance, reduce the risk of injury, and enhance the potential for adherence to life-long physical activity programs. As it takes years of training to achieve high-level performance, training should be viewed as a gradual process, and athletes should be provided with adequate time for rest and recovery. The art and science of training athletes involve modifying the training program to maintain an effective training stimulus, while recognizing individual differences in motivation and stress tolerance.

SUGGESTED READING

Achten J., Jeukendrup A.E. Maximal fat oxidation during exercise in trained men. *International Journal of Sports Medicine* 24: 603–08, 2003.

American College of Sports Medicine. *ACSM's Guidelines for Exercise Testing and Prescription*. 8th ed. Philadelphia, PA: Lippincott Williams & Wilkins, 2010.

American College of Sports Medicine. ACSM's position stand: Progression models in resistance training for healthy adults. *Medicine and Science in Sports and Exercise*, 41(3): 687–708, 2009.

Bachl N., Baron R., Smekal G. Principles of Exercise Physiology and Conditioning. In Frontera, W. et al., Editors, *Clinical Sports Medicine: Medical Management and Rehabilitation*, Philadelphia, PA: Elsevier Health Sciences, 2007.

Behm, D., Chaouachi, A. A review of the acute effects of static and dynamic stretching on performance. *European Journal of Applied Physiology*, 2011 (epub. ahead of print).

Bompa, T., Haff, G. *Periodization*, 5th ed. Champaign, IL: Human Kinetics, 2009.

Brooks G., Fahey T., Baldwin, K. *Exercise Physiology: Human Bioenergetics and its Application*. 4th ed. New York: McGraw-Hill, 2005.

Elliot, M., Wagner, P., Chui, L. Power athletes and distance training: Physiological and biomechanical rationale for change. *Sports Medicine*, 37(1): 47–57, 2007.

Faigenbaum A., Kraemer W., Blimkie C., et al. Youth resistance training: Updated position statement paper from the National Strength and Conditioning Association. *Journal of Strength and Conditioning Research*, 23: S60–S79, 2009.

Henriksson J., Sahlin, K. Metabolism during exercise – energy expenditure and hormonal changes. In Kjaer, M. et al., Editors, *Textbook of Sports Medicine*, Malden, MA: Blackwell Science, 30–48, 2003.

Kraemer, W., Fleck, S., Deschenes, M. *Exercise Physiology – Integrating Theory and Application*. Philadelphia, PA: Lippincott, Williams & Williams, 2011.

Mujika, I. *Tapering and Peaking for Optimal Performance*, Champaign, IL: Human Kinetics, 2009.

National Strength and Conditioning Association, *Essentials of Strength Training and Conditioning*, 3rd ed. Champaign, IL: Human Kinetics, 2008.

Stone, M., Stone, M., Sands, W. *Principles and Practice of Resistance Training*. Champaign, IL: Human Kinetics, 2007.

Wilmore, J., Costill, D., Kenney, L. *Physiology of Sport and Exercise*. 4th ed. Champaign, IL: Human Kinetics, 2008.

 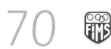

CHAPTER 5

SPORT NUTRITION

Norbert Bachl and Debra Wein

Nutritional recommendations for an athlete must take into consideration the specific energy requirements of the sport in question and the daily training volume, age, gender, and dietary preferences of the athlete. There is no single diet for optimal physical performance, but every diet should address the energy needs, macronutrient composition, micronutrient intake, and fluid balance of the athlete.

ENERGY NEEDS

The total daily energy requirement for athletes participating in endurance, strength, and team sports is between 2,500 and 4,000 kcal (10,460–16,736 kJ) for women and 3,000–6,000 kcal (12,552–25,104 kJ) for men. For less active individuals aged 18 to 35 years, the daily energy requirement is approximately 1,800–2,100 kcal (7,531.2–8,786.4 kJ) for women and 2,200–2,500 kcal (9,204.8–10,460 kJ) for men. The energy requirement may be even higher during growth, and there is a slight decrease with advancing age.

Certain activities require a larger energy intake during competition or periods of high-volume/intensity training. Saris reported an average energy expenditure of approximately 6,500 kcal (27,196 kJ) per day for nearly three weeks during the Tour de France, with daily variations between 3,000 kcal (12,552kJ) for a rest day and 9,000 kcal (37,656 kJ) when cycling over a mountain pass. Energy requirements for elite cross-country skiers can exceed 5,000 kcal (20,920 kJ) for women and 8,000 kcal (33,472 kJ) for men during high-volume training. During the Race Across America, male competitors need more than 14,000–16,000 kcal (58,576–66,944 kJ) per day when cycling 22–23 hours a day at an average speed of 29–31 km/h.

On the other hand, there are groups of athletes such as gymnasts, ballet dancers, and ice dancers, as well as certain weight-class athletes such as boxers, wrestlers, and participants of judo who must strive to maintain a low body mass and are therefore more likely to take in too few calories for their activity. In such situations,

Table 5.1 Equations for calculation of RMR in kcal/d (Burke, 2007)

Harris–Benedict (1919)

Male: RMR (kcal) = 66.47 + 13.75 (body mass in kg)
                        + 5 (height in cm)
                        − 6.76 (age in years)

Female: RMR (kcal) = 655.1 + 9.56 (body mass in kg)
                          + 1.85 (height in cm)
                          − 4.68 (age in years)

Table 5.2 Representative values for activity factor (Burke, 2007)

Activity category	Per unit of time of activity	Range
Resting Sleeping, reclining	RMR x 1.0	< 1.1
Very light Seated and standing activities, painting trades, driving, laboratory work, typing, sewing, ironing, cooking, playing cards, playing a musical instrument, billiards	RMR x 1.5	1.5–2.5
Light Walking on a level surface at 2.5–3 mph, garage work, electrical trades, carpentry, restaurant trades, tennis, ten-pin bowling, tennis (leisurely pace)	RMR x 2.5	2.0–4.0
Moderate Walking 3.5–4 mph, weeding and hoeing, carrying a load, cycling (slow), skiing, dancing, cricket, horse-riding, sailing, swimming (slow), stretching, tennis (moderate)	RMR x 4.0	3.0–5.0
Strenuous Jogging/running (7 km/h), tennis (fast pace), ice/roller skating, swimming (moderate pace), gymnastics, aerobic, basketball, football, squash, weight training, walking uphill with a load, soccer	RMR x 7.0	5.0–9.0
Very strenuous Swimming (race pace), rowing (race pace), cycling (race pace), squash (fast pace), running (10–15 km/h)	RMR x 10.0	7.0–13.0

Table 5.3 Methods for dietary assessments (Dunford, 2006)

Method	Coverage	Advantage	Disadvantage
Dietary history	All items or selected items	Long-term perspectives of dietary habits individual data	– Time consuming – Skilled interviewer needed – Memory demanding – Quantitative data difficult to obtain – Variations in dietary habits lost
24-hr recall	All foods	Relatively rapid and simple	– Selection of interview day critical – Quantitative data difficult to obtain – Skilled interviewer needed
Food frequency questionnaire (FFQ)	Only listed food items	– Rapid and simple – Easy to computerize – Large groups covered by mail	– Restricted number of food items – Memory demanding – No direct contact with interviewer
Weight food diary	All foods	Exact data on nutrient content possible (not dependent on accuracy of food tables)	– Dietary intake may be affected – Resource demanding – Requires reliable equipment – Collaboration necessary

where energy intake falls below the energy requirement, the result is a relative state of malnutrition with respect to micronutrients. Female gymnasts sometimes consume fewer than 1,200 kcal (5,020.0 kJ) per day, which may result in an especially low intake of micronutrients such as vitamins B_1, C, E, and folate, and minerals, including iron, magnesium, calcium, and zinc, and contribute to the female athlete triad. In addition to nutrition counseling regarding energy needs and performance, nutritional supplementation might be beneficial to these athletes.

Measurement of total daily energy expenditure:

- indirect calorimetry;
- doubly-labeled water;
- predicting total daily energy expenditure by multiplying resting metabolic rate (RMR) by an appropriate activity factor (Tables 5.1 and 5.2).

To evaluate/control the present energy intake and nutritional status of an athlete, there are various methods of assessment to choose from (Table 5.3).

MACRONUTRIENT COMPOSITION

MACRONUTRIENT COMPOSITION

Diets rich in whole grains, vegetables, and fruits (high-carbohydrate foods):

- help prevent disease;
- maintain body weight;
- optimize athletic performance.

Optimal nutrition includes a plant-based diet that is high in carbohydrate (55–60% of total calories), low in fat (< 30% of total calories), and adequate in protein (10–15% of total calories). Decades of research support that diets rich in whole grains, vegetables, and fruits (i.e. high-carbohydrate foods) help prevent disease, maintain body weight, and optimize athletic performance. Despite the popularity of fad diets, there is still no substantial evidence that supports a change in that recommendation. A carbohydrate-deficient diet would, in fact, deplete muscle and liver glycogen rapidly and compromise the capacity for both high-intensity anaerobic and long-duration aerobic exercise.

Carbohydrate recommendations can also be given in relative terms, such as grams of carbohydrates per kilogram of body weight. Most athletes need a carbohydrate intake of 4–6 g/kg body weight per day. A carbohydrate need of 70% of the

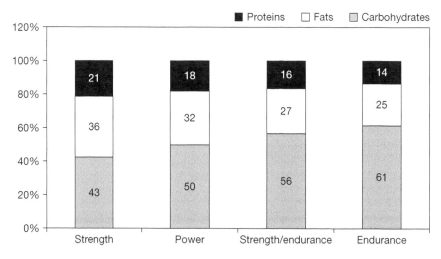

Figure 5.1 Contribution of proteins, fats, and carbohydrates to energy metabolism during various intensities of exercise

Source: From McArdle, Katch et al., 2009

74

norbert bachl and debra wein

daily energy intake (such as in a carbohydrate loading program, explained below) increases the amount to up to 7–8 g/kg body weight per day. When endurance training is particularly intense, or during special competitions of longer duration, a carbohydrate intake of 9–10 g/kg body weight per day may be necessary (Figure 5.1).

Carbohydrates are core

Carbohydrates are what the body relies on most for fuel during exercise, and the amount stored in the body will directly affect the athlete's stamina and endurance.

Carbohydrates are stored in limited amounts as glycogen in muscles and the liver. The muscle glycogen is the fuel for the muscles, whereas liver glycogen maintains a normal level of blood sugar to fuel the brain. Training and eating properly can increase glycogen stores.

Adequate carbohydrate intake is especially important for endurance athletes, because stored glycogen provides substantial energy during prolonged bouts of aerobic exercise. High carbohydrate intakes are also important for anaerobic training, as the body uses carbohydrates exclusively during very-high-intensity activities, and muscle glycogen depletion can occur. An understanding of the different types of carbohydrate and how the body metabolizes them will help explain the benefits of a high carbohydrate diet.

CARBOHYDRATES ARE CORE

- Carbohydrates are what the body relies on most for fuel during exercise.
- The amount of carbohydrates stored in the body directly impacts stamina and endurance.

Complex versus simple carbohydrates

Carbohydrates have traditionally been categorized as either simple or complex, based on their molecular weight. Simple carbohydrates include the common monosaccharides and disaccharides, such as glucose, fructose, sucrose, and galactose, which can be found in sweets and candies. Simple carbohydrates are also produced naturally in fruits and vegetables. Complex carbohydrates are polysaccharides, which include the digestible starches (pasta, bread, cereal, legumes, and starchy vegetables) and indigestible fibers.

Fiber

Fiber is defined as "plant cellular material resistant to digestion by human beings" and can be further classified as soluble, such as hemicellulose (bran, cereals, whole

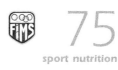

grains such as bulgur or brown rice), pectin (apples, citrus fruits, strawberries), and gums (oatmeal, dried beans, other legumes), or insoluble, such as cellulose (whole-wheat flour, bran, cabbage family, celery, peas, beans, root vegetables) and lignin (mature vegetables, wheat). Complex carbohydrates from "whole" foods such as whole-wheat bread, brown rice, fruits, and vegetables provide the fiber needed to keep the digestive tract running smoothly, as well as keeping a better balance of vitamins and minerals than the highly refined simple sugars. The 2010 Dietary Guidelines for Americans recommend at least 25 grams of fiber a day for women and 38 grams a day for men as part of a healthy diet, versus the 12–14 grams that the average American eats every day.

The glycemic index

More recently, carbohydrates have been looked at in relation to their glycemic effect, using properties such as texture, structure, and absorption rate rather than molecular weight. The glycemic effect of a food is how high and fast the blood glucose rises, and how quickly the bodily responses return the blood glucose to normal level.

Different foods have different effects on blood glucose, depending on the following factors:

- the digestibility of the starch in the food;
- interactions of the starch with the protein in the food;
- the amounts and kinds of fat, sugar, and fiber in the food;
- the presence of other constituents, such as molecules that bind starch;
- the form of the food (e.g. dry, paste, or liquid; coarsely or finely ground; how thoroughly cooked); and
- the combination of foods consumed at a given time.

Foods can now be classified by their glycemic index (GI) as either low, medium, or high. High-GI foods are absorbed quickly by the gut and can raise blood sugar levels rapidly, whereas low-GI foods are absorbed slowly and have a moderate effect on raising blood sugar levels. Some of the low fat or non-fat, heavily processed foods (i.e. non-fat cookies and cakes) tend to have a high GI because of the addition of simple sugars when the fat is taken out. In contrast, minimally processed, high-fiber foods with little fat (i.e. a slice of multigrain bread with peanut butter) tend to have a lower GI.

The United States Department of Agriculture (USDA) and Department of Health and Human Services (DHHS) have developed the "food guide pyramid" to assist in meal planning and food choices. The intent was to replace the concept of the four major food groups and give a better understanding of which foods were more appropriate in greater amounts. The food pyramid recommends numbers of servings for various daily caloric intakes. Most recently, with the release of the

76

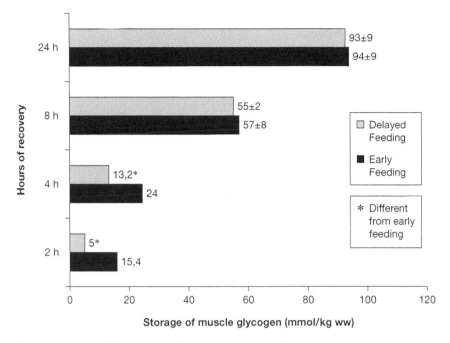

Figure 5.2 2010 Dietary Guidelines for Americans: Food group recommendations
Source: Department of Agriculture, 2010

2010 Dietary Guidelines for Americans, the USDA and DHHS took this one step further with the unveiling of the website www.ChooseMyPlate.gov. This new, simplified approach to nutrition and food-group recommendations breaks down food groups by balancing the correct portions of each food group on a plate. For example, fruits and vegetables make up one-half of the plate, grains take up one-quarter, and the final quarter of the plate is protein. Additionally, there is a glass of milk (or any dairy item) paired with the plate of food groups (Figure 5.2). Unlike the old food guide pyramid, new recommendations are now offered in a measureable quantity (ounces or cups) rather than servings. By logging on to www.ChooseMyPlate.gov, individuals can now receive personalized nutrition recommendations in their "Daily Food Plan," based on age, gender, weight, height, and physical-activity level. To appreciate the role of the personalized "Daily Food Plan" in helping an athlete to plan his/her daily intake of food, a 2,400-calorie diet is described below. In this example, the personalized "Daily Food Plan" is designed for a 23-year-old female who is 5' 4" and 125 lbs and who participates in more than 60 minutes of physical activity a day. This athlete should consume the following amount of food from each food group for her 2,400-calorie food plan:

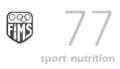

77

- 8 ounces of grains;
- 3 cups of vegetables;
- 2 cups of fruits;
- 3 cups of milk and dairy; and
- 6.5 ounces of protein foods.

To clear up any confusion, it is important to outline the appropriate serving sizes and food-group tips as described in the "Daily Food Plan":

- *Simplifying serving size*: Serving sizes are not designed to portray how much a person should consume as a meal or a snack, but to serve as a pattern with which to compare his/her intake.
- *Grains*: Make half your grains whole; 1 ounce is equivalent to 1 slice of bread, 1 cup of ready-to-eat cereal, or half a cup of cooked rice, cooked pasta, or cooked cereal. For more specific amounts, please visit www.ChooseMyPlate.gov.
- *Vegetables*: Vary your veggies. Make half your plate fruits and vegetables; 1 cup is equivalent to 1 cup of raw or cooked vegetables, or vegetable juice, or 2 cups of raw leafy greens. For more specific amounts, please visit www.ChooseMyPlate.gov.
- *Fruits*: Make half your plate fruits and vegetables; 1 cup of fruit is equivalent to 1 cup of fruit or 100% fruit juice or half a cup of dried fruit. For more specific amounts, please visit www.ChooseMyPlate.gov.
- *Dairy*: Switch to fat-free or low-fat (1%) milk; 1 cup of dairy is equivalent to 1 cup of milk, yogurt, or soymilk, 1.5 ounces of natural cheese, or 2 ounces of processed cheese. For more specific amounts, please visit www.ChooseMyPlate.gov.
- *Protein foods*: Choose lean proteins; 1 ounce of protein foods is equivalent to 1 ounce of meat, poultry or fish, one-quarter of a cup of cooked beans, 1 egg, 1 tablespoon of peanut butter, or a half ounce of nuts or seeds.

Carbohydrate loading

During preparation for a competition, a training period with high intensity, or sustained endurance competitions, carbohydrate intake can be increased to 65–70% of the daily energy intake for a few days. Table 5.4 indicates the factors affecting the decision to undertake carbohydrate loading. Numerous investigations have shown that the time to exhaustion during physical exercise increases with initial muscle glycogen content, and athletes are thus advised to maintain high carbohydrate intakes while decreasing the amount of training during the last 3–5 days before competition. This diet can nearly double the muscular glycogen content.

Table 5.4 Factors affecting the decision to undertake carbohydrate (CHO) loading
(Burke, 2007)

CHO loading should be considered if:	CHO loading is not necessary if:
Exercise is moderate intensity	Exercise ≠ endurance activity
Endurance activity where heavy demands are placed on glycogen stores (e.g., marathon, triathlon, cross-country skiing)	Activity < 60–90 min
Activity > 90 min of continuous exercise	High-intensity activity for short time (e.g., sprint events, field events)
Athlete currently eating less than 7–10 g CHO/kg BM/d and is motivated to follow a loading regimen	Athlete is already on a CHO diet (> 8–9 g/kg BM/d or more than 800 g CHO/d)
Sport allows athlete to devote 2–3 days to tapered exercise and high carbohydrate intake prior to event	Athlete suffers from unstable diabetes or is hyperlipidemic → very high CHO diet is contraindicated
No medical reasons contraindicating very high CHO intake for 3–5 days	Athlete competes in a sport that is weight sensitive, so he or she cannot afford the gain in body mass (~1–2 kg)
In previous events, athlete experienced overwhelming fatigue or "no fuel"	

Before exercise

Proper nourishment before exercise serves various purposes. The appropriate pre-exercise feeding should:

- prevent low blood sugar during exercise;
- provide fuel by topping off muscle glycogen stores;
- settle the stomach, absorb gastric juices, and prevent hunger; and
- instill confidence in the athlete's abilities.

It is important to remind athletes that fasting is detrimental to performance and is strongly discouraged before exercise. Unless observed for religious reasons, fasting is not recommended.

The pre-exercise meal should consist primarily of high-carbohydrate, low-fat foods for easy and fast digestion. A diet with high-glycemic carbohydrates within 1 hour before exercise, however, may negatively affect exercise performance, because the rapidly rising blood sugar causes an excessive release of insulin, which leads to a relative hypoglycemia and inhibits lipid mobilization from adipose tissue, both triggering an early depletion of the carbohydrate reserves. In contrast, low-glycemic carbohydrates will avoid these effects, as well as providing a steady supply of glucose available from the digestive tract during the exercise period. Low GI foods are thus generally recommended before activity (Table 5.5).

Table 5.5 Carbohydrates, calories, and glycemic index of commonly consumed foods

Food	Carbohydrates (g)	Total calories	Glycemic index
Spaghetti/macaroni/noodles (1 cup)	40	200	Medium
White/brown rice (1 cup)	35	160	Medium
Parboiled rice			Low
Baked potato (1 large)	55	240	High
Starchy vegetables			High
Corn (1/2 cup)	18	80	
Winter squash (1/2 cup)	15	65	
Carrots (1 medium)	10	60	
Peas (1/2 cup)	10	40	
Tomato sauce (1/2 cup)	10	80	
Legumes			Low
Baked beans (1 cup)	50	330	
Lentils (1 cup)	40	215	
Kidney beans (1 cup)	33	204	
Lima beans (1 cup)	28	140	
Garbanzo beans (1 cup)	27	287	
Split-pea soup (11 oz)	35	220	
Bread products			Medium to high
Bread, whole grain (2 slices)	25	150	
Submarine roll 8″ (1 large)	60	280	
Bagel (1)	30	210	
English muffin (1)	25	130	
Bran muffin (1 large)	45	320	
Corn bread (1 large slice)	29	198	
Graham crackers (2 squares)	11	60	
Cold/hot cereals			Medium to high
Grape nuts (1/2 cup)	46	200	
Shredded wheat (1 cup)	37	180	
Raisin bran (1 cup)	42	180	
All bran (1 cup)	27	180	
Oatmeal (1 oz)	30	140	
Cream of wheat (1 oz)	22	100	
Pancakes 4″ (2)	30	140	Medium
Waffles, Eggo (2)	34	240	Medium
Fruits			Medium
Apple/orange	20	80	
Banana	26	105	
Raisins (1/2 cup)	60	240	
Grapes (1 cup)	16	58	
Apple sauce (1/2 cup)	26	97	
Dried apricots (8 halves)	30	120	
Fruit yogurt (1 cup)	50	250	Low

In recovery after prolonged or heavy exercise, the most immediate nutritional priority is rehydration, closely followed by restoration of the body's carbohydrate stores. To enhance the rate of muscle and liver glycogen resynthesis, an immediate post-exercise carbohydrate intake of between 0.7 and 1.5 g/kg body weight in the first 2 hours and then 0.7–1 g/kg body weight per hour is generally recommended. This amount of carbohydrate intake will result in a muscle glycogen resynthesis rate of about 7% per hour. Although this rate decreases with increased muscular glycogen content, glycogen stores can be re-established within 24 hours after a glycogen-depleting bout of exercise, if a total carbohydrate intake of about 9–10 g/kg body weight is available in this period. Recent investigations show that, during the recovery period, carbohydrates with higher or moderate GI and a small amount of protein are the most effective method of replacing muscle glycogen

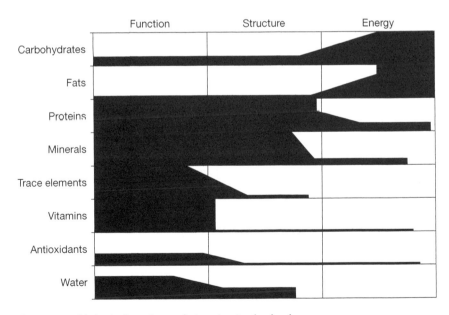

Figure 5.3 Biologic functions of vitamins in the body
Source: From McArdle, Katch et al., 2009

stores (Figure 5.3). When choosing a recovery meal or snack, choose food items or combinations in the ratio 3–4:1 for carbohydrates:protein.

Lipids

Lipids are a primary energy source, providing up to 70% of the total energy in rest and about 50% during light and moderate exercise. When exercise continues for more than 3 hours, the role of stored lipid becomes more important and may provide more than 80% of the energy requirements in prolonged exercise. Fat serves many other functions that are indirectly related to exercise performance – it is an essential component of cell membranes, and nerve fibers and vital organs are supported and cushioned by it; all steroid hormones in the body are produced from cholesterol; fat-soluble vitamins that gain entry into the body are stored in, and transported through the body, via fat; the insulating subcutaneous fat layer also helps preserve body heat.

Fat is stored mainly in the adipose tissue, and some in muscle cells. The metabolic mixture between carbohydrates and lipids is different during exercise of varying intensities. During exercises of light to mild intensity (40% VO_2 max), the main energy source is lipid, predominantly as plasma free fatty acid (FFA) delivered from adipose tissue depots. When the intensity of the exercise increases, the balance of fuel utilization crosses over – the energy for the more intensive exercise is provided predominantly by muscle glycogen and blood glucose. This pattern of energy use shows the important role of lipids during endurance exercises of light to mild intensity, and the role of muscle glycogen as the major energy source during high-intensity aerobic exercise. As the saying goes, "fat burns in a carbohydrate flame." Endurance training increases the capacity for fat metabolism in the muscles, so that, during submaximal exercises, fat metabolism will cover a greater proportion of the energy demands of the trained athlete than of an untrained person. This increased capacity is caused by an increased quantity of enzymes involved in b-oxidation, Krebs-cycle metabolism, and electron-transport chain, as well as an improved transport of fatty acids through the muscle fiber and within the muscle cell by the action of carnitine and carnitine-transferase.

Many athletes neglect their fat intake, fearing an increase in body fat. It is important to remind athletes that an intake of 20–25% of calories from fat is not only acceptable but also preferred. Allowing a misunderstanding of the role of fat

---

LIPIDS

- Many athletes neglect fat intake, fearing an increase in body fat.
- Remind athletes that an intake of 20–25% of calories from fat is not only acceptable but also recommended.

---

in the body can place the athlete at greater risk for the female athlete triad. A more detailed discussion can be found under the section "Female Athlete Triad" in this chapter.

Protein

Protein is a class of nitrogen-containing compounds formed by amino acids. Proteins are the major structural component of the cell and are used for growth, repair, and maintenance of body tissue, as well as maintaining the osmotic pressure in the plasma. Hemoglobin, enzymes, and many hormones and antibodies for protecting the body from diseases are produced from proteins. Protein can also produce energy for the body. Twenty amino acids have been identified as necessary for human growth and metabolism, eight of which cannot be synthesized in the body and must be consumed in the diet. These eight amino acids are therefore termed essential amino acids.

Protein catabolism during exercise becomes most apparent when the body's carbohydrate reserves are low. This catabolism can be seen especially in prolonged strenuous exercise, when the alanine–glucose cycle may account for up to 40–50% of the total glucose released by the liver.

Available evidence suggests that the daily protein requirements for a healthy adult are about 0.83 g/kg body weight, and, in adolescents, 0.9 g/kg body weight. The amount of protein required for strength and speed athletes is up to 1.2–1.8 g/kg body weight per day. Athletes engaged in endurance training are recommended to increase their protein intake to up to 1.2–1.4 g/kg body weight per day, which can be easily achieved by a normal balanced diet. Many athletes believe that supplementing the diet with amino acids such as arginine and ornithine will stimulate the release of growth hormone. After high-intensity exercise, nevertheless, the concentration of circulating growth hormone increases. The effectiveness of such supplements is thus debatable, and these supplements are therefore considered unnecessary. Similarly, many athletes turn to protein supplements to achieve the recommended protein requirement (1.2–1.8 g/kg body weight). However, it is important first to determine the regular protein intake of the athlete

---

PROTEINS

Protein catabolism during exercise is most apparent:

- when the body's carbohydrate stores are low;
- especially after prolonged, strenuous exercise;
- when the alanine–glucose cycle may account for 40–50% of total glucose released by the liver.

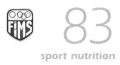

before suggesting a protein supplement. Many sports have high calorie demands, and it is likely that athletes involved in these sports are already taking in adequate protein.

The vegetarian approach

For various reasons, some recreational athletes and an increasing number of competitive and champion athletes have adopted vegetarianism. The true vegetarians, or vegans, eat only food from plant sources. Lacto-vegetarians additionally consume dairy products, and lacto-ovo-vegetarians eat plant foods, dairy products, and eggs. Vegetarian athletes who consume dairy products and eggs are at a lower risk of poor nutritional intake, because the diet is that much less restrictive.

How can athletes handle the vegetarian diet to maintain optimal performance? For athletes who are strict vegans, it is necessary to select their foods very carefully to provide a good balance of the essential amino acids, sufficient calorie intake, and adequate sources of zinc, riboflavin, vitamin B12, vitamin D, calcium, and iron (Tables 5.6 and 5.7). Poor planning or lack of knowledge has led some athletes to experience a decreased performance capacity after switching to a vegetarian diet. Vegan athletes should be referred to a qualified, registered dietitian for help in selecting foods and diets that maximize nutrient intakes.

BALANCE OF MICRONUTRIENTS

Vitamins and minerals have an important role in energy metabolism (Tables 5.6 and 5.7). The intake of vitamins and minerals is positively related to the energy intake, and a deficiency of one or several micronutrients may impair physical-exercise capacity. Vitamins and minerals are found in a wide range of foods, and deficiencies are rare in people with a well-balanced diet.

An athlete should try to ensure adequate vitamin and mineral intake mainly through a well-balanced diet. If an athlete uses micronutrient supplements, it is recommended not to exceed twice the RDA, because this dose seems to be both safe and adequate for optimal sports performance.

Vitamins are organic substances that neither supply energy nor contribute to body mass. Vitamins A, D, E, and K are fat-soluble and can accumulate to toxic levels in the body. C- and B-complex vitamins are water-soluble. Except in relatively

---

BALANCE OF MICRONUTRIENTS

- Vitamins and minerals are found in a wide range of foods.
- Intake of vitamins and minerals is positively related to energy intake.
- Deficiencies are rare in people eating a balanced diet.

norbert bachl and debra wein

Table 5.6 Summary of the most important effects of vitamins and minerals on body functions related to athletic training and performance (Burke, 2007)

	Cofactors and activators for energy metabolism	Nervous function, muscle contraction	Hemoglobin synthesis	Immune function	Antioxidant function	Bone metabolism
Water-soluble vitamins						
Thiamin	•	•				
Riboflavin	•	•				
Vitamin B6	•	•	•	•		
Folic Acid		•	•			
Vitamin B12		•	•			
Niacin	•	•				
Pantothenic acid	•					
Biotin	•					
Vitamin C				•	•	
Fat-soluble vitamins						
Vitamin A				•	•	
Vitamin D						•
Vitamin E				•	•	
Macrominerals						
Sodium		•				
Potassium		•				
Calcium		•				•
Magnesium	•	•		•		•
Trace elements						
Iron	•		•		•	
Zinc	•			•	•	
Copper	•				•	
Chromium	•					
Selenium					•	

85

sport nutrition

Table 5.7 Function and food sources of vitamins and minerals

Nutrient	Functions supporting exercise	Food sources
Water-soluble vitamins		
Thiamine (B1)	Coenzyme in cellular metabolism	Whole grains, legumes
Riboflavin (B12)	Component of FAD+ and FMN of the electron transport chain	Most foods
Niacin	Component of NAD+ and NADP+	Lean meats, grains, legumes
Pyridoxine (B6)	Coenzyme in metabolism	Meat, vegetables, whole grains
Pantothenic acid	Component of coenzyme A (e.g. acetyl-CoA, fatty acyl-CoA)	Most foods
Folacin	Coenzyme of cellular metabolism	Legumes, green vegetables, whole wheat
(B12)	Coenzyme of metabolism in nucleus	Muscle meat, eggs, dairy products
Biotin	Coenzyme of cellular metabolism	Meats, vegetables, legumes
Ascorbic acid	Maintains connective tissue, immune protection	Citrus fruits, tomatoes, green peppers
Fat-soluble vitamins		
beta-carotene (provitamin A)	Tissue maintenance and repair	Green vegetables
Retinol (A)	Sight, component of rhodopsin (visual pigment), maintains tissues	Milk, butter, cheese
Cholecalciferol (D)	Bone growth and maintenance, calcium absorption	Eggs, dairy products
Tocopherol (E)	Antioxidant, protects cellular integrity	Seeds, green leafy vegetables, margarine
Phylloquinone (K)	Role in blood clotting	Green leafy vegetables; cereals, fruits, meats
Minerals		
Calcium (Ca^{2+})	Bone and tooth formation, muscle contraction, action potentials	Milk, cheese, dark-green vegetables
Phosphorus (PO_3^-)	Bone and tooth formation, acid-base chemical energy	Milk, cheese, yoghurt, meat, poultry, grains, fish
Potassium (K^+)	Action potential, acid-base, body water balance	Leafy vegetables, cantaloupe, lima beans, potatoes, milk, meat
Sulfur (S)	Acid-base, liver function	Proteins, dried food
Sodium (Na^+)	Action potential, acid-base, osmolality, body water balance	Fruits, vegetables, table salt
Chlorine (Cl^-)	Membrane potential, fluid balance	Fruits, vegetables, table salt
Magnesium (Mg^{2+})	Cofactor for enzyme function	Whole grains, green leafy vegetables
Iron (Fe)	Component of hemoglobin, myoglobin, and cytochromes	Eggs, lean meats, legumes, whole grains, green leafy vegetables
Fluorine (F)	Bone structure	Water, seafood
Zinc (Zn)	Component of enzymes of digestion	Most foods
Copper (Cu)	Component of enzymes of iron metabolism	Meat, water
Selenium (Se)	Functions with vitamin E	Sea food, meat, grains
Iodine (I)	Component of thyroid hormones	Marine fish and shellfish, dairy products, vegetables, iodized salt
Chromium (Cr)	Required for glycolysis	Legumes, cereals, whole grains
Molybdenum (Mo)	Cofactor for several enzymes	Fats, vegetable oils, meats, whole grains

FAD+ = flavin adenine dinucleotide (oxidized form); FMN = flavin mononucleotide; NAD+ = nicotinamide adenine dinucleotide (oxidized form); NADP+ = nicotinamide adenine dinucleotide phosphate (oxidized form)

rare and specific instances, water-soluble vitamins are generally non-toxic. Vitamins regulate metabolism, facilitate energy release (several of the B-complex vitamins), and have a very important role in the process of bone and tissue synthesis. To avoid great loss of vitamins, it is recommended to use more gentle ways of food preparation, such as microwaving, pressure-cooking, or steaming.

Antioxidants

Many vitamins and minerals have antioxidant capacity, including vitamins such as alpha tocopherol (vitamin E), beta-carotene, ascorbic acid (vitamin C), as well as minerals such as selenium, iron, zinc, copper, and magnesium. Antioxidants are available in foods or produced by the body to combat oxidative stress. Oxidative stress occurs when the body produces excessive reactive oxygen species because of an increased production and decreased clearing. Consequences of oxidative stress may include premature aging, atherosclerosis, cancer, diabetes, muscular dystrophy, rheumatoid arthritis, Alzheimer's disease, Parkinson's disease, and muscle fatigue and injury.

Antioxidants may help reduce the amount of free radical damage by:

- preventing free radical formation;
- scavenging the radicals and changing them to less reactive molecules;
- assisting in the repair of damage caused by the radicals; and
- assisting with other agents that promote a healthy environment.

Regular physical activity produces a myriad of benefits for the body, including a decreased risk of contracting certain diseases and an increased aid for weight management. However, exercise may also result in a decrease in circulating antioxidant levels and a chronic state of oxidative stress. The intake of antioxidants can improve the antioxidant status of the body and may decrease the damaging effect of radical formation, especially during strenuous exercise.

The intake of antioxidants may also help prevent post-exercise oxidative stress. Antioxidant supplements protect the body against oxidative stress during physical activity and training at high altitudes, and may also diminish the effect of exercise on the immune system, protecting athletes against post-exercise infections. It is important to help athletes make appropriate decisions about antioxidants.

ANTIOXIDANTS

- Intake of antioxidants improves antioxidant status of body.
- Antioxidants may decrease damaging effect of radical formation, especially during strenuous exercise.

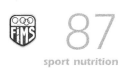

If supplements are chosen, the athletes should be advised to take them in moderate rather than excessive amounts. Again, the best sources of these nutrients are foods.

Minerals important for athletes

Macrominerals are minerals that the body requires in more than 100 mg/d; micro-minerals (trace elements) are those required at lower amounts. Approximately 4% of body mass is composed of different minerals, which are required for numerous physiological processes, including muscle contraction, oxygen transport, fluid balance, and bioenergetics. Minerals also serve as important parts of enzymes, provide structure in the formation of bones and teeth, and help in the synthesis of the biologic macronutrients glycogen, lipids, and protein.

Calcium

An adequate calcium intake in a well-balanced diet is needed to prevent bone mineral loss and reduce the risk of osteoporosis in later life. A prime defense against bone loss with age is an adequate calcium intake throughout life, and regular physical activity from childhood through adulthood. Paradoxically, women who train too intensively and those whose body weight has reduced to a point at which menstruation is adversely affected often show advanced bone loss at an early age (see "Female athlete triad" section). A well-balanced diet is necessary to meet an adequate calcium intake. Restricted energy intake, dietary extremism, fad diets, and a vegan eating pattern may limit the amount of calcium taken in. Athletes thus need to be counseled to ensure that their diet contains adequate amounts of calcium.

CALCIUM

Risk factors for women to develop premature osteoporosis include:

- intensive training;
- a reduced body weight to the point where menstruation is adversely affected.

Iron

An inadequate iron intake can result from a restricted energy intake, dietary extremism, fad diets, vegetarian diets, and a limited variety of food. It is not clear whether regular physical activity creates a significant drain on the body's iron reserves. Studies have shown that endurance athletes, especially middle- and long-distance runners, may be at greater risk for low iron stores, resulting in an increased risk for anemia. Athletes at risk for iron depletion should have their iron levels regularly monitored. Iron deficiency can be prevented by eating lean meats and chicken and by replacing coffee and tea at meals with a vitamin C drink to enhance iron absorption. When dietary interventions fail, iron supplements can be recommended after an evaluation of iron intake, hematological characteristics, and iron reserves.

Are vitamin or mineral supplements necessary?

It is generally accepted that an optimum nutrition status is important, not only for the maintenance of maximum performance but also for minimizing health risks, particularly muscular stress and inflammatory reactions after high-intensity exercise. A well-balanced diet meets the nutritional needs of the recreational athlete. Competitive athletes need higher levels of vitamins and minerals that reflect the increased energy needs. It is necessary to stress the importance of an optimum balanced diet during training, competition, and recovery period. Although there is no absolute evidence that supplementation with different vitamins and minerals enhances physical performance and shortens the recovery period, athletes often supplement with vitamins and minerals. It is important for the team physician to ensure that athletes do not take in excessive amounts of any vitamin or mineral supplement.

FLUID BALANCE

Excessive sweating during exercise may result in significant losses of body water and water-soluble minerals, thus decreasing physical performance capacity. Fluid should therefore be replaced during and following exercise. Water makes up 40–60% of total body mass. About 62% of total body water is intracellular, and 38% is extracellular (plasma, lymph, and other fluids outside the cell). The normal daily water intake ranges from 2.5 l in winter to 3. 5 l in summer. During exercise, the body loses fluid through the skin as perspiration and as water vapor in expired air. The amount of loss depends on the ambient air temperature, humidity, and altitude, with a range between 0.5 and 1.2 l; under extreme ambient conditions, fluid loss can be up to 2 l per hour or more. When dehydration exceeds 2% of body weight, a measurable deterioration of physical performance can be observed (Table 5.8).

As seen in Table 5.9, a severe dehydration is potentially fatal. Exercising while dehydrated causes body temperature to rise quickly and can lead to a heat stroke. For example, during a marathon race at high ambient temperatures, runners may lose about 8% of body weight, corresponding to about 13% of total body water. Even in shorter events, fluid losses of 2–4% body weight are possible. Electrolyte loss during exercise occurs primarily with water loss from sweating. The major elements lost with sweat are sodium and chloride, with smaller amounts of potassium and magnesium.

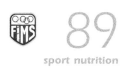

Site	Electrolytes (mEq/l)				Osmolarity (mOsm/l)
	Na+	Cl-	K+	Mg2	
Sweat	40–60	30–50	4–6	1.5–5	80–185
Plasma	140	101	4	1.5	295
Muscle	9	6	162	31	295

mEq/l = milliequivalents per liter (thousandths of 1 g of solute per liter of solvent)

To maintain performance capacity and prevent health risks caused by dehydration, it is necessary to replace water and some minerals during training and competition, especially during sustained exercise under hot and humid ambient conditions, as well as in the recovery period.

The body's need to replace lost fluid is greater than its need to replace lost electrolytes. The thirst mechanism alone, however, is not sufficient to maintain hydration during exercise, and more fluid should be consumed than the body apparently needs. Sufficient rehydration during and after exercise can only be achieved if the sodium lost in sweat is replaced as well as water. Drinking too much fluid with too little sodium may lead to hyponatremia (low plasma level of sodium), which can cause confusion, disorientation, and even seizures. Adding carbohydrates to drinks is a useful way of increasing energy supplies, which can enhance high-intensity endurance performance by maintaining blood sugar concentrations. Carbohydrate found in rehydration solutions can be used by the active muscles either to spare muscle glycogen, or to serve as reserve glucose for a period when muscle glycogen becomes depleted. Depending on the duration and intensity of exercise, as well as the ambient weather conditions, the composition of drinks should be adjusted according to the relative priority of the need to supply fuel or water, which in turn depends also on the individual athlete. Establishing a pattern of fluid intake should be part of training; this training allows individual athletes to develop a personal strategy of fluid rehydration and to get used to the sensations of fluid in the stomach. This is especially important for athletes who live and train in cold climates and who are not used to coping with an increased fluid need in training bouts and competitions in hot weather. Carbohydrate-containing rehydration solutions should contain a carbohydrate concentration of between 5 and 8% (the carbohydrate content (g) should be divided by the fluid volume (ml) and multiplied by 100 to determine the percentage of carbohydrate in a drink), with a moderate to high GI. Maintaining a relatively large fluid volume in the stomach throughout exercise enhances gastric emptying. The best regimen to reach this goal is consuming 400–600 ml of fluid in the 2 hours before exercise, followed by 200–300 ml every 10–20

Table 5.9 Recommendations for ingestion of fluids, carbohydrates, and electrolytes before, during, and after prolonged submaximal exercise*

Issues	Exercise < 60 min	Exercise 60–180 min	Exercise > 180 min
Exercise intensity	80–130% VO$_2$ max	80–90% VO$_2$ max	30–70% VO$_2$ max
Primary concerns	Dehydration, hyperthermia	Dehydration, CHO nutrition	Hyperthermia, dehydration, CHO nutrition, hyponatremia
Proposed formulation			
Pre-event[†]	30–50 g CHO	30–50 g CHO	30–50 g CHO
During exercise			
Initial 60 min	6% CHO Na+: 10–20 mEq/l Cl-: 10–20 mEq/l	6% CHO Na+: 10–20 mEq/l Cl-: 10–20 mEq/l	6% CHO
After 60 min		8–12% CHO	8–12% CHO
Recovery			
Initial 120 min	6% CHO Na+: 10–20 mEq/l Cl–: 10–20 mEq/l 8–12% CHO 8–12% CHO	12% CHO 0.7 g/kg/h Na+: 10–20 mEq/l Cl–: 10–20 mEq/l 8–12% CHO	12% CHO 0.7 g/kg/h Na+: 10–20 mEq/l Cl–: 10–20 mEq/l
After 120 min	6% CHO Na+: 10–20 mEq/l Cl-: 10–20 mEq/l 8 12% Cl IO	6% CHO Na+: 10–20 mEq/l Cl-: 10–20 mEq/l 8–12% CHO	6% CHO Na+: 10–20 mEq/l Cl-: 10–20 mEq/l 8–12% CHO
Volume[‡]			
Pre-event	300–500 ml	300–500 ml	300–500 ml
During exercise	500–1000 ml	500–1000 ml	500–1000 ml
Recovery	500–1000 ml	500–1000 ml	500–1000 ml

* A hyperhydration with glycerol solutions at low concentrations (1–4%) has also been shown to be beneficial.

† Carbohydrate can be in solid or liquid form. If solid, carbohydrate should be ingested with stated volumes of water.

‡ The frequency of ingestion is not stated. More frequent ingestion of smaller volumes is recommended to prevent gastric distress. CHO = carbohydrate

Source: Adapted from Gisolfi C.V., Duchman S.M. Guidelines for optimal replacement beverages for different athletic events. *Med. Sci. Sports Exerc.* 1992; 24:679–87

91

sport nutrition

minutes during exercise, depending on individual variations and climate conditions.

Pre-exercise feeding

A pre-competition meal should include foods that can be readily digested and contribute to the energy and fluid requirements of exercise. Such a meal should be high in carbohydrates and relatively low in lipids and proteins. With individual variations, 3 hours should be sufficient to permit digestion and absorption of the pre-competition meal. Commercially prepared liquid meals may offer a good approach to pre-competition feeding and also caloric supplementation. Such commercial liquid meals are usually well balanced with respect to macro- and micronutrients, contribute to fluid needs, and are absorbed rapidly, with no residuals in the digestive tract.

Suggestions for pre-event food and fluid intake (Burke, 2007):

- plain breakfast cereal with low-fat milk and fruit;
- oatmeal with low-fat milk and fruit juice;
- pancakes/pikelets with maple syrup, honey, or golden syrup;
- toast, muffins, or crumpets with honey/jam/syrup;
- baked beans and toast;
- creamed rice (with low-fat milk) and tinned fruit;
- spaghetti with low-fat tomato-based sauce;
- baked potato with low-fat filling;
- low-fat breakfast bar or muesli bar and banana;
- roll or sandwich with banana and honey;
- fresh fruit salad with low-fat yoghurt or fromage frais;
- smoothie based on low-fat milk or soy milk, low-fat yoghurt and mango/banana/berries.

PRE-EXERCISE FEEDING

- Mode and level of exercise generally should result in daily output of 300 kcal (1,255.2 kJ) of energy expenditure.

Techniques for weight loss and weight gain

To evaluate the normalcy of the body weight of an individual, most professionals use the body mass index (BMI), derived from body mass and stature and calculated as BMI = body mass/kg:stature/m^2. Individuals whose BMI ranges from 20 to 25 have the lowest health risk. The suggested desirable BMI range for women is

norbert bachl and debra wein

21.3–22.1; for men, 21.9–22.4. BMI values above 27.8 for men and 27.3 for women are associated with an increase risk of cardiovascular diseases and metabolic diseases. The surgeon general has defined being overweight as having a BMI between 25 and 30, whereas obesity is defined as a BMI exceeding 30. However, for athletes with a high lean body mass, the BMI may be an inappropriate measurement. Body composition measures via hydrostatic weighing or caliper testing may be a more appropriate measure of body-composition changes in athletes.

Weight loss

There is strong evidence that continuous exercise of moderate to high intensity, especially endurance exercise, is effective for weight reduction, if restricted energy intake is followed at the same time. The greater the energy expenditure, the greater the potential for fat loss. Although the weight-loss effect is independent of the mode of exercise, as long as there is a sufficient caloric deficit, best effects are achieved through endurance exercise of moderate intensity over a longer period of time. Moderate to strenuous running, bicycling, swimming, or walking will stimulate fat loss. Circuit resistance exercise or ball games can also be recommended, although, depending on exercise intensity, the caloric expenditure may be lower. In general, appropriate mode and level of exercise should result in a daily output of 300 kcal of energy expenditure through exercise. If an athlete reduces the caloric intake by 300 kcal per day and is exercising daily with an energy expenditure of 300 kcal, then he/she is able to reduce the body mass of about 0.5 kcal of adipose tissue.

The combination of exercise and diet offers a flexible and effective approach to losing weight. Exercise enhances the mobilization and utilization of lipids, thereby causing fat loss. Regular exercise also retards the loss of lean tissue. Studies show that the combination of exercise and diet is able not only to reduce body-fat mass but also slightly to increase lean body mass. A more pronounced increase in lean body mass can be achieved through diet and regular resistance exercise. The rapid weight loss during the first few days of a diet is primarily caused by a loss of body water and stored glycogen. When exercising and dieting for a longer period, with the weight loss continuing, a greater loss of fat per unit of body weight is exhibited. The responsiveness of weight loss to exercise and diet may be related to sex and genetic differences, with underlying differences in the distribution of body fat and sensitiveness to neurohumoral stimulation.

Weight gain

Gaining weight is attained by increasing calorie intake. In the past, physicians have recommended an increase in fat intake to help athletes increase their caloric intake and gain weight. It is now believed that, for athletes to gain weight, they should consume similar percentages of macronutrients as recommended for their sport, but in larger amounts. Thus, instead of consuming 2,500 calories as 65% from

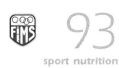

carbohydrates, 10–15% from protein, and 25–30% from fat, the original percentages should be used, but for a larger amount of total calories, such as 3,000.

If a person consumes approximately 3,500 kcal (14,644 kJ) per week in excess of need, the result is an increase in body mass of about 1 lb. If the person is not exercising, these excess calories are stored as body fat. Weight gain for athletes, however, should result in an increase in lean tissue. Heavy muscular overload (resistance training), supported by a well-balanced diet, may increase muscle mass and strength. Studies indicate that a weekly gain of about 0.5–0.75 kg lean tissue can be achieved when 700–1,000 kcal (2,928.8–4,184 kJ) is added to the daily diet, in addition to the extra energy required for training. Depending on the type, intensity, and frequency of training, as well as the hormonal characteristics and genetic preconditions of the athletes, variations in weight gain may occur. When an athlete aims to gain weight, it is important regularly to monitor their body mass and body fat using appropriate body-composition measurement tests.

SUPPLEMENTS

Aspartic acid

Aspartic acid is an amino acid involved in the conversion of ammonia to urea in the liver. Excess ammonia is associated with fatigue; it had been hypothesized that administering aspartates might facilitate the clearing of ammonia from the body, thereby delaying fatigue. Although there are no known risks associated with the use of aspartic acid, research on this topic is not conclusive. More controlled, systematic studies are needed to investigate the effects of aspartic acid on the physical capacity of athletes.

Buffering solutions

Sodium bicarbonate is an alkaline salt produced naturally in the body. When found in the blood, sodium bicarbonate is referred to as the alkaline reserve. The alkaline reserve is responsible for buffering lactic acid, which builds up in the muscles during intensive anaerobic exercise. Ingestion of agents that increase the bicarbonate concentration in the blood plasma makes it possible to increase blood pH level and leave the blood alkaline, thus allowing higher lactate concentrations in the blood to be tolerated, which theoretically should delay the onset of fatigue during short-term anaerobic exercise. Although there are controversial results from different studies, it appears that a bicarbonate ingestion of 300 mg/kg body weight, taken about 2–3 hours before exercise, may be effective and medically safe. However, there should be awareness that sodium bicarbonate can cause gastro-intestinal discomfort, including nausea, diarrhea, cramps, and bloating, as well as irritability and muscle spasms. In contrast, some studies have found similar effects of sodium citrate on buffering capacity, without gastrointestinal discomfort.

Caffeine

Caffeine is one of the most widely consumed drugs in the world, and it can be found in coffee, tea, cocoa, soft drinks, and various other foods. Caffeine is a stimulant to the central nervous system that increases mental alertness and concentration, elevates mood, and decreases fatigue and delays its onset. Caffeine also decreases the reaction time, enhances catecholamine release, increases FFA mobilization, and increases the use of muscle triglycerides.

In excessive amounts, caffeine can cause nervousness, restlessness, insomnia, tremors, and diuresis, as well as an increased susceptibility to heat injury. Caffeine may benefit endurance athletes by conserving the body's glycogen reserves to a small extent, but its diuretic effect may be harmful to athletes, especially when they are exercising in the heat. For power athletes, the diuretic effects of caffeine may help them lose weight. Caffeine in high doses, however, is not permitted in games and competitions, and anyone consuming an amount of caffeine that exceeds the permitted doses is liable to disqualification.

L-carnitine

Carnitine is essential for transportation of long-chain FFAs into mitochondria. During prolonged exercise, FFA concentrations in plasma are often elevated above the actual energy requirement. It has been hypothesized that an increase in the availability of L-carnitine may facilitate the oxidation of lipids. However, a number of studies have failed to find evidence for any ergogenic effect from L-carnitine supplementation.

Creatine

The use of creatine as a supplement is based on its role in skeletal muscle, where approximately two-thirds of its total is in the form of phospho-creatine (PCr). It is hypothesized that consuming creatine supplementation can increase the creatine content in skeletal muscle, enhancing the ATP–PCr energy system and thus performance in high-intensity exercise.

Results of research on this topic are conflicting. Improvement in the performance of strength and power athletes was noted when 15–20 g of creatine per day were administered for a period of 5–6 days, but the initial dose and the maintenance dose, which is usually lower, must be varied individually. However, it was found that, independent of the reaction to creatine supplementation, glucose ingestion together with creatine increases the creatine content of skeletal muscle.

Phosphate

Some early studies suggested that phosphate loading through the ingestion of sodium phosphate may have potential benefits during exercise, because the elevation of extra- and intracellular phosphate levels would increase the availability of phosphate for oxidative phosphorylation and PCr synthesis, thereby improving the energy-production capacity of the body. Supplemented phosphate may also result in a longer time taken to exhaust creatine phosphate stores during intensive exercise. Furthermore, added phosphate levels in the blood have been hypothesized to increase the production of 2,3-DPG, thus facilitating oxygen dissociation from hemoglobin. There are currently no known risks associated with phosphate loading, but conflicting results concerning its proposed ergogenic benefits were found. Further studies are needed to determine the effects and safety of phosphate loading.

FEMALE ATHLETE TRIAD

The female athlete triad refers to the interrelationship and often coexistence of disordered eating, amenorrhea, and premature osteoporosis. These problems represent a growing concern in sports medicine, because of their apparent increased incidence among athletes involved in appearance or esthetic sports, such as gymnastics, figure skating, dance, and distance running. Their constant focus on achieving or maintaining "an ideal body weight" and/or "optimal body fat" is often the underlying cause of the female athlete triad. Extreme pressure to attain good results, pressure from coaches, unrealistic expectations, pressure from society or self, low self-esteem, and poor body image may also contribute to the problem. A family history of disordered eating or substance abuse and family dysfunction may also be contributing factors.

The interaction between intensive training, disordered eating patterns, and hormonal disturbances may have a negative influence on the normal development and maturation of bone. The prevalence of menstrual dysfunction in female athletes varies among sports and with intensity of training. Compared with the rate of oligomenorrhea and amenorrhea in the general female population of 2–5%, the prevalence in female athletes increases to 3.4–66%.

The endocrine problems may involve menstrual dysfunction, premature osteoporosis, and growth and development effects. Malnutrition may lead to a multitude of problems, especially in the cardiovascular and gastrointestinal systems. In more severe cases, malnutrition can have a potentially negative effect on every organ system. The best "treatment" for disordered eating pattern is a sufficient prevention. It should be emphasized that both preventive and treatment efforts need a multidisciplinary team consisting of psychologists, nutritionists, physicians, and coaches to correct the problem. If not treated, the female athlete triad can increase the risks for short- and long-term health consequences, as well as psychological, medical, and orthopaedic repercussions.

Preventing the female athlete triad

The American Dietetic Association has suggested some guidelines for preventing the female athlete triad in Nutrition Intervention in the Treatment of Eating Disorders, 2011, and the Team Prevention Strategies of 1994:

The following techniques and strategies should be considered when working with each new athlete:

- Separate food- and weight-related behaviors from feelings and psychological issues. Having the athlete appreciate the difference can help her to learn to separate facts and move toward a better understanding of how to get better.
- Teach the connection between food intake and sports participation includes health and the requirement of nutrients in food for physical and mental health and the optimal functioning of our bodies.
- Incorporate education with behavior change. For example, teach the need for nutrients and energy before suggesting an increase in caloric intake.
- Work on small changes rather than making gross alterations in the athlete's lifestyle. Discourage an athlete from wanting to change everything at once. Small changes are more likely to be adapted and maintained.
- Explain that setbacks are normal and can be used as learning tools to resculpt responses to cues.
- Teach self-monitoring techniques such as a food diary and behavior records, so that the individual can feel a sense of control over her treatment and choices. You can include food, exercise, and behaviors such as frequency of bingeing and/or as soon as possible purging as well as weight gain/fluctuation
- Use weight and eating contracts, but avoid using these techniques if the individual becomes too over-involved and you feel that it may be counterproductive.
- Slowly increase or decrease weight to prevent the individual from feeling a loss of control and potentially causing her to withdraw from therapy.
- Teach the athlete to maintain a weight that is healthful. Encourage regular meal times, variety and moderation of intake, and gradual reintroduction of foods (typically those most recently excluded from the diet are best received).
- Evaluate and change your approach as necessary throughout treatment and with each individual.
- Strive, ultimately, for the individual to be comfortable in social eating situations where she does not have total control.

The following techniques and strategies should be considered by each female athlete:

- Monitor the menstrual cycle by using a diary or calendar.
- Consult a physician if experiencing menstrual irregularities, recent injuries, or stress fractures.
- Seek counseling if feeling overly concerned about body image or weight.
- Consult a sports nutritionist to help design an eating plan that will support micronutrient and macronutrient needs.
- Seek emotional support from parents, coaches, and teammates when needed.

Some important messages you can share with your athletes:

- Sports participation includes physical and mental health.
- Winning at all costs is not an ideal philosophy.
- Successful performance relates to optimal nutrient intakes of all of the macro- and micronutrients.
- Strength, stamina, and body composition are more important than body weight.
- Sexual maturation is normal.
- Changes in eating, activity levels, menstrual patterns, or performance should be addressed with an appropriate professional as soon as possible.

FEMALE ATHLETE TRIAD

The female athlete triad is the result of an unhealthy focus by female athletes on achieving and/or maintaining "ideal body weight" and/or "optimal body fat". The female athlete triad is caused by:

- pressure to attain good results;
- pressure from coaches;
- unrealistic self-expectations;
- societal pressures;
- low self-esteem;
- poor body image.

SUGGESTED READING

American College of Sports Medicine, American Dietetic Association, Dietitians of Canada. Nutrition and athletic performance [Position Statement]. *Med. Sci. Sports Exerc.* 2009; 41(3): 709–31.

Burke L.M. Dietary Carbohydrates, in *Nutrition in Sport* ed. by R.J. Maughan, 2000, pp 73–84.

Burke L.M. *Practical Sports Nutrition*. Champaign: Human Kinetics; 2007.

Campbel B., Spano M. Vitamins and Minerals, in *Textbook of NSCA's Guide to Sport and Exercise Nutrition* by Lukaski H.C., 2011, pp 87–108.

Choose My Plate. United States Department of Agriculture. September 7, 2011. www.choosemyplate.gov/

Dunford M. Fluid, Electrolytes and Exercise in *Textbook of Sports Nutrition, A Practice Manual for Professionals*, 4th ed. by B. Murray, 2006, pp 94–115.

Hamilton B. Vitamin D and Human Skeletal Muscle. *Scand. J. Med. Sci. Sports*. 2010; 20: 182–90.

Hoch A.Z., Pajewski N.M., Moraski L., Carrera G., Wilson C., Hoffman R.G., Schimke J.E., Gutterman D.D. Prevalence of the Female Athlete Triad in High School Athletes and Sedentary Students. *Clin. J. Sport Med*. 2009; 19(5): 421–8.

Ishijima T., Hashimoto H., Satou K., Muraoka I., Suzuki K., Higuchi M. The Different Effects of Fluid with and without Carbohydrate Ingestion on Subjective Responses of Untrained Men during Prolonged Exercise in a Hot Environment. *J. Nutr. Sci. Vitaminol*. 2009; 55: 506–10.

Kerksick C., Harvey T., Stout J., Campbell B., Wilborn C., Kreider R., Kalman D., Ziegenfuss T., Lopez H., Landis J., Ivy J., Antonio J. International Society of Sports Nutrition Position Stand: Nutrient Timing. *J. Int. Society of Sports Nutr*. 2008; 5(17).

Keul J., König D., Huonker M., Berg A. Ernährung, Sport und muskelzelluläre Belastbarkeit, *Dtsch Z. Sportmed*. 1996; 47: 228–37.

McArdle W., Katch F., Katch V. Macronutrient Metabolism in Exercise and Training in *Textbook of Sports and Exercise Nutrition*, 3rd ed., 2009, pp 154–69.

Ozier A.D., Henry B.W. American Dietetic Association: Nutrition Interventions in the Treatment of Eating Disorders [Position Statement]. *J. Am. Diet. Assoc*. 2011; 111: 1236–41.

CHAPTER 6

FIELDSIDE ASSESSMENT AND TRIAGE

Anthony C. Luke and William D. Stanish

This chapter reviews general concepts for the fieldside assessment of an injured athlete. Physicians who cover the sidelines understand that anything can happen in sport. The medical team covering the event should be familiar with the injuries that may occur in that sport and must be prepared to manage an athlete with a serious injury or medical emergency until the player can be transferred to a medical facility. If the injury does not require transfer, the team physician can manage the problems and decide on return to play. Typically, the physician will triage the athlete to a medical facility for more definitive care, withhold the athlete from play with further follow-up arranged, observe the athlete with potential return to sport in mind, or clear the athlete to go back to competition.

The key principles of event coverage are to be aware of, and be prepared to care for, the common and the unexpected injuries. Careful, early planning and practice of the emergency protocols avoid delays in providing proper medical care and facilitate transfer of an athlete to an appropriate medical center for more advanced treatment in the event of a serious and potentially life-threatening injury. Details of the emergency plans will depend on the sport covered, the event site, and the medical resources available.

The objectives of this chapter include reviewing an approach to managing the fallen athlete and discussing basic skills necessary for first aid fieldside care by a team physician. The chapter presents a stepwise "C–ABCDE" approach for performing the primary survey of an injured athlete. Details for the focused examinations carried out in a secondary survey for specific injuries are discussed in other chapters of this manual. The chapter also covers basic principles of initial stabilization, practical emergency procedures, and first aid fundamentals, as well as planning issues concerning event coverage, emergency protocol planning, and traveling with a team.

PROTOCOL FOR EMERGENCY ASSESSMENT

The primary survey

When an athlete collapses, the team physician must consider both traumatic and medical causes. The priority of the initial assessment is to identify any life-threatening injuries that can be reversed. These include cardiac arrest, airway, cervical spine, and breathing dangers. For example, if there is a problem related to the airway or circulation, the athlete may have a limited window of time, as short as 4 minutes, before irreversible cellular damage occurs from deprivation of oxygen. Once cardiorespiratory dangers are cleared, the athlete is checked for neurological and other life-threatening medical emergencies. Cardiovascular causes are the commonest reason for non-traumatic sudden death in the athlete. Dehydration, temperature-related illnesses, electrolyte imbalances, drug use, and other severe medical conditions can also be fatal.

The examination always begins with a primary survey, which is done on the field before moving the patient. Using aspects of popular acute cardiac and trauma protocols, a suggested algorithm is the "C–ABCDE" approach to provide a uniform method of examining the downed athlete. The "C–ABCDE" approach stands for cardiopulmonary resuscitation (CPR) and cervical spine (C), airway (A), breathing (B), circulation (C), disability (D), and exposure and environment (E). This approach is detailed in Figure 6.1.

During the primary survey, the athlete may not need to be moved immediately. The athlete should be left in the position in which he/she is found throughout the primary survey, unless there is immediate danger, cardiorespiratory emergency, or airway compromise that needs attention. Each step of the algorithm should be cleared before moving the player off the field, and it is important regularly to re-evaluate these steps of the protocols to make sure the evaluation has not changed since the initial examination. Practicing a consistent approach to the initial assessment of an injured athlete helps ensure that important aspects of the examination are not overlooked. The medical team should wear gloves whenever managing an athlete and practice universal body precautions to avoid unnecessary direct contact with body secretions and fluids.

Procedures

C – CPR

Assessment

- Upon encountering a downed athlete, the most immediate, but rare, life-threatening condition is cardiac arrest. A cardiac arrest may be suspected if an athlete is unresponsive and not breathing normally (disregarding occasional gasps). Concerns of sudden arrhythmia, myocardial infarction, shock, or blunt trauma to the chest causing commotion cordis should trigger immediate CPR with chest compressions without assessing the pulse. CPR rarely leads to harm in individuals found not to be in cardiac arrest, and so it should be initiated if cardiac arrest is presumed.

Management
Chest compressions should be administered without delay during CPR with evidence of improved patient survival. Checking the pulse and even protecting the cervical spine to turn the player over cannot delay initiation of chest compressions. Chest compressions should be carried out by hands with a suggested rate of 100 compressions per minute at a depth of 5 cm, allowing the chest to rebound. Cycles of 30 compressions can be performed, taking approximately

Primary Survey

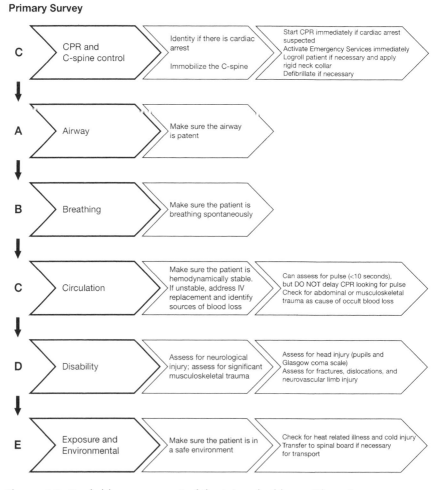

C	CPR and C-spine control	Identity if there is cardiac arrest Immobilize the C-spine	Start CPR immediately if cardiac arrest suspected Activate Emergency Services immediately Logroll patient if necessary and apply rigid neck collar Defibrillate if necessary
A	Airway	Make sure the airway is patent	
B	Breathing	Make sure the patient is breathing spontaneously	
C	Circulation	Make sure the patient is hemodynamically stable. If unstable, address IV replacement and identify sources of blood loss	Can assess for pulse (<10 seconds), but DO NOT delay CPR looking for pulse Check for abdominal or musculoskeletal trauma as cause of occult blood loss
D	Disability	Assess for neurological injury; assess for significant musculoskeletal trauma	Assess for head injury (pupils and Glasgow coma scale) Assess for fractures, dislocations, and neurovascular limb injury
E	Exposure and Environmental	Make sure the patient is in a safe environment	Check for heat related illness and cold injury Transfer to spinal board if necessary for transport

Figure 6.1 On-field management of the injured athlete – The primary survey

anthony c. luke and william d. stanish

18 seconds for each cycle. An automated external defibrillator (AED) has been shown to be a crucial intervention in the event of a cardiac arrest. Cardiac rhythms such as ventricular fibrillation and ventricular tachycardia can be converted to a stable rhythm following defibrillation. The present suggestion is to administer chest compressions for 2–3 minutes, most likely the time needed to prepare the AED to deliver a shock. The chance of successful resuscitation decreases rapidly with each passing minute, as vital tissue oxygenation decreases. The physician should be familiar with use of an automated external defibrillator, which commonly can identify shockable rhythms by administering the shock.

C – cervical spine precautions

Assessment
Because injury to the cervical spine can be overlooked and may have serious consequences, immobilization of the cervical spine should be done initially. Improper handling of an unstable cervical spine can cause spinal cord injury. If the mechanism of injury is consistent with possible neck injury, or the patient complains of persistent neck pain, a serious injury to the cervical spine should be assumed. Unless an immediate cardiopulmonary emergency is occurring, the athlete's neck should be protected with in-line manual support and moved in a controlled fashion.

Management
The helmet and any other equipment should be left in place unless it is necessary to remove it for airway access. It is usually best to have a designated person responsible for manually immobilizing the neck while other steps of the resuscitation are performed. Neck extension or flexion should be avoided, and in-line immobilization of the neck should be maintained until the cervical spine is cleared or stabilized with a rigid cervical spine collar and/or secured to a spine board.

The cervical spine must be protected throughout the primary survey, especially if the athlete is unconscious or agitated. The neck is typically secured by holding the head and providing in-line manual immobilization. In this maneuver, one person puts a hand on each side of the athlete's head to prevent sudden movement or rotation of the neck, or holds the top of the shoulders using their forearms to stabilize the head. Traction should not be applied. (See Figures 6.2A and 6.2B.)

A logroll maneuver is best avoided initially, especially if the athlete is stable. If an emergency condition exists, and the athlete needs to be turned over from a prone position, at least four people are suggested to perform a logroll maneuver (Figure 6.3). Three people kneel on one side of the player, while the leader provides in-line immobilization to the head. The leader coordinates the roll of the athlete on the "count of 3" toward the assistants. The team leader must make sure his/her hands are crossed before logrolling the patient, so that they are in the proper position when the patient is turned on to a supine position. Depending on what

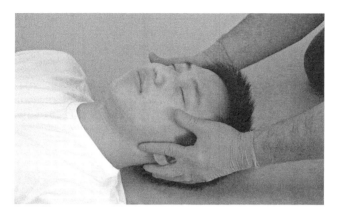

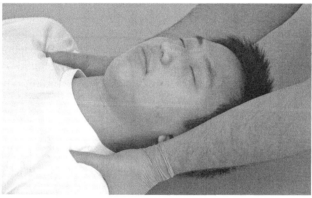

Figures 6.2 In-line immobilization techniques of the head and neck from above. (A) Hands should stabilize the head on both sides, with the third, fourth, and fifth fingers over the occiput. (B) Alternatively, stabilization can be applied using the forearms to stabilize the head, with the hands holding onto the shoulders

other injuries need to be addressed, the athlete may be moved afterwards onto a spineboard before transfer.

A – airway

Assessment

Airway and ventilation are other initial priorities in the approach to an injured athlete. Airway compromise is always a concern in the event of trauma around the head and neck. If the athlete is unconscious, a common cause of airway obstruction is the tongue falling back and occluding the airway. Oral trauma, facial trauma, direct injury to the neck, and foreign objects such as the player's mouth guard are other causes of airway obstruction.

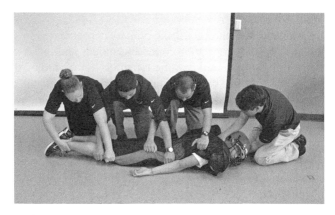

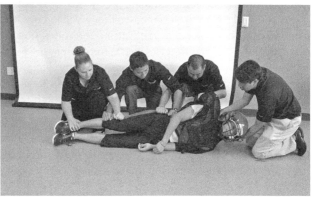

Figure 6.3 Logrolling an athlete. (A) The leader and three assistants position themselves at the head, torso, pelvis, and lower legs. The leader must ensure that his/her hands are placed appropriately on the head. (B) The leader counts to three and coordinates the logroll to 90°, and then indicates the completion of the roll to the supine position. Communication is important to successfully coordinate the logroll

When assessing the fallen athlete, a simple initial test is to ask the athlete a question, such as what his/her name is. If the athlete can respond clearly, the airway and ventilation should be secure. Abnormal breathing sounds, such as stridor, gurgling, whistling, and gasping sounds, suggest partial airway obstruction.

Signs of airway obstruction in the athlete include agitation and a decreasing level of consciousness. The athlete can be agitated because of difficulty breathing or insufficient oxygen. Intercostal retractions and use of accessory muscles for respiration indicate that there is an airway or breathing problem. Cyanosis is a sign of hypoxemia (low oxygenation) and can be seen as purplish discoloration over the nail beds and around the lips. Cyanosis is harder to distinguish if the athlete has dark skin.

Management

If the airway is compromised, the primary concern is to re-establish a secure, patent airway. The first steps are to open the mouth and make sure there is no foreign body in the mouth and that the tongue is not occluding the airway. This can be done by performing the chin-lift maneuver. To perform the chin lift, place an index finger under the athlete's mandible and gently pull the lower lip down with your thumb. It is important not to hyperextend or flex the neck when performing the chin lift. In cases of airway compromise by the tongue, the tongue will often fall forward with the chin lift and relieve the obstruction. However, if the tongue is still a concern, the jaw-thrust maneuver can be performed by placing each hand behind the angles of the lower jaw and displacing the mandible forward (Figure 6.4).

The team physician should examine the mouth for foreign objects, such as a mouth guard or dislodged teeth, and remove them with forceps. Otherwise, a finger sweep of the mouth may be performed, using the index finger to remove any foreign objects, taking care not to push objects further into the throat. Use extreme caution if placing your fingers inside the mouth of an athlete, as there is a risk of a serious finger injury if the athlete bites down. A suction device is extremely valuable if blood or vomit needs to be cleared from the mouth.

An oropharyngeal airway is a hollow, curved device, which can be inserted to provide a patent airway in an unconscious athlete. The size of the airway is estimated by measuring the distance between the front of the teeth and angle of the jaw from the side and comparing the length of the airway to match the distance.

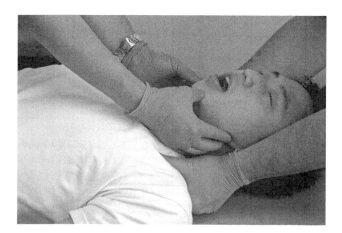

Figure 6.4 Jaw-thrust maneuver. The index finger and middle fingers lift the angle of the jaw forward on each side, while the thumbs pulls the lower lip and chin down, opening the mouth. In-line immobilization of the neck should be maintained

The airway is inserted by positioning the concavity upwards toward the roof of the mouth (upside down). The airway is slid along the roof of the hard palate until the soft palate is reached. The device is then rotated 180° so that the concavity is pointing down and positioned over the tongue.

A nasopharyngeal airway is a flexible hollow tube that can be inserted into the nostril of an awake patient and into the back of the mouth, by-passing the tongue. It should be lubricated well and inserted gently. A nasopharyngeal tube cannot be used if there is trauma to the nose or midface.

In most cases, it should be possible to ventilate an unconscious athlete with an oropharyngeal airway and bag–valve–mask device. However, if it is not possible to maintain the airway and ventilate the patient, a definitive airway, such as an orotracheal tube, a nasotracheal tube, or a surgical airway (cricothyroidotomy or tracheostomy) is required. Another indication for inserting a definitive airway is to protect the lower airways from aspiration of fluids. The physician should be experienced in establishing a definitive airway if it is to be performed. Management of the airway should not delay any CPR, but can be done in conjunction with other activities if trained staff are available.

B – breathing

Assessment
Sufficient oxygenation is necessary to maintain the vital organs. After the airway and cervical spine have been addressed, adequate ventilation should be checked. By leaning over the athlete, the team physician can listen for breath sounds from

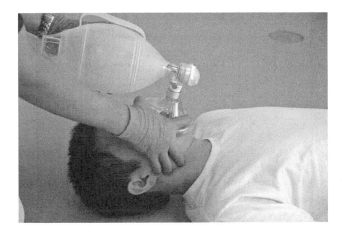

Figure 6.5 One-person ventilation with mask and bag. The third, fourth, and fifth fingers of one hand draw the mandible forward, while the thumb and index finger apply the mask to the face, creating a tight seal. The other hand ventilates the athlete by squeezing the bag firmly

the mouth and look for symmetric chest movements with breathing. Asymmetry of chest movement suggests chest wall injury. Using a stethoscope, satisfactory air entry with spontaneous breathing or assisted ventilation with a bag–valve–mask device can be auscultated over each lung field. Blood or air in the chest may block transmission of the breath sounds. The trachea can be palpated over the anterior neck to check whether it is deviated from the midline. A tension pneumothorax is suspected if an athlete has experienced severe trauma to the chest and is having difficulty breathing, and the trachea is deviated away from the side of the chest with decreased breath sounds (Figure 6.5).

Management
A bag–valve–mask device can be used to ventilate an athlete who is not breathing spontaneously. Chest compressions still take priority over ventilation efforts, although, if trained staff are available, ventilation can be delivered in conjunction with resuscitation efforts. Supplemental oxygen can be administered to the athlete through the mask. Bag–valve–mask ventilation is performed with one or two people. An appropriately sized mask is placed over the athlete's mouth and nose. If only one person is available, one hand is used to hold the mask in place, and the other hand is used to ventilate the athlete by squeezing the bag device. To maintain a good seal between the mask and the athlete's face, apply pressure by holding the mask in place with the thumb and index finger and draw the mandible forward by placing the remaining fingers under the angle of the jaw (Figure 6.5). If there is difficulty ventilating the athlete with this technique, suspect airway obstruction, an equipment problem, or poor technique. If the athlete cannot be ventilated, repeat the airway steps to rule out obstruction, check the equipment for malfunction, and reapply the bag–valve–mask device.

Two people can administer ventilation more effectively. One person uses both hands to apply the mask with a tight seal, while the second person ventilates the athlete by squeezing the bag with both hands. Ventilation should be performed at a rate of approximately one respiration every 5 seconds, or two respirations for every 30 chest compressions if they are being performed.

Alternative means of ventilation include a pocket mask and mouth-to-mouth resuscitation. A pocket mask has a mask to seal over the nose and mouth of the athlete and a mouthpiece, so that ventilation can be administered by breathing into the inlet. If there are no devices to ventilate the patient, then mouth-to-mouth resuscitation can be performed. With one hand, pinch the athlete's nose, and, with the other hand, secure the chin and hold the mouth open. There should be a tight seal between the administrator's and the athlete's lips, as the administrator exhales deeply to inflate the athlete's lungs.

Tension pneumothorax is a life-threatening injury. If a tension pneumothorax is suspected, a large-bore needle should be inserted immediately into the chest cavity anteriorly through the second intercostal space, to allow the air that is compressing the lung to escape from the pleural cavity. The athlete then needs to be transferred directly for definitive management, which includes chest-tube placement.

A pulse oximeter is a useful device that can assess the athlete's oxygen saturation and peripheral perfusion. The sensor is usually applied to a finger, toe, or earlobe. Oxygen saturation levels are normally close to 100% and become worrisome when they drop near or below 92%.

C – circulation

Assessment
Assessing of the pulse can be performed later in the primary survey, as it should not delay chest compressions, and pulse identification may be difficult even for an experienced professional. To assess quickly, the cardiovascular system can be reassessed first by feeling for the carotid pulse, which is easily checked by palpating under the angle of the jaw. The carotid artery is more easily felt at lower blood pressures than other peripheral pulses, such as the radial artery. If the carotid pulse is absent on either side, and the athlete demonstrates other signs of shock, suspect cardiac arrest or arrhythmia and consider initiating CPR immediately.

If there is a pulse, the athlete's heart rate and rhythm should be assessed. The rhythm should be regular, with no skipped or extra beats. The resting heart rate for an adult usually averages between 60 and 100 beats per minute (bpm). Exercising children can average 140 bpm or higher before 5 years of age and around 120 bpm before puberty. Trained athletes may have a lower resting heart rate than the average individual, sometimes as low as 40 bpm in endurance athletes. Therefore, a heart rate that suggests tachycardia may be deceptively lower for an athlete. Athletes have better compensatory mechanisms for hypovolemia, so it is even more difficult to recognize imminent shock.

Signs of shock other than tachycardia include peripheral vasoconstriction and decreased level of consciousness. Test capillary refill of the digits to assess peripheral circulation. If there is a high suspicion of shock, blood pressure measurement may be used to confirm a low blood pressure or narrowed pulse pressure. In the primary survey, measuring blood pressure, however, is not always practical.

An athlete who is tachycardic following a long period of exercise may be hypovolemic because of dehydration. However, in the event of trauma, bleeding must be considered as a cause of hypovolemia. Internal bleeding into third spaces such as the chest and abdomen, or from fractures of the long bones or pelvis, can lead to significant blood loss that results in shock. Causes of nonhemorrhagic shock include cardiogenic shock, tension pneumothorax, and neurogenic shock from a spinal injury.

Management
If there is obvious bleeding, apply pressure dressings to the wounds. Elevate the lower extremities above the level of the heart, unless there are complicating injuries to the lower extremities. Application of a commercial tourniquet can be applied to reduce blood loss from an injured extremity. Intravenous fluids can be administered as soon as possible. Normal saline (0.9%) is the fluid of choice.

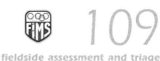

Ringer's lactate is an alternative. In cases of shock, 1–2 l of normal saline may be given, and the response assessed. If there is absolutely no response, then non-hemorrhagic causes of shock should be considered. If there is significant hemorrhage, the athlete may require blood transfusion at an appropriate medical facility.

D – disability

Assessment
Once the ABCs have been cleared, attention can be directed toward ruling out "disability," specifically intracranial, spinal cord, or peripheral limb injuries. While identifying possible injury to the head and neck, do not move the athlete or remove any athletic equipment, unless there are immediate life-threatening risks or danger of further injury. In-line immobilization of the neck still needs to be maintained throughout the assessment until a neck injury has been ruled out. Be aware that a second, painful injury or recent drug or medication use can distract the athlete from pain in the neck.

A significant head injury should be suspected if the athlete is unable to answer coherently or is confused, or if there is any sign of open, depressed, or basal skull fracture, two or more episodes of vomiting, and amnesia greater than 30 minutes. Always suspect a serious head and neck injury in an unconscious athlete. Do not try to revive the athlete by using smelling salts or ammonia, as the strong smell may cause the athlete to jerk his/her head.

Signs of bleeding from the ears, nose, or mouth, or bruising around the eyes or base of the skull, suggest a skull fracture and an underlying closed head injury (see Chapter 21, Head and neck injuries). If the athlete does not have a normal level of consciousness or has signs of head or neck trauma, he/she should be transferred for definitive medical care.

A rapid neurological screen includes checking the athlete's pupils with a penlight, asking the athlete a few questions, and assessing movement in each extremity. During the eye examination, look for spontaneous eye movement, size of the pupils, reactivity of the pupils to light, and symmetry of extraocular movements. Both pupils should react symmetrically to light. Dilation or sluggish light response of one pupil suggests an intracranial injury, usually on the side of the enlarged pupil. Abnormal extraocular movements suggest cranial nerve palsy and/or additional intracranial injuries. Asking the athlete the initial question – for example, "What is your name?" – can check the athlete's verbal response and basic cognitive function. Further questions, such as "Who are you playing today?", "What is the score?", and "What were you doing when you got injured?", can test the athlete's understanding and short-term memory. Motor function can be quickly evaluated by asking the athlete to squeeze the examiner's fingers and move the toes. This also checks the athlete's ability to follow commands.

By briefly performing eye, verbal speech, and motor testing, the Glasgow coma scale can be estimated. The Glasgow coma scale is commonly used in North

 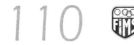

Table 6.1 Glasgow coma scale

Table 6.1 Glasgow coma scale

Eye opening

Spontaneous	4
To voice	3
To pain	2
None	1

Verbal response

Oriented	5
Confused	4
Inappropriate words	3
Incomprehensible sounds	2
None	1

Motor response

Obeys command	6
Localizes pain	5
Withdraws (pain)	4
Flexion (pain)	3
Extension (pain)	2
None	1

America to evaluate severity of head injuries (Table 6.1). If necessary, a more extensive neurological exam can be performed during the secondary survey (see Chapter 21, Table 21.1).

To assess further for cervical injury, ask the conscious athlete if there is any pain in the neck. The cervical spine can be felt very carefully and gently for tenderness. If there is a risk of moving the neck to accomplish this palpation, or reported pain, then this step should be deferred. Spasm of the neck muscles can result from direct injury of the muscle or as a protective mechanism in response to a serious, underlying injury to the neck.

An athlete who is unwilling to move the neck often has sustained a significant neck injury. If it seems that the athlete does not have much neck pain and no obvious serious neck injury, a simple screen is to ask the athlete who is lying in a supine position actively to rotate his/her neck left and right to 45° and then lift the head off the ground to touch the chin to the chest, if the pain is acceptable. This test should be avoided if there is high suspicion of a neck injury. A dangerous mechanism can include a fall from an elevation (five stairs or more), an axial load to the head, or a motor vehicle accident. If the athlete is unable to do so or is hesitant, avoid moving the neck and immobilize the spine until further investigations have cleared the neck of injury. If the athlete is comfortable moving the chin to the chest, and there are no signs of serious injury, the athlete can be removed from the event, and a more detailed examination to rule out causes of head or neck pain may be done on the sidelines.

The extremities can be quickly examined for fractures, dislocations, or wounds: look for areas of bleeding, swelling, and/or deformity. Palpating and logrolling each limb can screen for obvious injury. If there is an injury to an extremity, it is important to make sure that the athlete's neurovascular status is intact by checking sensation to light touch and pulses distal to the injury.

Management
In cases of both head and neck injuries, the stabilization procedures are similar, because a significant head injury may have associated neck injury, and vice versa. If an athlete complains of pain anywhere along the cervical spine, and/or a neck injury is suspected, the cervical spine should be manually immobilized and then protected mechanically with a rigid cervical spine collar, and the athlete should be transferred immediately to hospital on a spine board for further evaluation.

Extremity fractures may be immobilized with prefabricated or vacuum splints until they can be properly evaluated and treated. In the case of fracture causing serious neurovascular abnormality, reduction of the fracture may be attempted, if transfer of the athlete will be prolonged, and if the physician is experienced in the procedure. Alternatively, the injured limb may simply be splinted in a position that decreases tension on the compromised vessels and/or nerves. If there is an obvious dislocation, an experienced physician may try to relocate the joint on the field. However, if the attempt fails, the extremity should be immobilized in a comfortable position, as the dislocation may be complicated by a fracture or soft-tissue imposition. Associated vascular injury requires emergent transfer for further evaluation and treatment.

E – environment or exposure

Assessment
The environment should be safe for the athlete and the caretakers while the assessment is carried out; otherwise, the athlete should be moved to a safer

---

PRIMARY SURVEY TIPS

- Identify and reverse any life-threatening injuries in a stepwise fashion.
- Use the "C–ABCDE" approach (see Figure 6.1).
- If a cardiac arrest is suspected, start chest compressions immediately.
- Always suspect a cervical spine injury and provide in-line immobilization of the neck until it is cleared from injury.
- Practice universal body precautions.

---

environment as soon as possible. Temperature, altitude, weather, and environmental dangers can adversely affect the athlete further. One may suspect a heat or cold injury to the athlete, based on the recent activity and the weather. Signs of heat stroke include confusion, decreased level of consciousness, and hot, dry skin, rather than profuse sweating. Signs of hypothermia are decreased level of consciousness and cold, pale, cyanotic skin. Temperature illnesses are further complicated if the athlete is dehydrated and/or has metabolic problems, for example, acidosis, rhabdomyolysis, or hyponatremia.

Management
Heat or cold injuries should be addressed in the primary survey, and the patient should be transferred to a medical facility if symptoms are severe. Accurate core temperature is difficult to assess using oral, tympanic, or other external thermometers. Re-establishing proper circulation with fluids by mouth or intravenously will help the athlete correct a temperature-related illness. In cases of heat illness, the athlete may need to be cooled down quickly by the removal of any heavy clothing and equipment and the use of ice bags, water mist, or a water bath. In athletes suffering from hypothermia, wet clothing and equipment should be removed and replaced with warm blankets or other heating devices (such as air-warmers).

Indications for emergency transfer

Abnormalities that are identified by the primary survey almost always require transfer. Table 6.2 provides examples of serious problems that warrant transfer to an appropriate medical care facility, but it is not exhaustive. The recommended emergency protocol for "immediate transfer" requires that the athlete be stabilized using the "ABCDE" approach and be taken to the appropriate medical facility. Emergency transportation should be dispatched immediately after the injury occurs, and the medical center should be contacted in order to inform the medical staff of the condition of the athlete and any treatment administered so far, once the athlete is being transferred. Conditions requiring "urgent transfer" should be assessed at an appropriate medical care facility as soon as possible, ideally within 4 hours of injury. If surgery or a procedure requiring sedation is anticipated, the athlete should not take any fluids or food orally to facilitate anesthesia.

Transferring an athlete
It is important to move the athlete in a controlled fashion, particularly if there is a concern about possible spinal injury. Avoid rushing the athlete off the field or allowing unsupervised assistance by other players. If serious injury to the head, spine, or lower extremities is suspected, it is safer to transport the athlete from the field via a spine board or stretcher with a rigid cervical collar. Applying in-line immobilization of the neck, a lift-and-slide technique should be used, where six

Table 6.2 Conditions requiring emergency transfer

Problem	Recommended course of action following "ABCDE" protocol
Airway	
Airway compromise	Immediate transfer (to an appropriate medical facility); provide secure airway before transfer if possible
Anaphylaxis	Administer epinephrine injection intramuscularly; immediate transfer
Breathing	
Respiratory arrest	Start CPR; immediate transfer
Drowning	Start CPR; immediate transfer
Tension pneumothorax	Decompress pneumothorax with large-bore needle in second intercostal space on affected side; chest tube if possible; immediate transfer
Circulation	
Cardiac arrest	Start CPR; defibrillation with AED; immediate transfer
Severe dehydration	Administer fluids; immediate transfer
Internal organ injury (ruptured spleen, liver laceration, fractured kidney)	Administer fluids intravenously; immediate transfer; NPO; may require surgery
Hidden (internal) bleeding (retroperitoneal bleeding, third space bleeding, pelvic or long-bone fractures)	Administer fluids intravenously; immediate transfer; NPO; may require surgery
Severe bleeding	Control bleeding; ± administer fluids; immediate transfer
Myocardial infarction	Administer aspirin; immediate transfer
Disability	
Suspected cervical spine injury	Cervical spine immobilization; immediate transfer on spinal board; may require neurosurgical or orthopaedic consultation
Any suspected spine injury	Cervical spine immobilization; immediate transfer on spinal board; may require neurosurgical or orthopedic consultation
Loss of consciousness, declining level of consciousness	Cervical spine immobilization; immediate transfer on spinal board; may require CT scan
Confusion, neurological symptoms, worsening headache	Urgent transfer; may require CT scan
Fractures involving skull, pelvis, long bones	Splint the injured extremity; administer fluids if necessary; immediate transfer; NPO; will likely require specialist consultation

Table 6.2 continued

Problem	Recommended course of action following "ABCDE" protocol
Open fracture	Splint the injured extremity with a sterile dressing over the wound; administer fluids if necessary; immediate transfer; NPO; likely requires orthopaedic consultation; needs antibiotic coverage
Dislocations	Splint/support the injured extremity; immediate transfer if dislocated; urgent (as soon as possible) transfer if reduced; may require orthopaedic consultation
Possible fracture or multiple ligament injury	Splint/support the injured extremity; urgent transfer; may require orthopaedic consultation
Neurovascular injury in the extremities	Reduce fracture or dislocation; splint/support the injured extremity; urgent transfer; NPO; may require surgical or orthopaedic consultation
Acute compartment syndrome (in an extremity)	Splint/support the injured extremity; urgent transfer; NPO; may require orthopaedic consultation
Environment/exposure	
Heat illness	Cool patient (water, ice bags); administer fluids; remove excess clothing; immediate transfer
Hypothermia	Warm patient (blankets, dry clothes, use body heat if necessary); remove wet clothing; immediate transfer; avoid rapid rewarming if severe hypothermia
Other emergency problems	
Hypoglycemia/diabetic insulin shock	Administer glucose by mouth or intravenously; immediate transfer; may require glucagon injection intramuscularly
Hyponatremia	Fluid-restrict athlete; transfer immediately to obtain labs for sodium level and possible hypertonic saline solution
Seizure	Logroll patient on side to avoid aspiration; immediate transfer; administer benzodiazepine rectally or intra-venously (if prolonged seizure of more than 30 minutes)
Dental injury	Urgent transfer for dental consultation; place any loose teeth or fragments in an appropriate transport medium
Eye injury	Apply eye shield for protection; avoid increasing intraocular pressure; immediate transfer; may require ophthalmology consultation

Notes:
Immediate transfer = athlete should be transferred emergently without delay; the athlete should be sent to an appropriate medical facility with services available to manage the specific injury (i.e. trauma center).
Urgent transfer = athlete should be transferred on an urgent basis and evaluated at an appropriate medical facility as soon as possible, ideally within 4 hours.
CPR = cardiopulmonary resuscitation; AED = automated external defibrillator; CT scan = computed tomography scan; NPO = "nil per os" – no oral intake of fluids or food.

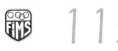

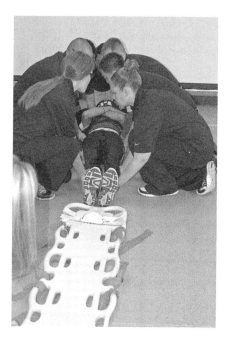

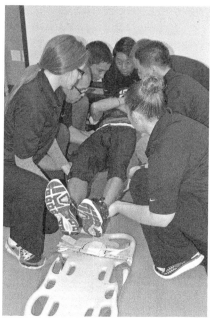

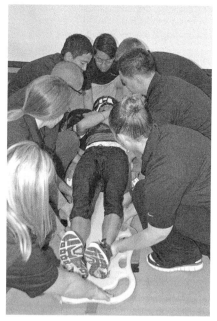

Figure 6.6

The lift-and-slide technique, ideally performed with six or more persons but can be done with four.

(A) A leader provides cervical spine immobilization, while other staff are positioned on each side at the shoulders and thorax, hips and legs, respectively.

(B) The leader counts to three, and all assistants lift the athlete approximately 6 inches off the ground, while an individual slides the spine board beneath the athlete.

(C) On a second count of three, the staff lower the athlete on to the spine board.

or more people lift the supine athlete and slide a spine board underneath (Figure 6.6). This method has been reported to produce less motion at the head and in the cervical spine than the logroll technique, during which the athlete can be tilted 45° to the side and a spine board can be slid underneath the player. Either should be used in appropriate situations. An appropriately sized, rigid neck collar should be applied to the patient to immobilize the neck in a neutral position (Figure 6.7). Indications for application of a rigid collar include significant trauma to the neck or upper back, head injury, post-traumatic loss of consciousness, post-traumatic shock, neurological deficits consistent with central nervous symptom dysfunction, intoxication, inability to speak, or another injury that may be "distracting" the athlete away from the neck. The occiput of very young children is prominent, related to their proportionately larger head size. In this situation, padding (around 1 inch) may be needed under the shoulders to bring the cervical spine into neutral position. Similarly, adjustments in the height of the head or shoulders should be made with padding to ensure proper alignment of the neck in an athlete wearing a helmet or shoulder pads. The forehead, chin, trunk, and pelvis are secured to the board with straps. Supports, sandbags, or intravenous fluid bags are placed next to the athlete's head and secured with tape or straps. The athlete should be kept on the spine board until transferred to an appropriate medical facility for testing and definitive management.

Ideally, a secure airway should be established before the athlete is transferred. In most cases, unless there is impending airway compromise, the head protection should be left in place. However, anything obstructing access to the airway, such as a face mask, should be removed. The medical team should be aware of how the equipment is removed in an acute situation without causing further injury. The equipment should be cut away rather than unnecessary time being spent to preserve the equipment. Remember that the most important concern is the health of the athlete. If possible, the team physician or certified health professional should accompany the athlete to the hospital.

The secondary survey

The secondary survey is performed on the sidelines, or preferably in a designated room that is private and quiet, with adequate lighting. The purpose of the secondary survey is to identify all musculoskeletal or organ injuries resulting from

---

SECONDARY SURVEY TIPS

- Perform the survey in a controlled environment.
- Carry out detailed examinations of any injured system or joint; rule out associated injuries.
- Administer first-aid treatments.

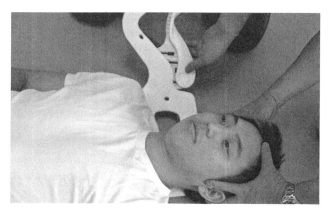

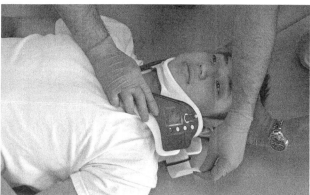

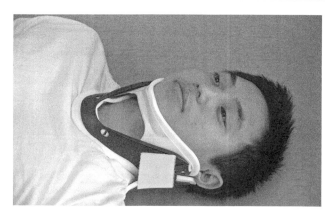

Figure 6.7 Application of rigid neck collar. (A) In-line immobilization is maintained as the collar is passed behind the neck. (B) The back of the collar is positioned behind the neck. (C) The front of the collar is wrapped anteriorly under the chin and secured with straps, thus immobilizing the cervical spine

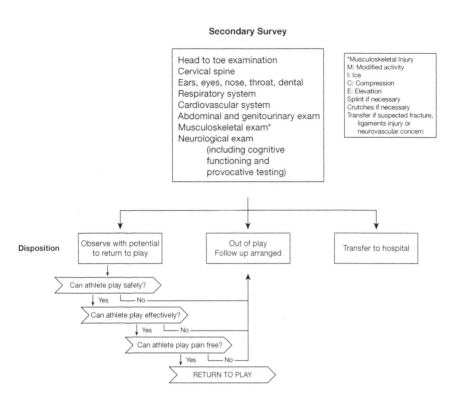

Secondary Survey

Head to toe examination
Cervical spine
Ears, eyes, nose, throat, dental
Respiratory system
Cardiovascular system
Abdominal and genitourinary exam
Musculoskeletal exam*
Neurological exam
(including cognitive
functioning and
provocative testing)

*Musculoskeletal Injury
M: Modified activity
I: Ice
C: Compression
E: Elevation
Splint if necessary
Crutches if necessary
Transfer if suspected fracture,
  ligaments injury or
  neurovascular concern

Disposition

Observe with potential
to return to play

Out of play
Follow up arranged

Transfer to hospital

Can athlete play safely?
Yes — No
Can athlete play effectively?
Yes — No
Can athlete play pain free?
Yes — No
RETURN TO PLAY

Figure 6.8 On-field management of the injured athlete – The secondary survey

the injury. A thorough examination is carried out, including a detailed examination of any apparently abnormal system or joint. More first aid treatments can be administered at this time. The athlete can be observed and functionally tested if there is consideration of a return to competition.

First aid

Beyond identifying life- and limb-threatening injuries and stabilizing the patient, the team physician should be comfortable administering first aid. The athletes benefit greatly when the physician is able to manage minor problems that allow the athlete to return to competition. However, it is important for the physician to recognize his/her limitations in terms of skills and resources. The physician should decide in a timely fashion whether transfer to a medical center for appropriate investigation or more definitive medical care is necessary. In cases where there is remote access, or if partial evaluation and treatment can be safely done on-site, with plans for early follow-up and further care, the physician may decide to manage the problem or perform procedures on-site at the sports event.

Skills that are useful on the sidelines include suturing and wound care; taping and splinting joints; applying pressure bandages; applying protective devices such as eye shields and protective padding; and maneuvers such as application of ice and heat, stretching the athlete, and simple massage. It is also helpful to understand the roles and skills of the other medical team members in order to direct care of the athletes appropriately.

Suturing and wound care

The physician may be required to treat lacerations and wounds, especially in contact sports. A physician should be familiar with sterile suture techniques in order to repair simple lacerations. Antiseptic or other cleansing solution, local anesthetic, suture materials, a needle driver, scissors, forceps, and gauze are supplies needed to repair a laceration. Small or superficial wounds may be closed with sterile adhesive strips or surgical glue.

Before closing a laceration, clean the wound with irrigation with a large amount of sterile saline or antiseptic solution. Avoid using hydrogen peroxide or iodine unless the wound is extremely dirty or there are no other solutions available. Debride any dead tissue or uneven edges and remove any foreign bodies. Wounds that are dirty and have a high risk of infection may be left open until they can be more definitely treated at a medical facility. Local anesthetic may be infiltrated in the wound edges or in the appropriate nerve block location to decrease sensation in the area. Do not inject epinephrine near fingers, toes, or other body appendages. Remember to check the status of the athlete's immunizations, as tetanus prophylaxis is usually necessary every ten years.

Proper application of bandages, dressings, and padding is important for managing open wounds. For persistent bleeding, apply a compressive, pressure bandage to the wound, using adequate amounts of absorptive, sterile gauze or pads. Bandages that are wrapped circumferentially around a limb should not be applied too tightly. Cyanosis or pallor of the limb distal to a circumferential compressive dressing may indicate a tourniquet effect, and the circumferential wrap may need to be removed if transfer is delayed. A circumferential wrap may be used to wrap dressings around the head. If a pressure bandage cannot be applied, hold the gauze over the wound with firm, constant pressure to stop bleeding.

Abrasions should be cleansed with sterile gauze and normal saline. All debris, such as dirt and gravel, should be removed from the wound. Affected areas should be covered and protected with a bandage.

Athletic taping

Knowledge of basic athletic taping and splinting can be useful for managing and protecting soft-tissue and joint injuries. Taping can be helpful in the event of mild sprains, particularly of the ankle, wrist, and fingers, as well as in cases of patello-femoral pain and various foot problems.

Splinting and protection

If there is a significant injury to a bone or joint, splinting may be required. To splint a bone or joint, immobilize the joint above and below the area of injury to prevent movement. Preformed or commercial splints can be useful in the event of an injury requiring rapid immobilization.

To protect a tender area, such as a deep muscle contusion, a doughnut-shaped pad helps avoid direct pressure over the injured area. A circular-shaped pad made of foam or other viscoelastic material, with the center cut out, can be secured to the injured area to reduce contact and pain. To protect an eye injury from further damage, secure an eye shield over the eye using three long strips of tape, from the forehead to the cheek, on the affected side.

Reducing dislocations

Joint dislocations are usually the result of a high-impact trauma. Oftentimes, the dislocation can be safely reduced at the fieldside. Dislocated joints can be more easily reduced early, before pain, muscle spasm, and swelling become too significant. Dislocations can have associated neurovascular injuries and require emergency evaluation. Reduction of a dislocation can be complicated by soft-tissue imposition in the joint or by fracture, particularly in skeletally immature athletes. Therefore, reduction attempts should be limited, if success is not achieved initially. The physician should be familiar with joint reduction techniques before attempting these maneuvers.

The shoulder is the commonest large joint to be dislocated. More than 90% of shoulder dislocations are anterior. Several techniques are described to reduce the shoulder. Hip dislocation requires emergent reduction to decrease the chance of avascular necrosis of the femoral head. Hip dislocation is very often associated with fracture of the acetabulum and/or femoral head and usually requires heavy sedation or general anesthesia for reduction at an appropriate facility. A knee dislocation may be reduced on the field. However, it requires further emergency evaluation because of the high risk of associated neurovascular injury. The patella, which typically dislocates laterally, often can be reduced on the sideline by extending the knee and manually moving the kneecap into its normal position in the trochlear groove. After reduction, the knee should be evaluated for any associated ligament, neurovascular, or osteochondral injury. The elbow, ankle, or foot may be reduced before urgent transfer to a medical care facility, depending on the training and experience of the physician. Dislocations of the interphalangeal joints of the fingers may be assessed, reduced, and protected with athletic taping or a lightweight aluminum-foam splint. The injured finger can be buddy taped to an adjacent finger, which is used as a natural splint. Return to play should be decided on an individual basis. Dislocation injuries are accompanied by ligament injury and sometimes fractures, and so further evaluation should be considered, even if the athlete is allowed to return to the contest.

Physical therapy

The team physician should be familiar with some therapeutic maneuvers for treating early sports injuries, especially if no trainer or therapist is available. Simple massage techniques, icing, stretching maneuvers, and rehabilitation exercises can be useful for acute soft-tissue injuries, such as sprains, strains, and contusions.

Return-to-play guidelines

Return-to-play decisions are usually made on an individual basis. To clear an athlete for return to play, the physician must determine if the individual can play the sport safely and effectively and can perform pain free (Figure 6.1, B). If safety is a concern, play is not allowed. However, if it is felt that the athlete can play safely, albeit with pain, the contraindications for return to play become relative. The effectiveness of play, often in consultation with the coach, then becomes a determining factor. Finally, if the athlete is experiencing significant pain with competition, the physician, coach, and athlete should seriously consider not returning him/her to play, as the injury may be underestimated. The rule of thumb is, "when in doubt, sit it out."

RETURN-TO-PLAY TIPS

- The athlete should be safe from further injury, effective in participating, and relatively pain-free before returning to play.
- "When in doubt, sit it out."

An athlete should be tested functionally to ensure that he/she is fit to compete. The athlete should be asked to perform sport-specific drills to test balance, absence of symptoms, pain tolerance, and effectiveness in sport. Examples of useful sideline drills are a 40-m sprint, five push-ups, and five sit-ups, or other common sport-specific maneuvers. If the athlete is unable to demonstrate reasonable effectiveness on the sideline, he/she has limited ability to compete and may be at risk of making the injury worse.

PRE-EVENT PLANNING

Whether it is a local community sports event or a professional-level competition, the principles for event coverage are the same. However, the risk of injuries, resources, budget, and expectations following decisions vary. The nature of the sport, the number of participants, and the environment are important considerations. For the sports physician, management of the collapsed athlete begins before the injury occurs, with proper preparation.

Appropriate staff should be organized to meet the demands of the event. The number and type of caregivers should be adequate, based on the number of participants, the risk of injury in the sport, and past experience of the event organizers. It is important that physicians and other qualified staff be trained in basic cardiac life support or CPR techniques. Staff members with experience or courses in trauma management are extremely beneficial.

Depending on the location and level of the event, resources can be limited. The physician should arrange to have easily accessible communication, medical supplies, and, most importantly, a means of transport for the athlete to a medical facility. Table 6.3 outlines some basic, recommended supplies for event coverage. The necessary supplies can vary, depending on the nature of the sport, the number and severity of injuries expected, the number of athletes participating, and the experience of the physician. A team physician should be familiar with the use of all the equipment in the medical bag.

The physician should carefully study the competition venue. Medical care areas should be strategically placed to facilitate quick and easy access to an injured athlete, in locations where injuries will likely occur. For example, in planning a marathon, the team physician should consider the course and anticipate most injuries and hydration problems to occur at, or near, the finish of the race. The most practical access route for ambulance transfer of an athlete to a medical facility should be planned in the event of an emergency. It is important to practice emergency protocols, so that all staff members are familiar with their roles, and any potential problems in the plan can be corrected. A communication network among staff, the transport team, and the hospital should be planned for well before the event begins. Cellular phones and two-way radios are extremely useful means of communication.

Weather on the day of the event is an important factor. The physician needs to determine the safety of holding the event and estimate the risk of temperature illness for the athletes on the given day. When the ambient temperature increases over 23°C (> 73°F), there is a higher risk for heat illnesses. Temperatures above 28°C (> 82°F) can be hazardous. Hypothermia becomes a concern as ambient temperatures drop, depending on the sport and clothing worn. For aquatic events, particularly outdoors, the physician must be aware of the water temperature. Water below 10°C is hazardous. The athletes should be made aware of weather warnings and recommended clothing before the event begins.

PRE-EVENT PLANNING TIPS

- Proper preparation is the key to successful event coverage.
- At minimum, the physician must be able to communicate with further medical staff and have adequate medical supplies to initially treat, and a means of transferring, an athlete to an appropriate medical facility.
- Study the competition venue for areas of potential injury and access to injured athletes.
- Practice the emergency protocols.
- Consider temperature, weather, and environment as potential risks.

Table 6.3 Suggestions for a medical bag and supplies

CPR and Cervical Spine

Automatic External Defibrillation device

Rigid cervical spine collar of appropriate sizes for the athletes

Airway and ventilation supplies

Bolt cutters or heavy scissors to remove equipment if necessary
Oropharyngeal (Oral) airways, various sizes
Nasopharyngeal (Nasal) airway
Pocket mask for ventilation
Bag-valve-mask (masks and ventilation bag)
Intubation equipment (Endotracheal tubes with stylet, large forceps (McGill

forceps), laryngoscope with blade (and batteries))
14 gauge catheter for tension pneumothorax
Cricothyroidotomy kit
Syringe (10 mL)
Lubricant
Portable suction (manual)
Oxygen tank and reservoir

Circulation supplies

Intravenous catheters
Intravenous fluids (Normal saline or Ringer's lactate)

Intravenous line tubing
Tape to fix IV catheter in place
Rubber tubing for tourniquet

Miscellaneous

Exam gloves (non-sterile and sterile pairs; latex and non-latex)
Bandage/trauma shears (to cut through clothes, tape)
Absorbent 4x4 gauze, sterile
Sterile dressings and bandages
Band-Aids
Tongue depressors
Cotton tip applicators
Athletic tape
Alcohol swabs
Antiseptic solution
Disinfectant
Lubricant
Salt packets ± electrolyte powder/ solution
Ice
Syringes and needles
Suture kit (needle driver, forceps, scissors, scalpel, suture material, flexible skin closure strips)
Sharps box

Red biohazard bag
Penlight
Stethoscope
Blood pressure cuff
Oto/ophthalmoscope with blue filter
Oral/rectal thermometer
Reflex hammer
Rapid Splint (for arm or leg)
Eye shield
Mirror
Fluorescein eye drops and cobalt blue light
Tooth transport medium
Foil blanket
Urine dipsticks
Tampons
Plastic bags for ice, biohazard
Prescription pad/forms/paper/pen
List of banned substances
For Transport
Spineboard with side head supports
Stretcher
Crutches (± wheelchair)

Medications

Injectable Epinephrine (1: 1000 solution, prefilled syringes)
Dextrose (50%, prefilled syringes)
Nitroglycerine (spray or tablets)
Aspirin chewable tablets
Beta Agonist inhaler
Aerochamber
Analgesic medications

Anti-inflammatory medication
Antibiotic medication
Local anesthetic solutions
Oral glucose paste or tablets
Topical medications (antibiotic, steroid cream, sunscreen)
Other medications

TRAVELING WITH A TEAM

When traveling with athletes, the team physician should study the country and location in which the competition is being held. The physician should investigate the common illnesses, the local communicable diseases, and any immunizations that may be necessary to enter the country or are recommended for foreign travelers. This should be done several weeks, or even months, in advance to properly administer immunizations.

Time change and high altitude are also issues that can affect athletic performance. Athletes often need at least 24–48 hours to acclimatize to a time change. In cases of climate or altitude changes, the acclimatization process may take anywhere from one to three weeks.

It is useful for the physician to learn and inform the athletes of some of the customs of the area visited. The team physician should be aware of the local food and water safety, and the level of hygiene. Athletes should be advised to carry bottled water and some food supplies if they are not accustomed to the food and drink in the location visited. The physician should be aware of the travel arrangements, accommodations, and modes of transportation in the destination country. The commonest cause of death in foreign countries is from motor vehicle accidents.

Finally, it is important for the team physician to be familiar with the athletes and their individual medical problems. Meeting with them before travel and competition helps the physician develop a rapport with the athletes and anticipate any special needs or medications required. A conscientious, well-prepared team physician can provide a healthy environment, which may increase the confidence of the athletes in their performances and reduce the consequences of sports injuries if they occur.

SUGGESTED READING

American College of Sports Medicine Expert Panel: Sideline preparedness for the team physician: consensus statement. *Med. Sci. Sports Exerc.*, 2001; 33: 846–9.

Armstrong L.E., Casa D.J., Millard-Stafford M., et al. American College of Sports Medicine position stand. Exertional heat illness during training and competition. *Med. Sci. Sports Exerc.*, 2007; 39(3): 556–72.

Committee on Trauma. *Advanced Trauma Life Support for Doctors: Student Course Manual* (8th ed.). Chicago, IL: American College of Surgeons; 2008.

Everline C. Application of an online team physician survey to the consensus statement on sideline preparedness: the medical bag's highly desired items. *Br. J. Sports Med.*, 2011; 45(7): 559–62.

Hazinski M.F., Nolan J.P., Billi J.E., et al. Part 1: Executive summary: 2010 International Consensus on Cardiopulmonary Resuscitation and Emergency Cardiovascular Care Science With Treatment Recommendations. *Circulation*, 2010, Oct. 19; 122(16 Suppl. 2): S250–75.

Hodge D.K., Safran M.R. Sideline management of common dislocations. *Curr Sports Med. Rep.*, 2002; 1: 149 55.

Swartz E.E., Boden B.P., Courson R.W., et al. National Athletic Trainers' Association position statement: acute management of the cervical spine-injured athlete. *J. Athl. Train.* 2009; 44(3): 306–31.

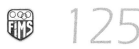

CHAPTER 7

DRUG TESTING AND DOPING

Eduardo Henrique De Rose and
Marco Michelucci

The personal and financial rewards of modern sport can create unhealthy desires to win at all costs. To gain a competitive advantage, some athletes may use ergogenic aids, which enhance sporting performance beyond that attainable through genetic ability and training. Ergogenic aids can be grouped into five categories:

- pharmacological (performance-enhancing drugs, e.g. anabolics or stimulants);
- physiological (e.g. blood doping);
- psychological (e.g. hypnosis);
- mechanical (e.g. clothing or equipment);
- nutritional (dietary supplementation).

Pharmacological and physiological aids are often referred to as "doping." To ensure a level playing field, doping is controlled by sports governing bodies. Sports governing bodies, international and national sports federations, and national Olympic committees have agreed to follow the rules established by the World Anti-Doping Agency (WADA) and its World Anti-Doping Code, approved in 2003. Since its foundation in 1999, WADA is the non-governmental agency responsible for publishing and revising the International Testing Standards (ITS) and the annual List of Prohibited Substances and Methods.

The World Anti-Doping Code was created to reach harmonization in the world of anti-doping, in terms of procedures and sanctions. The code established a new definition for doping, and the following constitute anti-doping rules violation (ADRV):

- the presence of a prohibited substance or its metabolites or markers in an athlete's body specimen;
- use or attempted use of a prohibited substance or prohibited method;
- refusing, or failing without compelling justification, to submit to sample collection after notification as authorized in applicable anti-doping rules or otherwise evading sample collection;

- violation of applicable requirements regarding athlete availability for out-of-competition testing, including failure to provide required whereabouts information and missed tests that are declared based on reasonable rules;
- tampering, or attempting to tamper, with any part of doping control;
- possession of prohibited substances and methods;
- trafficking in any prohibited substance or method;
- administration or attempted administration of a prohibited substance or method to any athlete, or assisting, encouraging, aiding, abetting, covering up, or any other type of complicity involving an anti-doping rule violation or any attempted violation.

The new concept of doping establishes that not only enhancing substances should be considered as such, but also substances that affect the health of the athlete or are against the spirit of the game. When two of these three conditions are present, we may have an ADRV.

Today, the problem of doping in sports concerns not only the Olympic Movement and public authorities, but also associations that bring together sports specialists, including the oldest of these, FIMS. The number of positive cases of doping has increased considerably during the past several years. This increase is no doubt related to the huge amounts of money involved in professional sport, as well as the increasing number of competitions around the world – a situation that forces athletes into year-round training and multiple competitions.

These factors make it impossible for athletes to find adequate rest periods, which is the reason for many stress traumas and for athletes' attempts to improve their metabolism using forbidden substances or doping methods.

The team physician must have a keen knowledge of banned substances and techniques, as well as drug testing procedures. He/she should also be aware of the adverse effects of performance-enhancing drugs, which may require medical treatment. In this context, the team physician has a number of roles, acting as:

- educator
- healer
- detective and
- counselor.

PROHIBITED CLASSES OF SUBSTANCES AND METHODS

WADA has a Foundation Board formed of an equal number of members from the Olympic Movement and from the public authorities of the five continents. The List of Prohibited Substances given in this chapter is the one published by WADA in October 2011 and is valid for the year 2012.

The prohibited list is currently classified in pharmacological groups and methods. Some of the substances are prohibited only in specific sports.

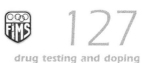

Substances and methods prohibited at all times (in- and out-of-competition)

Prohibited substances

S0. Non-approved substance

Any pharmacological substance that is not addressed by any of the subsequent sections of the list and with no current approval by any governmental regulatory health authority for human therapeutic use is prohibited at all times.

S1. Anabolic agents

This class of substances includes the anabolic androgenic steroids and the Beta$_2$-agonists.

1. *Anabolic androgenic steroids*: Examples of androgenic steroids are androstenediol, androstenedione, bolandiol, bolasterone, boldione, clostebol, dehydrochlormetyltestosterone, epiandrosterone, dihydrotestosterone, testosterone, fluoxymesterone, methandienone, methenolone, nandrolone, 19-norandrostenediol, 19-norandrostenedione, oxandrolone, stanozolol, and other substances with similar chemical structure or similar biological effect(s).
2. *Exogenous anabolic androgenic steroids*: Examples of exogenous anabolic steroids are androstenediol, androstenedione, dihydrotestosterone, and testosterone and their metabolites and isomers.
3. *Other anabolic agents*: Examples of other anabolic agents are clembuterol, selective androgen receptor modulators (SARMs), tibolone, zeranol, zilpaterol.

It is important to note that some dermatological creams used for gynecological and urological reasons, and for better healing of the skin, may include anabolic agents such as clostebol in their formula.

Some birth-control pills must not be used in athletes. For example, the use of pills that contain norentindrone may result in a positive test for 19-norandrosterone.

S2. Peptide hormones, growth factors, and related substances

The following substances and their releasing factors are prohibited:

1. *Erythropoiesis-stimulating agents*.
2. *Chorionic gonadotrophin* (CG) and *Luteinizing hormone* (LH) in males.
3. *Insulins*.
4. *Corticotrophins*.
5. *Growth hormone* (GH) and *insulin-like growth factor* (IGF=1), as well as any growth factor affecting muscle, tendon, or ligament protein synthesis or degradation, vascularization, energy utilization, regenerative capacity or fiber type switching, and other substances with similar chemical structure or similar biological effect(s).

Although the use of synthetic hormones is growing among athletes, their cost is still very high, limiting widespread use. On the other hand, standardized methods for laboratory detection in urine samples do not exist for all hormones, as techniques for the manufacture of these synthetic hormones, employing genetic engineering, are capable of producing molecules identical to endogenous hormones.

Erythropoietin (EPO) regulates the number of red cells in the blood. It is mainly produced by the kidneys and travels to the bone marrow, stimulating the production of red cells. The use of EPO increases the percentage of reticulocytes, the hematocrit, and the count of hemoglobin in the blood. Athletes use it to increase muscle oxygenation. Thus, it is particularly important in endurance sports.

It is known that administration of human CG and similar components leads to an increase in the endogenous production of androgen steroids. It acts in a similar way to LH, present in the physiologic path of production of male hormones. These are prohibited in men only.

Insulin is permitted only to treat insulin-dependent diabetes, after approval of the Therapeutic Use Exemption (TUE) by the international sport federation concerned.

The effect of corticotrophin administration is considered analogous to that of oral, intramuscular, or intravenous use of corticoids.

GH stimulates growth, promotes protein synthesis, and breaks down fat, thereby increasing lean body mass. There is great concern about GH use among athletes. It is possible to detect GH in blood, but the window is not very large.

The presence of an abnormal concentration of an endogenous hormone or its diagnostic markers in the urine of a competitor constitutes a doping offense, unless it has been conclusively documented to be solely due to a physiological or pathological condition.

S4. Hormone and metabolic modulators

The following are prohibited:

1. *Aromatase inhibitors*.
2. *Selective estrogen receptor modulators* (SERMs), including, but not limited to, raloxifeno, tamoxifeno, and toremifeno.
3. *Other anti-estrogenic substances*, including, but not limited to, clomiphene, cyclofenil, and fulvestranto.
4. *Agents modifying myostatin function(s)*, including, but not limited to, myostatin inhibitors.
5. *Metabolic modulators*: Examples are peroxisome profilator activated receptor (PPARo) agonists and PPARo–AMP-activated protein kinase (AMPK) axis agonists.

S5. Diuretics and other masking agents

Masking agents include diuretics, desmopressin, plasma expanders such as glycerol, intravenous injection of albumin, dextran, hydroxyethynil starch, and manitol.

Diuretics include acetazolamide, amiloride, bumetanide, canrenone, chlorthalidone, ethacrynic acid, furosemide, indapamide, metolazone, spironolactone, thiazides, and other subsrtances with similar chemical structure and similar biological effect(s).

It is important to note that a TUE for diuretics is not valid if an athlete's urine contains a diuretic in association with prohibited substances.

Prohibited methods

M1. Enhancement of oxygen transfer

The following are prohibited:

1. *Blood doping*, including red cell products of any origin.
2. *Artificially enhancing the uptake, transport, or delivery of oxygen*, including perfluorochemicals, efaproxiral (RSR13), and modified hemoglobin products, but excluding supplemental oxygen.

Blood doping includes the transfusion of autologous, homologous, or heterologous blood and red blood cell products of any origin, other than for medical treatment (hemorrhage or acute anemia). If such a situation occurs, the team physician may submit the case to the TUE committee of the international sports federation concerned, and an exception may be granted.

M2. Chemical and physical manipulation

The following are prohibited:

1. *Tampering*, or attempting to tamper, in order to alter the integrity and validity of the samples collected during a doping control is prohibited. This includes urine substitution and adulteration.
2. *Intravenous infusion* and/or injections of more than 50 ml per 6-hour period are prohibited, except for those legitimately received in the course of hospital admission or clinic investigations.
3. *Sequential withdrawal, manipulation, or reintroduction of whole blood*, in any quantity in the circulatory system.

M3. Gene doping

The following, with the potential to enhance sport performance, are prohibited:

1. *The transfer of nucleic acids or nucleic acid sequences.*
2. *The use of normal or genetically modified cells.*

SUBSTANCES PROHIBITED IN-COMPETITION ONLY

Stimulants

All stimulants are prohibited, except imidazole derivates for topical use and those stimulants included in the 2012 Monitoring Program.

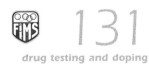

Stimulants included:

(a) *Non-specific stimulants*
Adrafinil, amfepamone, amiphenazole, amphetamine, anphetaminil, benfluorex, benzphetamine, benzylpiperazine, bromantano, clobenzorex, cocaine, cropopamide, crotetamida, dimethylanphetamine, ethilanphetamine, famprofazona, femproporex, fencamina, fendluramine, fenethyline, furfenorex, mefenorex, mephentermine, mesocarbo, methamphetamine, methylanphetamine, methylenedioxyamphetamine, methylenedioxymethamphetamine, modafinil, norfenfluramina, phendimetrazine, phenmetrazine, phentermine, 4-phenylpiracetam, prenylamine, and prolintano. A stimulant not listed in this section is a specified substance.

(b) *Specified stimulants*
Adrenaline, cathine, ephedrine, etamivan, etilefrina, fenbutrazato, fencmfamin, heptaminol, isometheptene, levmetamfetamine, meclofenoxato, methylephedrine, methylhexaneamine, methylphenidate, nikethamide, norfenefrina, octopamina, oxilofrina, parahydroxyamphetamine, pemolina, pentetrazola, phenpromethamine, propylhexedrine, pseudoephedrine, selegilina, sibutramine, strychnine, tuaminoheptano, and other substances with similar chemical structure or similar biological effect(s).

Table 7.1 Threshold of urinary concentrations for report of an adverse analytical result, according to the prohibited list of WADA (2012)

Substance	Concentration
Cathine	> 5 µg/ml
Ephedrine	> 10 µg/ml
Methylephedrine	> 10 µg/ml
Pseudoephedrine	> 15 µg/ml

Some specific stimulants have a minimum threshold in urine to be considered as an adverse analytic result, as shown in Table 7.1.

The following substances included in the 2012 Monitoring Program (bupropion, caffeine, nicotine, phenylephrine, phenylpropanolamine, pipradrol, and synephrine) are not considered as prohibited substances.

Local administration of adrenaline (nasal or ophthalmologic) or co-administration with local anesthetics is not prohibited.

S7. Narcotics

The following are prohibited: Buprenorphine, dextromoramide, diamorphine (heroin), fentanyl, hydromorphoine, methadone, morphine, oxycodone, oxymorphone, pentazocine, and pethidine.

S8. Cannabinoids

Natural (cannabis, hashish, marijuana) or synthetic delta 9-tetrahydrocannabinol (THC), and cannabimimetics (Spyce and HU-210) are prohibited.

S9. Glucocorticosteroids

All glucocorticosteroids are prohibited when administered by oral, intravenous, intramuscular or rectal routes.

SUBSTANCES PROHIBITED IN PARTICULAR SPORTS

- P1. Alcohol
- P2. Beta-blockers

The sports where they are prohibited are shown in Tables 7.2 and 7.3.

Table 7.2
International federations that have banned alcohol

Federations	
Aeronautic	FAI
Archery	FITA
Automobile	FIA
Karate	WKF
Motorcycling	FIM
Skiing	FIS

The doping violation threshold for alcohol (hematological value) is 0.10 g/l, according to the prohibited list of WADA (2012)

Table 7.3
Sports where beta-blockers are prohibited in-competition, according to the prohibited list of WADA (2012)

Aeronautic	FAI
Archery	FITA*
Automobile	FIA
Billiards	WCBS
Bobsleigh	FIBT
Boules	CMSB
Bridge	FMB
Darts	WDF
Golf	IGF
Nine-pin bowling	FIQ
Power boating	UIM
Shooting	ISSF*
Skiing	FIS+

Notes:

* Also prohibited out-of-competition.

+ In sky jumping and free style/and snowboard.

Table 7.4 Specified substances in agreement with Art. 4.2.2, from the World Anti-Doping Code and according to the 2012 prohibited list

S3.	Beta$_2$-agonists
S4.1	Aromatase inhibitors
S4.2	Selective estrogen receptor modulators (SERMs)
S4.3	Other anti-estrogenic substances
S5.	Diuretics and other masking agents
S6.b	Specified stimulants
S7.	Narcotics
S8.	Cannabinoids
S9.	Glucocorticosteroids
P1.	Alcohol
P2.	Beta-blockers

Specified substances

According to the prohibited list of 2012, there are some substances that are particularly susceptible to unintentional anti-doping rule violations because of their general availability in medical products or that are less likely to be successfully abused as doping agents.

A doping violation involving specific substances listed in Table 7.4 may result in reduced sanctions if it is established that there was no intention to enhance sport performance when the substance was used.

SAMPLING PROCEDURES

It is the duty of the team physician or his/her delegate to attend the doping test of his/her athletes and to assist in the collection of their samples. For this reason, it is important to know the main phases of the process very well.

Selection of athletes

During Olympic and regional games, the representative of the international sports federation in question selects the athletes. They may be medalists or athletes selected at random. The team physician, in the case of a written notification from doping control, should always be advised and should also go with the athlete to the doping station. Please note that the athlete will be required to provide a piece of photographic identification – perhaps the accreditation of the championship, if it bears a photo, or the athlete's passport.

Sometimes, athletes are tested on an out-of-competition basis. This means that an athlete may be asked to provide a urine sample anywhere, anytime, and without any advance notice. It's important to know that an accredited doping control officer (DCO) must identify him/herself to collect a urine sample, as well as show a letter of authorization of the respective international sport federation.

Sample-taking procedures

As soon as the athlete is notified of selection for doping control, the team physician should permit the athlete to drink only from sealed-closed bottles or cans. It is important to let the athlete select his/her own drink and also the kit for the collection of the sample. The team physician should always carefully verify that the collection vessel and the doping kit chosen are perfectly closed and clean before the athlete is allowed to use it.

The athlete has the right to handle his own sample or may ask the team physician to do it for him. The DCO, if allowed, may also handle the samples. The team physician should help the athlete inform the proper authorities concerning medication used in the preceding days. Experienced athletes have a list of medications ready in case of a control. It is also proper to ask to which accredited laboratory the sample will be sent, and what is the chain of custody of the sample before it reaches the laboratory. The athlete should receive a copy of the notification and the doping control form at the end of the procedure.

It is important to know that, if the athlete is a minor, the team physician should have the right to observe the doping officer during the passing of the urine.

WADA-accredited laboratories

In accordance with the World Anti-Doping Code, only WADA-accredited laboratories may carry out doping analysis for the Olympic Movement and the public authorities. The analysis will be performed in accordance with the routines defined by WADA, and the result of the "A" sample will be sent to the sports federation and to the medical authority concerned. In case of an adverse analytical result (AAR) or atypical (AT) result during Olympic or regional games, the Chief-of-Mission will be informed, and the athlete will be called for a hearing. The athlete has the right to be accompanied by three people. It is a task of the team physician to perform the preliminary analysis of the case and to assist the athlete in this eventuality.

Appeals

In the case of an AAR that is considered a violation of the anti-doping rule (VADR), there are always at least two opportunities for appeal. The first is to the sports federation concerned, which may discuss the case again in a doping panel. The second is the Court of Arbitration in Sport (CAS), which is headquartered in

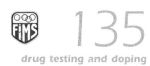

135

Substance group		Number	Adverse analytical findings (%)
S1.	Anabolic agents	3,374	60.8
S6.	Stimulants	574	10.3
S8.	Cannabinoids	533	9.6
S5.	Diuretics and other masking agents	396	7.1
S9.	Glucocorticosteroids	234	4.2
S3.	Beta$_2$-agonists	209	3.8
S2.	Hormones and related substances	86	1.6
S4.	Hormone antagonists and modulators	75	1.4
P2.	Beta-blockers	30	0.5
S7.	Narcotics	20	0.4
P1.	Alcohol	9	0.2
M2.	Chemical and physical manipulation	6	0.1
M1.	Enhancement of oxygen transfer	—	0.00
Total		5,546	

Lausanne, Switzerland. The CAS has the final word in any legal dispute involving athletes, including problems related to doping.

EPIDEMIOLOGY OF DOPING

The accredited laboratories are obliged to report every AAR or AT result case, not only to the international sports federations concerned, but also to WADA. Periodically, this information is released as statistics for the laboratory on the WADA website (www.wada-ama.org). This makes it possible to see the number of doping controls performed in all sports, as well as the substances detected and the incidence of VADRs (Table 7.5).

Incidence of adverse analytical results in Olympic and non-Olympic sports

Table 7.6 shows the total number of controls done in 2010 and the incidence of positive cases in Olympic and non-Olympic sports. Although the majority of the controls are done in the Olympic arena, the percentage of AARs is very similar among these different areas of sport.

Some experts believe that in-competition doping control is illogical, as the athlete can anticipate testing, but reality shows otherwise, probably because it is more

136

Table 7.6 Doping control results in 2010, according to WADA laboratory statistics

Sport	Samples	Adverse analytical findings	%
Olympic sports	180,584	1,624	0.90
Non-Olympic sports	77,683	1,666	1.50
Total	258,267	2,790	1.08

universalized. It seems that out-of-competition doping control always reaches the same athletes, located in the main cities of the world, and fails to test athletes who are in isolated areas.

Breakdown of the AARs by prohibited substances

The analysis of the positive cases presented in Table 7.5, expressed by the prohibited classes of substances and masking agents, shows a clear predominance of anabolic agents, particularly anabolic steroids. The use of stimulants, cannabis, and diuretics is very similar, but the percentage is much lower compared with anabolic steroids.

The participation of the team physician in the athlete's educational process may help to reduce the risk of self-medication and the use of recreational drugs. Periodic, unannounced doping control tests may also help to reduce the number of AARs and AT results in these areas.

MEDICAL ASPECTS OF THE USE OF PROHIBITED SUBSTANCES

Although the most important reason sports physicians should not prescribe doping agents is because they are immoral or unethical, it is also important to stress the medical risks associated with the use of doping agents. Athletes have the right to know all the risks related to wrong choices, and addressing these topics with them is also an important responsibility of the team physician.

Anabolic steroids

The main effect of anabolic steroids, and the reason athletes sometimes use them, is their enhancement of protein synthesis and consequent increase of muscle mass and force. This effect is more evident in boys and women of any age than in sexually mature men. The increased aggressiveness caused by anabolic steroids is also considered advantageous in some sports. The main clinical indication for androgenic therapy in males is primary hypogonadism, where the correction of

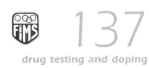

testosterone serum levels reproduces all testicular functions except that of spermatogenesis. Considering the risk–benefit ratio, other situations where prescription of androgens is medically justified are rare. These include certain forms of refractory anemia and angioneurotic hereditary edema. Recently, analogs of testosterone have been tested in patients with severe muscle wasting, of the type seen in acquired immunodeficiency syndrome (AIDS), and in autoimmune-related rheumatologic diseases. However, there is no condition where androgens should be prescribed in healthy subjects.

The use of androgens can provoke a feminization effect in men, particularly gynecomastia. This effect is caused by the conversion (aromatization) of some forms of androgens to estradiol, an estrogen hormone, by extra-glandular tissues, through a natural metabolism route of the androgen hormones. Other adverse effects of these hormones used in men are inhibition of hypothalamus/hypophysis gonado-trophin secretion, with resulting lack of spermatogenesis stimulation, and testicular trophism. Consequently, testicular atrophy, azoospermia, and infertility can occur, remaining present for some months after cessation of use, or even becoming permanent.

With regards to toxicity, the regular use of testosterone analogs can cause, among other conditions, water and salt retention, with edema and sometimes hyper-tension; increase of low-density lipoprotein (LDL)-cholesterol and reduction of serum high-density lipoprotein (HDL)-cholesterol; thyroid dysfunction; mood and sleeping alterations; and psychiatric disease in susceptible people. Alterations of hepatic function, with jaundice and sometimes hepatic adenocarcinoma, can occur after prolonged use of testosterone analogous with alteration of the 17-alpha position. This molecular chemical modification diminishes the drug's breakdown by the liver and allows its oral administration, but it can result in liver hepatotoxicity with prolonged use.

Adverse effects take three main forms: virilization (in women and boys), feminization (in men and boys), and toxic effects (in all users). All androgynous hormones cause virilization when used by women, with acne, facial hirsutism, menstrual irregularity, and deepening of the voice. Generally, almost all symptoms disappear if use is discontinued. On the other hand, continuous and extended use can cause additional effects, such as male-pattern baldness and growth of the clitoris, besides leading to the non-reversibility of effects such as voice changes. Serious growth defects and bone development beyond deep virilization occurs when androgen hormones are administered to children.

It is important to remember that intermittent use of anabolic androgen, known as "cycling," can diminish or delay the appearance of certain adverse effects, especially those that depend on a continuous and prolonged use. On the other hand, this system of administration still involves, not only the enhancement of muscle mass, but also the toxic effects noted above. Thus, the use of these hormones in healthy individuals cannot be justified, whatever the mode or sequence of administration.

Peptide hormones, growth factors, and related substances

The most used substances of this group are no doubt growth hormone and EPO. The former is used to increase power, and the latter to increase aerobic capacity.

The use of growth hormone in sport is considered unethical and dangerous, owing to adverse effects including allergic reactions, diabetogenic effect, and acromegaly or gigantism. In addition, the use of this hormone may lead to heart disease, problems in the ligaments and joints, increase of fat tissue, and muscle weakness.

EPO is used to treat anemia, mainly in patients with chronic kidney diseases, because they lose the capability to produce this hormone. The synthetic EPO that is used by athletes can only be injected. It will elevate arterial blood pressure and is also a potential cause of thrombosis. Pain and discomfort in the site of the injections are not uncommon, and using needles and syringes that are not sterile may lead to infections, including AIDS.

Impairing the ability of the blood to circulate may decrease the delivery of oxygen to the muscles, which may decrease performance, and also may cause hypertensive encephalopathy. Other side effects of EPO may be heart palpitations, skin rash, myalgias, nausea, and iron deficiency.

Beta$_2$-agonists

Beta$_2$-agonists are prescribed medically to treat asthma symptoms. The most potent beta$_2$-agonist is clembuterol, which is included in the prohibited list as an anabolic agent. Like salbutamol, it is most often used to produce larger muscular mass and reduce fat. The reported toxicity of these substances is associated with anxiety, tremor, nervousness, headaches, increase in blood pressure, and arrhythmias. In the prohibited list of 2012, salbutamol, salmeterol, and formoterol are permitted without TUEs, as the anti-doping laboratories are now able to detect, based on the urinary concentrations of the substances, if the use was just therapeutic by aerosol, or if it was used by an oral, intramuscular, or intravenous route, aimed at an increase in performance.

Diuretics

Diuretics are prohibited substances for two main reasons. First, they increase the urinary stream and the free water fraction in urine, which serves as a masking agent because it diminishes the concentration of other substances besides accelerating elimination. Diuretics may also promote fast weight loss, which is desired in sports that have weight classes (such as wrestling and martial arts).

Beyond the unethical aspects of urine or rule manipulation (in the case of artificial weight reduction), there is the concern to protect athletes from problems

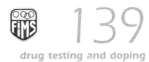

such as induced dehydration and serious electrolyte disorders such as loss of potassium, which may cause muscle cramps and decrease the work capacity of the muscle.

Stimulants

The effect of stimulants on the central nervous system is responsible for improved performance and causes an increase in aggressiveness and strength. On the other hand, the increased adrenergic activity produced by these agents can increase arterial blood pressure and cardiac irritability, which may result in cardiac arrhythmias, coronary spasm, and myocardial ischemia in susceptible individuals.

Use of stimulants may also cause agitation, tremors, loss of coordination, and sleeplessness. Particularly in hot and humid weather, there is always a risk of a death caused by cardiac failure. One should also consider the possibility of addiction and drug dependence resulting from the use of stimulants.

Narcotic analgesics

The main effect of these components is central analgesia. Their medical indications are precise and limited to treating postoperative pain, the terminal stages of carcinoma, or severe pain associated with trauma. The reason they are prohibited is to prevent the harmful inhibition of pain in injured athletes; inhibiting pain can seriously aggravate an injury and affect an athlete's long-term health. In addition, the potential for dependence makes this substance class particularly dangerous when used without correct medical indications. Another possible effect of the use of narcotics is physical dependence, which may begin after a short period of use. After that, the main problems are withdrawal symptoms, including restlessness, aching joints, sweating, nausea, and pain.

Cannabinoids

Cannabis may evoke a subjective feeling of relaxation, altering visual images and impairing psychological and physical performance, which can be demonstrated by objective tests. The ability to learn tasks declines, as well as memory. Decreased levels of testosterone and lowered heart rates are encountered with prolonged use.

Beta-blockers

Athletes use these substances to reduce anxiety and tremor, as well as to produce reduction of the heart rate and of arterial blood tension, which may improve performance in certain sports. Beta-blockers are particularly popular among shooters, because a slower heartbeat gives the shooter more time to aim between heartbeats.

eduardo h. de rose and marco michelucci

Blood transfusion

Blood transfusions to increase athletic performance are also unethical and may carry risk of allergic reaction, acute hemolytic reaction, homodynamic overload, metabolic unbalance, and the transmission of infectious diseases (viral hepatitis and AIDS).

CONCLUSION

The new millennium has been witness to profound modifications in the legislation, the coordination, and the technology of the fight against doping in Olympic and non-Olympic sports, as well as in all levels of national and local sports activities.

Effective since 2003, the World Anti-doping Code replaced the Anti-doping Code of the Olympic Movement, which up until that time had been the document that defined the list of forbidden substances and methods. It also describes the procedures for collection of samples (International Standard for Testing (IST)) and systemizes the sanctions for the positive cases, as well as the procedure for appeals in case of sanctions.

The new code will govern out-of-competition tests and competitions organized by the participants in the Olympic Movement: international sports federations and national Olympic committees, represented by entities including the Association of the Summer Olympic International Federations (ASOIF), the Association of International Olympic Winter Sports Federations (AIOWF), and the Association of National Olympic Committees (ANOC).

WADA was established on November 10, 1999, and had its first meeting on January 13, 2000. WADA is now responsible for the elaboration of the List of Prohibited Substances and Methods, for the accreditation and technical control of the laboratories, and for financing and managing research in this field. Because WADA is composed equally of representatives of the Olympic Movement and public authorities, the decisions made should be more effectively enforced, thus complementing the international campaign against doping in sport.

This is undoubtedly the most important development in doping control since the beginning of this process in 1967. The active participation of public authorities, made possible through the International Convention against Doping in Sport, should greatly help to reduce the use of drugs in sport. This UNESCO Convention was created in the 33th General Assembly in October 2005, and 158 of the 193 member countries adopted this convention.

To conclude, it is important to understand that doping control and doping problems are highly dynamic subjects, and it is the responsibility of the team physician always to be very well informed and up to date, and also to supervise and educate the multidisciplinary team that assists athletes in their preparation for competition.

141

SUGGESTED READING

Australian Sports Drug Agency: www.ausport.gov.au/asda

Bueno C.R. *Dopaje*. Madrid: Interamericana; 1992.

Canadian Centre for Drug-Free Sport. Doping Control – Standard Operating Procedures. Gloucester, Canada: Canadian Centre for Drug-Free Sport; 1994.

Clasing D. *Doping*. Stuttgart: Gustav Fischer; 1992.

Combs R.H., West L.J. *Drug Testing: Issues and Options*. New York: Oxford University Press; 1991.

Council of Europe. *Explanatory Report on the Anti-Doping Convention*. Strassbourg, France: Council of Europe; 1990.

Council of Europe: www.coe.fr/fr/txtjue/135fr.htm

De Rose E.H., Aquino Neto F.R., et al. Anti-doping control in Brazil: results from the year of 2003 and prevention activities. *Rev. Bras. Med. Esporte* 2004; 10: 294–8.

De Rose E.H., Feder M.G., et al. Informações sobre o uso de medicamentos no esporte, 2005; available at www.cob.org.br

De Rose E.H. Doping in athletes – an update. In L. Micheli (ed) *Clin. Sports Med.*, 2008: 27, 1.

Elliot D., Goldberg L. Intervention and prevention of steroids use in adolescents. *Am. J. Sports Med.* 1996; 24: 41–7.

Evans N.A. Gym and tonic: a profile of 100 male steroid users. *Br. J. Sports Med.* 1997; 31: 54–8.

Fuentes R.J., Rosemberg J.M., Davis A. *Athletics Drug Reference*. Triangle Park: Clean Data; 1995.

Goldberg L., Elliot D., Clarke G.N., et al. Effects of a multidimensional anabolic steroids prevention intervention. The adolescent training and learning to avoid steroids (ATLAS) Program. *JAMA* 1996; 276: 1555–62.

International Olympic Committee. *Doping*. Lausanne, Switzerland: International Olympic Committee; 1999.

International Olympic Committee. *Olympic Movement Anti-Doping Code*. Lausanne, Switzerland: International Olympic Committee; 1999.

Lamb D. Anabolic steroids in athletics: how well do they work and how dangerous are they? *Am. J. Sports Med.* 1984; 12: 31–8.

Lombardo J.A., Hickson R.C., Lamb D.R. Anabolic androgenic steroids and growth hormone. In Lamb D.R., Williams M.H. (eds), *Ergogenics: Enhancement and Performance and Exercise in Sport*. Carmel: Brown and Benchmark; 1991.

Melia P., Pipe A., Greenberg L. The use of anabolic-androgenic steroids by Canadian students. *Clin. J. Sports Med.* 1996; 6: 9–14.

Mottram D.R. *Drugs in Sports*. Champaign: Human Kinetics; 1988.

New Zealand Sports Drug Agency. *Drugs in Sport – Information Series*. Auckland, New Zealand: New Zealand Sports Drug Agency; 1993.

Ringhofer K.R., Harding M.H. *Coaches' Guide to Drug and Sport*. Champaign: Human Kinetics; 1995.

Segura J. Doping control in sports medicine. *Ther. Drug Monit.* 1996; 18: 471–6.

Strauss R.H. *Drugs and Performance in Sports*. Philadelphia: WB Saunders; 1987.

Tricker R., Connoly D. Drug education and the college athlete: evaluation of a decision making model. *J. Drug Educ.* 1996; 26: 159–81.

Wilson J.D., Griffin J.E. The use and misuse of androgens. *Metabolism* 1980; 12: 1278–95.

World Anti-doping Agency, International Standard for Therapeutic Use Exemptions, in force January 2005; available at www.wada-ama.org

World Anti-doping Agency, World Anti-doping Code, 2003. Available at www.wada-ama.org

www.jeunesse-sport.gouv.fr/francais/mjs.luttedop.htm

www.nodoping.org

Yesalis C.E. *Anabolic Steroids in Sports and Exercise*. Champaign: Human Kinetics; 1990.

CHAPTER 8

MEDICAL AND OTHER CONDITIONS AFFECTING SPORTS PARTICIPATION

Martin P. Schwellnus and Wayne Derman

A team physician is frequently faced with the problem of the diagnosis and management of medical conditions that may affect the health and exercise performance of an athlete. A team physician may encounter the interaction between illness in almost every system in the human body and exercise. The purpose of this chapter is to discuss some of the more common illnesses affecting different organ systems, and their interaction with exercise.

One of the principal roles of the team physician is to accompany athletes who travel long distances to compete in a tournament. Therefore, "jet lag" has also become one of the common issues the team physician has to deal with. The team physician is also often obliged to address issues outside the realm of "common medical conditions." The team physician may sometimes need to step in and address lifestyle habits of the athlete that might impact performance. These may include athletes' sexual activity and use of "social drugs." These issues will also be discussed briefly in this chapter.

EPIDEMIOLOGY OF MEDICAL CONDITIONS IN ATHLETES

In recent years, there has been an increasing focus on protection of the health of the athlete. Early data reported from one team at two Summer Olympic Games show that medical conditions in athletes are more common than injuries. This finding has, in part, stimulated more research to determine the incidence and nature of the medical conditions that a team physician is likely to encounter during a tournament. Collectively, data from these studies consistently show that illness accounts for at least 30–50% of all the medical encounters during a variety of international tournaments. Furthermore, these data show that respiratory illness, gastrointestinal (GIT) illness, and dermatological conditions are very common in athletes. Finally, these data show that infections account for the majority of these illnesses. Therefore, in this chapter, illness in these systems will be discussed in some detail.

EXERCISE AND INFECTIOUS DISEASES

Athletes are not immune to developing infections. In fact, during intensive training and competition and international travel, athletes appear to be more prone to developing infections. The relationship between exercise and changes in the immune system has recently been reviewed. Furthermore, depending on the nature of the sports in which athletes participate, they may be exposed to infections transmitted through direct skin contact, contaminated water, blood, or tissue products via respiratory droplets.

The more common infections in athletes that will be discussed briefly in this chapter include:

- respiratory tract infections (upper and lower respiratory tract);
- skin infections (contact sports);
- GIT infections (traveling and contact sports);
- waterborne infections (water sports);
- other infections related to international travel (SARS, bird flu, and HIV).

PRACTICAL CLINICAL POINT 1

Common infections in athletes

- Upper and lower respiratory tract infections (endurance athletes).
- Skin infections (contact sports).
- GIT infections (traveling and contact sports).
- Waterborne infections (water sports).
- Genitourinary infections.
- Blood-borne infections.

Practical guidelines for the administering of vaccinations in athletes will also be discussed briefly.

Respiratory tract infections

Respiratory tract infections (RTIs) can be divided into infections of the upper and lower respiratory tracts. Data clearly show that symptoms of upper respiratory tract infections (URTIs) are more common. Therefore, the majority of this section will focus on infections of the upper respiratory tract (URT). A URTI can be defined as an acute illness affecting the nasopharynx that results in localized and sometimes systemic symptoms, usually caused by a number of different viruses or bacteria. URTIs are the commonest infections that affect the adult population, including athletes. An average adult contracts between two and five URTIs per year.

There is some scientific evidence to support the hypothesis that high-intensity (> 80% of maximum ability) and prolonged exercise (> 60 minutes) is associated with a depressed immunity, which lasts for up to 24 hours after exercise. During this period, there appears to be an increased risk of developing a URTI. Athletes engaged in regular, intense, prolonged training may therefore be at a higher risk of developing symptoms of URTIs.

Conversely, exercising at a lower intensity (< 70% of maximum ability) appears to protect the body against URTIs. Although there is some evidence to suggest that vitamin C, 500 mg/d, also protects against URTIs during sport, recent data show that vitamin C can reduce the duration of the URTI. However, it is important to note that, in recent years, evidence has accumulated to show that not all symptoms of URTIs in athletes (during training or after sports events) are infective in nature. In particular, it has been documented that allergies affecting the URT are very common in athletes. Therefore, the team physician must also consider non-infective causes of URT symptoms in athletes.

PRACTICAL CLINICAL POINT 2

Precautions for athletes to decrease the risk of developing URTIs

- Space high-intensity and prolonged exercise sessions and race events as far apart as possible.
- Avoid overtraining and chronic fatigue.
- Maintain a well-balanced diet and consider nutritional supplements if indicated.
- Get adequate sleep.
- Take vitamin C during periods of infection to reduce the duration of the infection.
- Ensure adequate carbohydrate intake during intense, prolonged exercise.

Return-to-play guidelines following a URTI

In general, if the URTI is associated with systemic symptoms, sports participation must be avoided until the symptoms have disappeared. Systemic symptoms include fever, myalgia, resting tachycardia, malaise (excessive fatigue), chest pain, cough, and lymphadenopathy.

If the URTI is not associated with any of the above symptoms, low-intensity (< 70% maximum ability) and short-duration (< 20 minutes) exercise may be permitted in some cases during the URTI, with the approval of the physician. Moderate exercise may be resumed as soon as the symptoms have subsided.

martin p. schwellnus and wayne derman

Skin infections

Skin infections are common in athletes. Cutaneous infections and their importance in sports have been reviewed. Therefore, a detailed discussion of the diagnosis and management of each of the skin infections is beyond the scope of this chapter. However, the team physician has to be aware of the common fungal infections (*tinea pedis, cruris, capitis, corporis*), bacterial (*staphylococcus aureas, streptococcus pyogenes, pseudomonas aeruginosa, corynebacterium minutissimum*), viral (*herpes simplex virus type 1, papilloma virus, molluscum contagiosum*), and parasitic organisms that can cause skin infections. In particular, the team physician must be aware of infections such as herpes and staphylococcus, which, although less common, can be transmitted in contact sports such as wrestling and rugby.

In most cases, after diagnosis, application of a topical antimicrobial agent can treat skin infections, and the athlete can continue full activity without a detrimental effect on exercise performance. However, in the case of contagious skin infections, such as herpes, contact with others needs to be restricted until the infective period is over.

Although not specifically classified as a skin infection, tetanus has to be considered in athletes who may sustain an open wound. Inoculation into the tissues with the spores of the anaerobic organism *clostridium tetani* can result in germination of the spores and subsequent toxin production, which interferes with the release of inhibitory neurotransmitters.

Following an incubation period of 4–21 days, tetanus can present with trismus (lock jaw), dysphagia, and facial spasms. Death can result from respiratory failure. Diagnosis is by clinical criteria and demonstration of Gram-positive bacilli and/or isolation of *C. tetani* from a wound. Treatment requires hospital admission and intensive-care support. Benzodiazepines can be used to treat muscle spasm, human tetanus immunoglobulin can neutralize the toxin, and metronidazole is the antibiotic of choice.

Water-borne infections

Bilharzia (schistosomiasis)

Schistosomiasis is a tropical infection caused by a digenetic trematode. The two predominant species are Schistosoma mansoni and S. haematobium. Less commonly, infection is by S. intercalatum. Human infection in athletes has been documented principally in Africa and involves athletes who participate in water sports where the trematode is prevalent. Human infection occurs on entry into shallow fresh water that contains the schistosome larvae. These larvae penetrate the skin, and the immature parasites migrate via the lungs to the portal circulation. Here they develop into adult worms, which migrate to the veins of the intestines (S. mansoni) or bladder (S. haematobium). After 7–12 weeks, the worms produce eggs, which are excreted and can be observed in the feces or urine.

Table 8.1 Tetanus prophylaxis in wound management of athletes

History of tetanus vaccination	Tetanus vaccine administration	Tetanus immunoglobulin administration
Not immunized or immunization not known with certainty	Administer full 3-dose course	Yes – if tetanus-prone wound
Last dose > 10 years ago	Reinforcing dose	Yes – if tetanus-prone wound
Last dose < 10 years ago	No	No, unless risk of infection is very high

Prevention of bilharzia in athletes

- Be aware of endemic bilharzia areas.
- Water sports should avoid areas of shallow or static (not flowing) water.
- If water sports are conducted in fresh water in endemic areas, inquire if molluscicide treatment of the water has been undertaken.
- Athletes should perform vigorous toweling and drying or application of alcohol immediately after water contact.
- Athletes who have been exposed should be assessed clinically and tested for the presence of bilharzia (eggs in stools or urine, serological test).

Clinical presentation of bilharzia is as a cercarial dermatitis (swimmer's itch), acute infection (Katayama fever), and later as chronic schistosomiasis. Laboratory diagnosis is by microscopy (urine or stool) or through a serological test. Once diagnosed, treatment is by single-dose Praziquantal (40 mg/kg).

Otitis externa in swimmers (swimmer's ear)

The term "swimmer's ear" has been used to describe any inflammatory condition of the ear that commonly occurs in athletes participating in water sports. This single term describes a variety of conditions that affect the external auditory canal or the middle ear in swimmers. The commonest disease of the external auditory canal associated with water sports is otitis externa. Other conditions include bony exostoses of the external auditory canal and infections of the middle ear (otitis media).

Risk factors for developing otitis externa in swimmers

- Spending long periods in water with the ears submerged, swimming in unchlorinated, fresh, hot, or contaminated water.
- Not removing water from the ears after swimming.
- Introducing bacteria by inserting a dirty finger, contaminated swabs, or other objects into the ear.
- Contact with water containing sensitizing agents to which the athlete is allergic, or agents that are known irritants such as chemicals.
- Constant use of over-the-counter ear drops that denude the ear canal further.

Otitis externa is an inflammatory condition of the external auditory canal, which can be caused by chemical irritation, allergies, or infections. Infections can be either bacterial or fungal. The main reason for an increased risk of otitis externa in swimmers is because water that repeatedly enters the canal washes cerumen out. Water that remains in the canal for some time causes maceration of the skin, leaving the damaged epithelium unprotected against invading organisms such as bacteria and fungi.

The diagnosis of otitis externa is made clinically. The swimmer with otitis externa will initially complain of ear fullness, ear discomfort, and hearing loss. Pain becomes prominent if the condition persists, and discharge from the ear may be observed. An allergic-type otitis usually presents with severe pruritus (itch).

On examination of the ear canal, there may initially only be erythema and edema observed. Other signs such as a discharge, absence of cerumen, a dull tympanic membrane, and hyperkeratotic epithelium are characteristic of otitis externa at a later and chronic stage. Cultures of otitis externa show that pseudomonas aeruginosa is the commonest bacteria and aspergillus is the commonest fungus causing the infection. Fungal infections are characterized by a fuzzy lining dotted with black specks and a discharge with a musty odor. A qualified medical practitioner should manage otitis externa. The first step is to clean out the canal thoroughly by irrigation or the use of instruments (only if experienced). Topical anti-infective agents must be used with caution. In case of bacterial infections, drops containing neomycin or polymyxin B may be used. Acidification of the canal will discourage bacterial growth; provided there is no perforation of the eardrum, topical acidifiers such as 2% acetic acid may be used. Fungal infections can be treated with a 1% tolnaftate solution. Pain and pruritus must be relieved by analgesics and hydrocortisone, respectively. Hydrocortisone drops must be used with care and only after the infection is controlled. The swimmer should ideally abstain from water sports for 7–10 days. Athletes with less severe infections can return to swimming after 2–3 days, provided the necessary precautions are taken.

PRACTICAL CLINICAL POINT 7

Preventing otitis externa in swimmers

- Dry the ear after swimming by tilting the head vigorously, jumping up and down, or drying gently with a towel.
- Avoid touching or scratching the ear.
- Use newer, silicone-type earplugs for protection.
- Wear a hood when surfing or sail-boarding.
- Put a dropper full of drying agent into the ear after each swim.

Other water-borne infections

A number of other microbial agents may infect athletes who come into contact with contaminated water sources. These include leptospirosis, aeromonas hydrophilia, giardiasis, and cryptopsoridiosis.

Leptospirosis is a spirochetal infection that presents with a flu-like illness, 2–20 days following water contact. After a few days, this progresses to a syndrome characterized by fever, aseptic meningitis, skin rash, and uveitis. Weil's disease is severe leptospirosis, which is characterized by progression to hepatitis, jaundice, renal failure, and coagulopathy. Treatment is by penicillin or doxycycline.

Aeromonas hydrophilia is an infection of the soft tissue following exposure to contaminated water (swimmers, skiers, paddlers). Giardiasis and cryptosporidiosis, as well as other GIT infections, may be acquired through water exposure during swimming and paddling in contaminated water. A wide range of GIT symptoms can occur, which require specific diagnosis and treatment. Giardiasis requires antibiotic treatment, typically oral metronidazole.

Genitourinary infections

A detailed discussion of sexually transmitted infections is beyond the scope of this chapter. However, team physicians need to be aware that localized infections of the genitourinary tract can occur in athletes, in particular female athletes. The correct choice of underwear is important to prevent infections such as vaginitis or urethritis. Localized vaginitis, without signs of pelvic inflammatory disease, can be treated by local or topical application of antimicrobial agents. Full athletic activity can be continued throughout the treatment period. In the case of more regional infections, such as cystitis or pelvic inflammatory disease, systemic, antimicrobial agents are indicated, and athletic activity should be restricted until full resolution of symptoms.

Blood-borne infections

There are a number of important blood-borne infections of which team physicians must be aware. These are hepatitis (B, C, and D) and the human immunodeficiency virus (HIV).

Viral hepatitis infection

Viruses causing hepatitis include hepatitis A (spread by fecal–oral route), hepatitis B, C, and D (spread by blood, perinatal transmission, and through sexual contact), and hepatitis E (fecal–oral transmission). Infections by hepatitis B, C, and D are associated with a high risk of chronicity (15–80%) and a higher risk of mortality (1–2%) once infected. Athletes participating in contact sports may be exposed to blood and blood-borne products and, therefore, may be at risk for acquiring hepatitis infections. Although the risk of transmission of hepatitis through contact sport is very low, athletes traveling to, or living in, areas where hepatitis (in particular hepatitis B) is endemic should be vaccinated. Furthermore, the general guidelines for decreasing the risk of blood-borne infections in contact sports should be followed.

HIV infection

The most important consideration regarding HIV infection and sports is whether there is a risk of HIV transmission during sports participation. HIV is transmitted through sexual intercourse, blood or blood products, and from mother to fetus.

Athletes are at risk of contracting HIV if they engage in high-risk sexual behaviors or use drugs intravenously. However, there is also a small but real risk of HIV transmission in contact sports. Transmission may occur if blood from an infected player contaminates an open, bleeding wound of a non-infected player. In sports such as rugby, soccer, boxing, wrestling, and synchronized skating, where the transmission of HIV is possible, players, coaches, and administrators need to ensure that open, bleeding wounds are treated before participants return to the sports field. Surfaces such as wrestling mats that are potentially contaminated by blood or tissue should be appropriately cleaned before the contest resumes. In some sports, such as boxing, compulsory testing of competitors has been instituted.

Malaria

Although not strictly speaking a blood-borne infection, malaria is a tropical protozoal vector-borne infection. The female Anopheles mosquito, which is a voracious nocturnal blood feeder, transmits malaria. It is the most prevalent

PRACTICAL CLINICAL POINT 9

Preventing HIV transmission during sports

General guidelines

- In general, the risk of HIV transmission during sports is higher in contact sports, where there is a risk of transmission through contamination of open lesions, wounds, or mucous membranes of a non-infected individual with infected blood or blood products.

Specific guidelines for sportspeople

- An athlete who engages in high-risk behavior is advised to seek medical attention regarding possible HIV infection.
- Athletes with known HIV infection should seek medical and legal counseling before considering further participation in sport.
- Athletes with known HIV infection should inform medical personnel of their condition if they sustain an open wound or skin lesions during sports participation, so that these can be managed appropriately.

Specific guidelines for sports administrators

- Sports administrators, including coaches and managers, have special opportunities for meaningful education of athletes with respect to HIV disease and should encourage athletes to seek counseling.

Specific guidelines for medical personnel attending to athletes

- Treat all open skin lesions sustained during sports participation appro priately before allowing the athlete to return to the playing field.

The following treatment of open skin lesions is recommended:

- Immediately clean the wound with a suitable antiseptic such as hypo-chloride (bleach, Milton), 2% gluteraldehyde (Cidex), organic iodines, or 70% alcohol (ethyl alcohol, isopropyl alcohol).
- The open wound should be covered securely so that there is no risk of exposure to blood or blood products prior to return to the playing field.
- All first aid and medical personnel attending to athletes with open wound lesions should wear protective gloves to decrease the risk of HIV transmission.

153

vector-borne disease and is endemic in 92 countries. In Sub-Saharan Africa, 95% of malaria is caused by *Plasmodium falciparum*, the remainder mainly by P. *vivax*.

Malaria is a disease associated with a considerable morbidity and mortality. Athletes may have to travel frequently to attend events held in areas where malaria is endemic, and this means that malarial prophylaxis must be taken. A number of specific guidelines for preventing malaria in traveling athletes have been issued.

PRACTICAL CLINICAL POINT 10

Prevention of malaria in traveling athletes

- Be aware of endemic malarial areas.
- Chemoprophylaxis is recommended (inquire at WHO website or local travel clinic).
- Wear clothing with long sleeves and long trousers at dusk and dawn.
- Use mosquito repellents containing 15–30% diethylmetatoluamide (DEET) on exposed skin and clothing.
- Use sleeping nets that are treated with insecticide.
- Spray rooms with insecticide aerosol/surface spray.
- Use mosquito vapor mats/burning coils at night.

It is recommended that athletes who travel to areas where malaria is endemic take malarial chemoprophylaxis. The effects of common malarial prophylactic agents on exercise performance have not been evaluated in scientific studies, but anecdotal reports indicate that these agents can have negative effects on exercise performance. Current advice to athletes should thus be to: (1) use the common agents beforehand when in training, to establish whether the agents are tolerated; (2) use agents that are prescribed only once a week if possible; and (3) schedule the first dose in such a way that the competition date is on day 6 after administration, rather than on the first or second day.

Vaccination of athletes

There are a number of important considerations with respect to vaccinations in athletes. First, it is important that all athletes are properly vaccinated when traveling to countries for competition; vaccination against cholera and yellow fever is particularly important. Second, all athletes, in particular those participating in contact sports, must be vaccinated against tetanus and hepatitis A and B. Athletes should also be well educated about HIV transmission. Finally, athletes must be aware that it is advisable to restrict athletic activity for 2–3 days after vaccination because of minor systemic inflammation.

154

EXERCISE AND ASTHMA, INCLUDING EXERCISE-INDUCED BRONCHOSPASM (EIB)

The relationship between asthma and exercise has recently been reviewed, and, therefore, the purpose of this chapter is not to review exercise and asthma in detail. However, in the context of medical conditions in athletes, this area will be briefly discussed.

Pathophysiology of EIB

The pathogenesis of EIB has been reviewed. Currently, the view is that the pathogenesis of EIB is multifactorial and is not completely understood. It is generally believed that EIB results from breathing relatively dry air in large volumes, which causes the airways to narrow by osmotic and thermal consequences of evaporative water loss from the airway surface. The hyperosmolar environment, which is created by evaporative water loss, may result in the release of mediators such as histamine. Histamine is a potent bronchoconstrictor, from mast cell degranulation. Inflammation is a characteristic of asthma, and, hence, the inflammatory process plays a role in the development of EIB in asthmatic patients. However, the role of inflammation in the pathogenesis of EIB in subject with no asthma is not clear.

Sports associated with EIB

Athletes participating in sports associated with high ventilation, particularly of cold and dry air (winter), are at higher risk of developing EIB.

Environmental pollutants may also increase the risk of developing EIB. These include chlorine in pools, chemicals related to ice-resurfacing machines, carbon monoxide, and nitrogen dioxide.

Diagnosis of EIB

The approach to the diagnosis of EIB involves a detailed medical history, a comprehensive clinical examination, and the use of special investigations, and a number of diagnostic algorithms have been suggested. Clinically, EIB may present with mild impairment of performance, or symptoms and signs of severe bronchospasm and respiratory failure. The commonest symptoms of EIB are cough, chest tightness, breathlessness, and wheezing. These symptoms normally develop 5–15 minutes after exercise and last for 20–60 minutes. In some patients, a delayed reaction resulting in airway obstruction of 4–10 hours after exercise can occur, which is the so-called "late-phase" EIB. It is important to inquire whether these symptoms also occur on exposure to cold air or in the presence of airborne irritants. Athletes with EIB may also experience hay fever, sinusitis, postnasal drip, drug allergies, or urticaria.

Sports associated with higher risk of EIB (high-ventilation sports)

- Cross-country skiing.
- Ice hockey.
- Track athletics.
- Cross-country running.
- Field hockey.
- Soccer.
- Swimming.

Bronchoprovocation tests for EIB

Exercise challenge test

- Type of exercise (treadmill running).
- Intensity > 80% maximum heart rate.
- Duration > 7 minutes.
- Spirometry before, immediately after, and for up to 30 minutes after.

Eucapnic voluntary hyperventilation test

- Gas mixture of 5% CO_2, 21% O_2.
- 85% of maximum voluntary hyperventilation for 6 minutes.
- FEV1 before (3 times) and after test (immediately, 5, 10, 15, and 20 minutes after).
- High specificity for EIB.

Metacholine challenge test

- Not recommended first line test.
- Low sensitivity.

Histamine challenge test

- Not recommended first line test.
- Low sensitivity.

Mannitol inhalation test

- High sensitivity and specificity for EIB.
- Test does not simulate exercise.

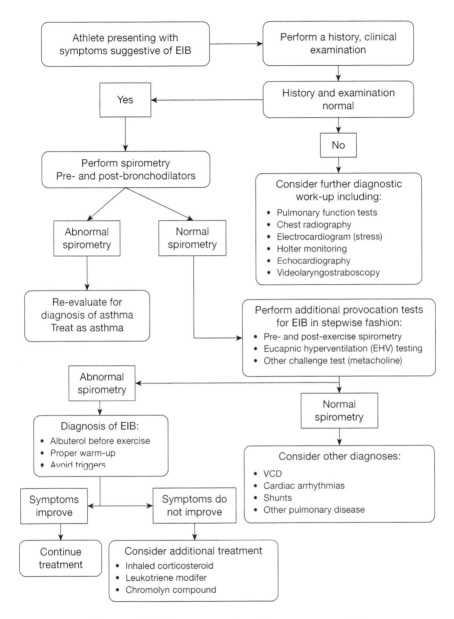

Figure 8.1 Evaluation of athletes presenting with symptoms of EIB

conditions affecting sports participation

The diagnosis of EIB is confirmed when there is a > 10% decrease in the maximal amount of air a person can forcefully exhale in 1 second, FEV1, following a bronchoprovocation test.

Management of EIB

The aim of treatment is to prevent or reduce the severity of EIB so that the athlete can participate normally in exercise. It is important to give the athlete practical advice on the non-pharmacological treatment of EIB. The team physician can take a major role in this area.

PRACTICAL CLINICAL POINT 13

Non-pharmacological management of EIB in athletes

- Perform a warm-up (15 minutes light intensity, followed by 15 minutes moderate to high intensity) before trainings or competitions.
- Be well trained for the sport.
- Avoid training in cool or dry weather conditions.
- Avoid training in areas such as forests or grass fields where there may be pollen that precipitates bronchospasm.
- Avoid training in polluted air.
- Wear a facemask to warm and humidify air when training in dry cold weather.
- Nutritional measures (low dietary salt intake, fish oil (Omega-3 poly-unsaturated fatty acids) supplementation).

The first line of pharmacological treatment is the use of inhaled corticosteroids and β_2-adrenergic agonists. The athlete can also be instructed to use two puffs of the inhaled β_2-adrenergic agonist 15–30 minutes before exercise (i.e., at the start of the warm-up). Cromolyn sodium is another drug that can be combined with a β_2-agonist, and is particularly effective in preventing late-phase EIB. Other medications that can be considered by the prescribing doctor include the following: inhaled anticholinergic medication, oral theophylline, leukotriene modifiers, and, in some cases, antihistamine medication.

It is important for the team physician to remember that medications for controlling EIB require notification, and the team physician must be aware of the requirements of WADA and the sports federations. In some cases, the rules may differ between the federation and WADA.

martin p. schwellnus and wayne derman

RESPIRATORY ALLERGIES IN ATHLETES

In recent years, there has been an increased recognition that many upper and lower respiratory tract symptoms in athletes can be attributed to allergies rather than infections. The current hypotheses on the etiology of respiratory tract symptoms in athletes have recently been reviewed. In this review, the allergic hypothesis for the etiology was reviewed. There is increasing evidence that allergies are very common in athletes and, in some instances, more common that in the general population. It has also been documented that allergies can lead to a decrease in exercise performance. The sports physician therefore needs to consider allergies as part of the screening of athletes and to consider allergies as a possible cause of respiratory tract symptoms. A questionnaire has recently been developed to assist the team physician in the screening of athletes for allergies.

GASTROINTESTINAL SYMPTOMS IN ATHLETES

Many athletes have experienced the extreme frustration of a poor performance in an important sports event caused by GIT symptoms. Others have experienced the inability to train optimally because of a chronic, nagging GIT problem. The team physician is often the person that a frustrated athlete consults to alleviate such a "trivial" problem.

PRACTICAL CLINICAL POINT 14

Gastrointestinal symptoms during exercise

- GIT symptoms may interfere with training or competition.
- They usually originate in the lower GIT tract.
- Causes can be unrelated to exercise, such as infection, cancer, gastric or duodenal ulcer.
- Possible etiologies are relative ischemia of mucosal lining, mechanical "bouncing" of intestines, and release of hormones.
- Medication may be considered – be certain it is not on the banned list.
- Once symptoms are attributed only to exercise and not to any organic disease, provide practical advice to athletes.

Causes of GIT symptoms in athletes

It is unlikely that there is one single cause for all GIT symptoms during exercise. The risk factors for GIT symptoms in athletes have been reviewed. First, it must first be emphasized that GIT symptoms during exercise can result from causes unrelated to exercise. These causes would include infections, cancers, gastric or

159

Table 8.2 The frequency of GIT symptoms associated with exercise

Symptom	Frequency (%)
Upper GIT tract:	
Loss of appetite	12–50
Heartburn	8–11
Belching	12–36
Nausea	4–21
Vomiting	4–31
Lower GIT tract:	
Abdominal pain	25–67
Urge to defecate	30–63
Bowel movement	13–51
Diarrhea	10–30
Rectal bleeding	2–12

duodenal ulcers, and a variety of other well-documented GIT tract diseases. Therefore, the team physician must advise the patient, particularly the older patient or the patient with chronic symptoms, to seek medical help in establishing a correct diagnosis.

For symptoms that are related only to exercise and not to organic disease, three main etiological mechanisms have been proposed. First, blood diverted away from the GIT tract to the contracting muscle during high-intensity or prolonged exercise may result in a relative ischemia of the mucosal lining of the GIT tract, which may cause rectal bleeding in some athletes. This hypothesis has recently been tested for the first time in a prospective cohort study in Ironman triathletes. The results

---

PRACTICAL CLINICAL POINT 15

Risk factors for GIT symptoms during exercise

- Female gender.
- Younger age.
- Poorly conditioned.
- Running, jumping sports.
- Motion sickness.
- Downhill running.
- High-intensity exercise.
- Dietary factors.
- Dehydration.
- Lactose intolerance.
- Previous abdominal surgery.
- Medication.

---

of this study do not support the reduced blood flow hypothesis. Further research to test this hypothesis is therefore required. Second, mechanical movement or "bouncing" of the small and large intestines, particularly during running or jumping, may cause lower GIT tract symptoms. Finally, high-intensity or prolonged exercise is associated with the release of a number of specific GIT hormones, which may have a role in the development of symptoms.

In studies conducted in groups of athletes, a number of possible risk factors for developing GIT symptoms have been identified, which are listed in Practical clinical point 15. Athletes are advised to consult this list and identify those factors that can be changed. The team physician can be of help by discussing these factors with the athlete.

Management of GIT symptoms in athletes

In the first instance, management should depend on establishing a correct diagnosis. It is important to consult a gastroenterologist or a sports physician to establish the cause of the problem. If the symptom is attributed only to exercise and not to any organic disease, specific advice should be given to the athlete. There is some practical advice that the team physician can give to athletes with GIT symptoms (see Practical clinical point 16).

There are three important considerations when prescribing medication for an athlete who presents with GIT symptoms during exercise. First, a clear diagnosis of the condition must be established, so that an underlying pathology, such as cancer, is not missed. A correct diagnosis is most important, particularly in the older athlete, and will determine what medication could be prescribed.

Second, any medication that is prescribed to an elite athlete must not contain substances in the banned list of drugs. In most cases, medications for GIT symptoms are not on the banned list and can thus be prescribed safely. The exceptions are appetite suppressants, which contain stimulants.

Third, medication should not interfere with the athlete's ability to perform optimally. Few studies have examined the relationship between GIT medication and exercise performance. In a study, loperamide HCl was shown not to affect exercise performance (endurance performance and isokinetic muscle strength). Anecdotal evidence suggests that topical antacids, H_2-antagonists, and proton pump inhibitors, which are all used to control heartburn, do not affect exercise performance. However, medications for controlling nausea, such as prochlorperazine, cyclizine HCl, and metoclopramide, have the side effect of causing drowsiness and thus may impair sports performance, although these are not results from scientific studies.

PRACTICAL CLINICAL POINT 16

Practical advice the team physician can give an athlete with GIT symptoms

Heartburn
- Avoid large meals 2–3 hours before training/racing.
- Use a topical antacid if necessary.

Nausea/vomiting
- Avoid large meals 2–3 hours before training/racing.
- Avoid high-intensity or prolonged exercise, particularly if you are not well trained.
- The use of an anti-emetic 1–2 hours before training or racing is not encouraged, because the effects of anti-emetics on performance, as well as their safety during exercise, have not been well established.

Abdominal cramps
- Be well trained for races.
- Avoid training at too high intensities if you are not accustomed to it.
- Avoid a very high dietary fiber intake in the 24 hours before a race.
- Avoid dehydration during training/racing.
- The use of an anti-spasmodic 1–2 hours before training or racing is not encouraged, because the effects of anti-spasmodics on performance, as well as their safety during exercise, have not been well established.

Urge to defecate/diarrhea
- Avoid a very high dietary fiber intake in the 24 hours before a race.
- Avoid dehydration during training/racing.
- Attempt to stimulate a bowel movement before training/racing (caffeine can be used, e.g., a cup of tea or coffee).
- Avoid hill running or running at high intensities.
- If severe and persistent, think about switching to gliding sports (cycling, swimming).
- The use of an anti-diarrheal medication 1–2 hours before training or racing is not encouraged, because the effects of anti-diarrheals on performance, as well as their safety during exercise, have not been well established.
- Probiotics have recently been used in the management of lower GIT symptoms in athletes.

NEUROLOGICAL CONDITIONS IN ATHLETES

Exercise and epilepsy

Epilepsy can be defined as a convulsive disorder characterized by sudden, brief, repetitive, and stereotyped alterations in behavior, which are presumed to be due to paroxysmal discharge of cortical and subcortical neurons. Epilepsy is a common neurological disorder, and about 10% of the population will at some time in their life have a seizure. Epilepsy is, therefore, also common in children and young adults who are physically active and wish to participate in sport.

Does regular exercise increase the risk of seizures?

It is common for patients with epilepsy to inquire whether regular exercise increases the risk, or perhaps decreases the risk, of precipitating seizures. In a recently published study, the exercise habits in a sample of adult outpatients with epilepsy were compared with those in the general population of the same age and sex. The results of the study showed that, in the majority of patients with epilepsy, physical exercise had no adverse effects, and a considerable proportion (36%) claimed that regular exercise contributed to better seizure control. However, in approximately 10% of the patients, exercise appeared to be a seizure precipitant, and this applied particularly to those with symptomatic partial epilepsy. The risk of sustaining serious seizure-related injuries while exercising seemed modest.

The effect of participation in a structured program of fairly intensive leisure activity on seizure occurrence was also investigated in adults with medically intractable epilepsy. The relative risk of seizures did not differ significantly during activity days (0.71 (95% confidence interval: 0.38–1.33)) compared with days of relative rest. Cognitive exertion including physical exercise therefore had no adverse effect on seizure control.

Patients with chronic epilepsy (without visual sensitivity) were studied to determine if exposure to video-game material is a risk factor for seizures. The results of this study showed that seizure occurrence was similar during periods of video-game play and during alternative leisure activities, including physical exercise.

Physical activity, alone or combined with other leisure activities, therefore does not appear to increase the risk of seizure occurrence. The only exception may be in patients with an underlying structural brain lesion, where there may be an increased risk of seizures during physical exercise.

PRACTICAL CLINICAL POINT 17

Special considerations for sports participation in athletes with epilepsy

Contact sports

▓ It has been suggested that contact sports, in which there is an increased risk of head injury, may be contraindicated in patients with epilepsy.

▓ There is no evidence to suggest that there is a greater risk for immediate or early seizures after a head injury in epileptic patients.

▓ Epileptic patients can safely engage in contact sports, provided normal precautions are taken in contact sports to protect against head injury, such as wearing protective headgear.

Swimming and water sports

▓ Recreational swimming by epileptic patients compared with the general population carries a four-fold increase in the risk of drowning.

▓ This risk is higher in children, and most drowning occurred when there was no supervision.

▓ Swimming for epileptic patients is not contraindicated, provided there is adequate (qualified lifeguard) supervision during swimming.

▓ Scuba diving is not permitted in athletes with epilepsy.

▓ Competitive underwater swimming and diving should be avoided.

High-risk sports

▓ There are sports where there may be a substantially increased risk of injury or even fatalities if a seizure occurs during the activity.

▓ These would include sports such as competitive motor sports, rock climbing, parachuting, and hang gliding.

▓ Legal and ethical issues require careful consideration when participation in these sports is discussed with an athlete.

ENDOCRINE CONDITIONS IN ATHLETES

Diabetes mellitus

Diabetes mellitus is not one disease but a group of metabolic diseases characterized by hyperglycemia resulting from defects in insulin secretion, insulin action, or both. Although the American Diabetes Association classifies diabetes into four clinical categories, most cases of diabetes mellitus fall into two broad categories, namely (1) those where there is an absolute deficiency of insulin secretion (Type I – insulin-dependent diabetes mellitus, or IDDM), and (2) those where there is either resistance to insulin action (insulin resistance) or inadequate insulin secretion or both (Type II – non-insulin-dependent diabetes mellitus, or NIDDM). Type II NIDDM accounts for the majority (> 90%) of patients with diabetes mellitus.

The focus of this section will be the role that physical activity plays in the prevention and management of both Type I and Type II diabetes mellitus.

Physical activity and the prevention of diabetes mellitus

In Type I diabetes mellitus, the primary disorder is lack of insulin following destruction of the pancreatic ß islet cells. This destruction is thought to occur as a result of an autoimmune process, but can also be secondary to pancreatic disease. Lack of physical activity is therefore not related to the cause of this disease.

It has been well established that regular participation in physical exercise reduces the risk of developing Type II diabetes mellitus and is important in the management of this disease. Although the actual mechanisms have not been well identified, it appears that physical activity acts both directly by improving insulin sensitivity, and indirectly by inducing favorable changes in body mass and body composition. A number of important specific adaptations to exercise training have been shown to be of benefit in the prevention of Type II diabetes mellitus. These include:

- increased muscle mass and decreased body fat (central area);
- increased muscle glucose uptake during exercise;
- increased skeletal-muscle blood flow;
- conversion of fast-twitch glycolytic II-b muscle fibers to fast-twitch oxidative II-a fibers (which are more insulin-sensitive and have greater capillary density);
- increased insulin-regulatable glucose transporters (GLUT4);
- improved control over hepatic glucose production.

The exact "dose" of physical exercise required for the prevention of Type II diabetes mellitus has not been well established. In one study, it has been shown that, for every additional weekly energy expenditure of 500 kcal, the risk of Type II diabetes is reduced by 6%. Data also indicate that the intensity of exercise is important, with greater reductions in risk if exercise training is conducted at a higher intensity. It has also been shown that the effects of exercise training are short lived, and this implies that a long-term commitment to perform regular exercise training is necessary to reduce the risk of this disease.

Finally, it is important to emphasize that there are other general health benefits of regular exercise training, which can also reduce the risk of complications from Type II diabetes mellitus, in particular, the additional benefits for the cardiovascular system.

Physical activity and the management of diabetes mellitus

Exercise training is an important component of the management of Type I diabetes mellitus. During an acute exercise bout, muscle contraction results in increased glucose uptake and increased insulin sensitivity, which can continue for 4–6 hours after exercise. This insulin-like effect of exercise has been shown to reduce the insulin requirements in these patients, but has not convincingly resulted in improved glucose control. Other beneficial effects of regular exercise training in patients with Type I diabetes mellitus are:

- increased functional capacity;
- improved blood lipid profile;
- reduced risk of cardiovascular complications;
- increased skeletal-muscle capillary density;
- increased general well-being.

Exercise prescription for athletic patients with diabetes mellitus (Types I and II)

In general, the exercise prescription is similar for patients with Type I and Type II diabetes mellitus. Prior to starting regular exercise, all patients should undergo

---

PRACTICAL CLINICAL POINT 19

General guidelines for exercise prescription in patients with diabetes mellitus

- Patients should ideally start the training program in a supervised setting where medical staff are in attendance.
- Exercise training should be conducted three times or more per week.
- Exercise sessions should be at least 30–60 minutes and be preceded by an adequate warm-up and followed by a cool-down.
- Activities can include brisk walking or jogging (unless complicated by injuries to feet), cycling, swimming, rowing, or aerobics.
- Exercise training at higher intensities is encouraged.

---

martin p. schwellnus and wayne derman

a comprehensive medical assessment (history and physical examination). This examination should place emphasis on establishing that there is good blood glucose control, and identifying any complications of the disease (myocardial ischemia, peripheral vascular disease, retinopathy, microalbuminuria, peripheral and/or autonomic neuropathy). All patients should also undergo an exercise stress ECG, consult with a nutritionist, and be informed of the potential risks of exercise training, such as hypoglycemia, hyperglycemia, orthopedic injuries related to peripheral neuropathy, increases in blood pressure during exercise, and the risk of cardiac complications.

MUSCULAR CONDITIONS IN ATHLETES

Exercise-associated muscle cramps

About 30–50% of all endurance athletes will experience cramping at some stage in their running careers. The causes, diagnosis, and treatment of cramping are still not well understood. Muscle cramps can be a manifestation of some underlying medical disease, but the majority of these medical diseases are rare, and most athletes with cramping suffer from exercise-associated muscle cramping (EAMC).

167

EAMC is defined as a "painful spasmodic involuntary contraction of skeletal muscle that occurs during or immediately after muscular exercise."

Early observations have led to the belief that cramps in athletes are caused by shortages of "electrolytes" (sodium, chloride, magnesium), "dehydration," or heat. However, there is a lack of scientific support for these theories, and it appears that EAMC is caused by a disturbance in the normal control of the nerves that cause muscle contraction. The development of abnormal neuromuscular control appears to be associated with the etiology of EAMC, possibly as a result of muscle fatigue resulting from increased exercise intensity and possible muscle damage.

Important observations from prospective cohort studies are that EAMC is associated with a past history of EAMC, increased exercise intensity, and possible pre-exercise muscle damage. Muscles most prone to cramping are those that span two joints (hamstring muscles, one of the front thigh muscles, some of the calf muscles, and foot muscles). These are also the muscles that are often contracted in a shortened position during exercise.

The clinical features of EAMC are skeletal-muscle fatigue followed by twitching of the muscle ("cramp prone state"). This progresses to spasmodic spontaneous contractions and eventual frank muscle cramping with pain. Relief from the "cramp prone state" occurs if the activity is stopped or if the muscle is stretched passively. Once activity is ceased, episodes of cramping are usually followed by periods of relief from cramping. Cramping can be precipitated by contraction of the muscle in a shortened position (inner range).

The clinical examination of an athlete with EAMC typically shows obvious distress, pain, a hard, contracted muscle, and visible fasciculation (twitching) over the muscle belly. In most instances, the athlete is conscious, responds normally to stimuli, and is able to conduct a conversation. Vital signs and a general examination usually reveal no abnormalities. In particular, most runners with acute cramping are not dehydrated or hyperthermic. An athlete who has generalized severe cramping or is confused, semi-comatose or comatose should be treated as an emergency and requires immediate hospitalization, where full investigation is required.

The immediate treatment for acute cramping is passive stretching of the affected muscle groups and then holding the muscle in stretched position until fasciculation (twitching) ceases. Supportive treatment involves keeping the athlete at a comfortable temperature and providing oral fluids if required. Athletes with recurrent acute EAMC should be investigated fully to exclude other medical conditions.

The key to the prevention of cramps is to protect the muscle from injury and from developing premature fatigue during exercise by being well trained, performing regular stretching, ensuring adequate nutritional intake (carbohydrate), and performing activity at a lower intensity and a shorter duration.

RENAL CONDITIONS IN ATHLETES

Hematuria in athletes

Athletes may complain of "dark urine" or even frank blood in the urine after activity. This is known as exercise associated hematuria (EAH). Both gross and microscopic hematuria has been reported in a variety of sports and in both trained and novice athletes. The incidence of EAH is variable and depends on the type, intensity, and duration of the sports, as well the sensitivity of the techniques that were used to diagnose hematuria. In general, hematuria is more common after high-intensity or prolonged exercise.

The prevalence of EAH in athletes participating in the Commonwealth Games was 11.4%. The incidence of hematuria after a standard marathon was reported as 18%, and after a 96-km road race was 63%. The precise etiology of EAH is not known. It is likely that EAH can be caused by a number of different pathologies at different sites in the renal tract (Table 8.3).

The earliest reports implicated the kidney as the source of hematuria. The decrease in renal blood flow, in particular in the vessels that supply the renal papillae, has been implicated in EAH.

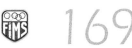

Table 8.3 Possible sites and causes of exercise-associated hematuria

Site of pathology	Cause
Kidney	Ischemia
	Acute renal failure
	Increased vascular fragility
	Trauma
	Nephroptosis
	Calculi
Ureter	Calculi
Bladder	Contusion
	Calculi
	Infection
Urethra	Contusion
	Calculi
	Infection
	Trauma
	Cold

Mechanical trauma to the kidney has also been implicated in EAH. In one case report, jogging was described as a cause of nephroptosis in a patient with weak ligamentous attachments of the kidney. It was suggested that jogging causes excessive displacement of the kidney, with resultant trauma. Furthermore, in contact sports, direct trauma to the kidney has been implicated as the cause of so-called "athletic pseudonephritis," which is a triad of hematuria, proteinuria, and casts in the urine post exercise. However, this is unlikely as the only cause of this clinical picture, as it also occurs in non-contact sports such as swimming and rowing.

Currently, the consensus of opinion is that the lower urinary tract is the most likely site of pathology in benign EAH. Runners with hematuria after a 10-km race were examined by cystoscopy and found to have contusions of the bladder mucosa. Contracoup lesions were demonstrated in the lower posterior bladder and the trigone. It was postulated that the cause of hematuria in these athletes was repetitive trauma of the anterior bladder mucosa against the fixed posterior wall.

EAH is benign in most cases and resolves after 24–48 hours. Initial investigation of the athlete who presents with EAH should include a comprehensive history to identify (1) the type, duration, and frequency of exercise; (2) fluid intake during exercise; (3) history of medication use; (4) family history of renal disease; and (5) systemic medical disease.

170

The athlete should undergo a systematic physical examination, including a urinalysis. If there are no identifiable causes for the EAH, the athlete should be re-assessed in 48 hours. If the hematuria has cleared and there are no other abnormalities on examination, the athlete can be followed up once more in 6 months' time. If the repeat urinalysis is abnormal, further investigations are required. These would include an intravenous pyelogram (IVP) and a cystoscopy. Further renal function tests are also indicated.

Proteinuria in athletes

In man, there is a normal daily excretion of protein in the urine of about 40–80 mg (usually less than 150 mg). The incidence is of exercise-associated proteinuria (EAP) is variable and depends on the sensitivity of the testing, and the type, intensity, and duration of the exercise. The incidence of EAP varies 11–100% after a bout of strenuous exercise.

The severity of EAP can be expressed as the protein excretion rate post exercise. Post-exercise excretion rates vary considerably, and values ranging from 86 μg/min (123 mg/day) to 5,100 μg/min (7.34 g/day) have been documented. The maximal protein excretion rate occurs in the first 20–30 minutes after stopping exercise. The protein excretion rate declines after exercise and returns to normal after approximately 4 hours.

At similar intensities of exercise, running appears to result in higher urinary protein excretion rates than swimming or cycling. In general, higher-intensity exercise increases the protein excretion rate. There is some evidence from early studies that lack of conditioning may be associated with EAP. However, recent studies have shown that, if exercise is performed at the same absolute intensity, the rate of protein excretion is not affected. In one study, protein excretion during exercise was documented in 73 pairs of mono- and dizygotic twins. The results indicate that there may be a genetic predisposition to the development of EAP.

The mechanisms that may be responsible for EAP include metabolic acidosis, renal hypoxia, renal vasoconstriction, increased rennin activity, and a loss of negative charge on the glomerular membrane.

An athlete will not usually present with any symptoms of proteinuria. Dipsticks may detect proteinuria incidentally during a pre-season medical assessment. Alternatively, dipsticks may detect proteinuria within 24–48 hours after strenuous exercise. In most cases, proteinuria in otherwise healthy athletes is benign and has no long-term effects. However, it does require a sound clinical approach to rule out serious renal disease.

A detailed medical history and a physical examination to exclude clinical evidence of renal or systemic disease should be performed. The history should include the intensity, duration, and type of exercise, the time span between the last exercise bout and the examination, fluid intake, environmental conditions, and previous history of proteinuria.

On examination, it is important to exclude associated renal or systemic disease, such as hypertension, edema, or anemia. If there is clinical evidence of renal or systemic disease, further blood tests, renal function tests, renal imaging, and eventually a renal biopsy may be required to establish the diagnosis. A nephrologist is the best person to perform these.

If there is no clinical evidence of renal or systemic disease, qualitative tests for proteinuria should be repeated two or three times. If no proteinuria is detected in well-concentrated urine specimens, the proteinuria can be ascribed to transient or functional proteinuria. The athlete can be reassured, and no further tests are required.

If proteinuria is detected each time during repeat tests, further investigation is required. This would include serum urea, electrolytes and creatinine, creatinine clearance, a postural proteinuria test, a 24-hour urine protein excretion test, and a renal ultrasound.

If the renal function tests and the renal ultrasound are normal but the proteinuria is not postural, the 24-hour urine protein test should be repeated two or three times to exclude intermittent proteinuria. If the proteinuria is intermittent, young patients (< 30 years) should be followed up annually, and older patients should be followed up every 6 months. Persistent proteinuria requires specialist investigation to exclude renal or systemic disease.

Acute renal failure in athletes

Acute renal failure is a most serious renal complication that may occur after exercise. The incidence of acute renal failure after physical exercise is not known. It is likely to be very variable, specifically with regard to (1) different types of exercise; (2) intensities and duration of exercise; (3) environmental conditions; (4) state of hydration of the participants; and (5) the use of medication during exercise.

Acute renal failure in the setting of exercise is precipitated by a number of possible factors, including dehydration, hyperpyrexia, myoglobinuria, hemoglobinuria, and the use of nephrotoxic medications during exercise. These factors usually cause acute renal failure during exercise in combination.

In severe dehydration, the renal blood flow is reduced, resulting in renal ischemia, which can cause acute tubular necrosis. Strenuous exercise that is performed in hot, humid environmental conditions can cause hyperpyrexia, which can damage a variety of organ systems. In particular, it can cause skeletal-muscle damage, directly or indirectly, by decreasing blood flow to muscles. Skeletal-muscle damage (rhabdomyolysis) is associated with the release of nephrotoxic substances, in particular myoglobin.

Hyperpyrexia can also be associated with intravascular hemolysis and resultant hemoglobinemia. The effects of these two pigments (myoglobin and hemoglobin) on the kidney require further discussion. Rhabdomyolysis is associated with the release of myoglobin, which is a globin chain containing a haem pigment. In acidic media such as during metabolic acidosis, and during bicarbonate absorption in the proximal tubule, globin dissociates from this ferrihemate compound. This ferrihemate compound is directly nephrotoxic as it interferes with renal tubular transport mechanisms.

PRACTICAL CLINICAL POINT 23

Guidelines for athletes to decrease the risk of developing acute renal failure after exercise

- Drink enough fluid during exercise, particularly in hot, humid environmental conditions.
- Acclimatize to hot, humid environmental conditions if possible.
- Do not use any form of medication during exercise unless advised by your doctor.
- Do not use any pain killers or anti-inflammatory drugs for at least 48 hours before prolonged strenuous exercise.
- Do not ignore blood in the urine after exercise.
- Make sure that you drink enough fluid in the first few hours after exercise.
- Seek medical advice urgently if you have not passed any urine 12 hours after exercise.

Other factors that may cause renal failure during rhabdomyolysis are (1) fibrin deposition in the glomeruli, (2) intravascular volume depletion secondary to muscle damage, and (3) release of purines resulting in a surge of uric acid production.

Clinical experience suggests that rhabdomyolysis leads to myoglobinuric renal failure only when other factors, such as intravascular volume depletion, hemoconcentration, renal vasoconstriction, or exposure to other nephrotoxins, are present.

In general, hemoglobin has less dramatic effects on the kidney, and clinical experience indicates that hemoglobinuria compromises renal function only in the presence of other factors, such as volume depletion, acidosis, or hypotension.

The use of non-steroidal anti-inflammatory drugs (NSAIDs) by athletes, particularly during ultra-distance events, should be strongly discouraged, because they may lead to acute renal failure. The mechanisms by which NSAIDs interfere with normal renal function involve inhibiting the synthesis of prostaglandins, which are important renal vasodilators. In the presence of high renin levels (such as during exercise), they can cause interstitial nephritis.

If the athlete has not passed urine in the first 12 hours post exercise, it is important to encourage increased fluid intake, particularly if there is evidence of intravascular volume depletion. Intravenous fluids may be indicated if this depletion is severe.

If the athlete has not passed urine 12 hours or longer after the exercise, further investigation is required. This may include:

- hospitalization for investigation and observation;
- urine examination (microscopy and electrolytes);
- blood tests, including serum urea and electrolytes;
- renal function tests (creatinine clearance);
- renal ultrasound.

GYNECOLOGICAL CONDITIONS IN FEMALE ATHLETES

Exercise-related menstrual abnormalities and the female athletic triad

Competitive sports participation in female athletes has increased in the last decades. There is thus an increasing need to understand the specific medical conditions related to sports participation in female athletes. One of these areas is related to exercise-related menstrual abnormalities, as well as the female athletic triad in female athletes.

The normal female menstrual cycle varies greatly in length from 22 to 36 days in women between the ages of 20 and 40 years. Typically, the cycle is divided into

174

the menstrual phase (coinciding with menstrual bleeding), followed by the follicular phase (dominated by estrogens), and the last phase, which is dominated by progesterone and is known as the luteal phase. The regulation of these phases is complex and involves the hypothalamus, pituitary gland, and ovaries. Positive and negative feedback from hormones regulate this cycle. Pulsatile release of gonadotropin-releasing hormone (GnRH) from the hypothalamus controls the release of follicle-stimulating hormone (FSH) and luteinizing hormone (LH) from the anterior pituitary gland. FSH stimulates growth and development of the primary follicles in the ovary leading to ovulation, and LH is responsible for estrogen production and secretion from the corpus luteum, which in turn releases progesterone for the maintenance of the endometrium. This is a highly complex and intricate control system, and intense or prolonged exercise training has been associated with disturbances of the normal menstrual cycle.

The following menstrual abnormalities have been observed in female athletes:

- athletic amenorrhea (defined as 0–3 periods per year);
- oligomenorrhea (defined as 4–9 periods per year);
- anovulation and shortened luteal phases (duration of less than 14 days);
- delayed menarche (no occurrence of menses before 16 years age);
- dysmenorrhea (pelvic pain or cramps at any time during the menstrual cycle).

There are no precise data on the prevalence of menstrual abnormalities in female athletes. This is owing to the wide variation of menstrual abnormalities in the general population and the wide variation of the physical demands of different sports. Also, very few well-conducted studies have been carried out to document the epidemiology of these conditions. However, it has been shown that the prevalence of menstrual abnormalities is higher in athletes (ranging 1–66%) than in non-athletes (ranging 2–5%). It is also evident that menstrual abnormalities are more common in sports in which there is a high physical demand (high intensity and increased duration of training), as well as sports where body-weight control and aesthetics are important (ballet, gymnastics).

Amenorrhea, oligomenorrhea, anovulation, short luteal phase, and delayed menarche

Amenorrhea, oligomenorrhea, anovulation, short luteal phase, and delayed menarche are common. The precise causes for these abnormalities are not clear. It appears that these conditions represent a continuum rather than separate entities. There appears to be consensus that the main abnormality in these conditions is that exercise alters, in some as yet unknown way, the pulsatile release of GnRH, which then has a concomitant effect on LH release and consequently affects estrogen and progesterone concentrations. The mechanisms possibly responsible for the altered pulsatile release of GnRH are numerous and relate to increased physical stress during exercise, nutritional deprivation, physical illness, and mental stress.

Guidelines for the clinical assessment of the female athlete with exercise-related menstrual abnormalities

- Obtain a careful history and examination before the condition is ascribed to exercise training.
- Rule out other systemic conditions, including pregnancy, thyroid disease, reproductive system abnormalities, diabetes mellitus, and other endocrine diseases.
- Carefully evaluate the athlete's exercise program, psychological status, and dietary and eating habits.
- If the clinical evaluation is normal, and the only suspected cause is an increased training load, advise the athlete to reduce training intensity and duration for 2–3 months.
- If menses resume following a reduction in training, generally no further evaluation is required.
- A full endocrine and gynecological evaluation is required if menses do not resume on reducing exercise training load and intensity.

Effects of menstrual abnormalities on exercise performance

Fluctuations in female athletic performance have been attributed to alterations in the menstrual cycle. However, recent reviews of the literature show that there is no significant effect of the phases of the menstrual cycle on physiological determinants of endurance performance.

Effects of menstrual abnormalities on fertility

Female fertility can be affected by many factors that affect normal reproductive function. Broadly, these factors fall into four categories: (1) nutritional deprivation, (2) physical illness, (3) psychological stress, and (4) rapidly increasing or excessive

Advice for the female athlete with possible infertility

- Decrease the exercise intensity by 10–20%.
- Gain 1–2 kg body weight.
- Monitor basal body temperature for 3 months.
- Seek psychological counseling to deal with any excessive emotional stress.

exercise. Exercise-related menstrual abnormalities that can negatively affect fertility are amenorrhea, anovulatory cycles, and shortening of the luteal phase. It is, however, important to emphasize that other factors, such as emotional stress, nutrition, and physical illness, must be excluded. These factors are often present in high-level athletes.

Further investigations and the use of medication may be required if ovulation has not returned to normal within 3–4 months.

Dysmenorrhea

Although there is anecdotal evidence that dysmenorrhea is less common in highly trained female athletes, this has not been confirmed in well-conducted scientific studies. Possible mechanisms for the decrease in dysmenorrhea have been linked to increased opioids circulating during exercise, as well as decreased levels of progesterone after ovulation.

Osteopenia and osteoporosis

High training loads and restricted energy intake are often seen in female athletes in an attempt to retain low body mass. This, together with the development of exercise-related menstrual abnormalities, in particular amenorrhea, has led to the description of a syndrome known as the "female athletic triad." The female athletic triad is composed of the following three conditions: amenorrhea, disordered eating, and osteoporosis. The female athletic triad has significant negative health consequences for the female athlete and requires investigation and treatment.

A young athlete who presents to the physician with delayed menarche requires a full, normal gynecological and endocrine evaluation to determine the cause, before it is ascribed to increased exercise training.

DERMATOLOGICAL CONDITIONS IN ATHLETES

Exercise-associated skin allergies

In certain susceptible individuals, physical exercise can act as the stimulus for an allergic reaction, which can manifest as a skin-related allergy. These reactions are known as exercise-associated skin allergies. An allergic reaction is an immunological response to the exposure to a physical or chemical stimulus. Exposure to the stimulus results in the release of vasoactive substances from activated cells (mast cells, basophils, mononuclear cells) or from enzymatic pathways (complement system). Vasoactive substances include histamine, bradykinin, prostaglandins, leukotrienes, and complement factors C3a, C4a, and C5a. These substances are responsible for vasodilation and bronchospasm, which present clinically as skin rashes and wheezing, respectively.

Urticaria

Urticaria is an allergic reaction characterized by an itchy, red, patchy skin rash (usually 10–15 mm in diameter) that develops 2–30 minutes after the start of exercise. The rash usually starts in the upper thorax and neck and may spread to other areas of the body. Various types of urticaria have been described:

- Cholinergic urticaria, which is much smaller (1–3 mm in diameter) than so-called classical urticaria, occurs in response to other physical stimuli such as anxiety, heat, and sweating, and it is treated with H1-histamine antagonists, in particular hydroxyzine or cyproheptadine. An exercise program with gradually increased load can induce tolerance to the condition.
- Cold urticaria occurs in response to exposure to cold and can affect athletes participating outdoors on cold winter days, or swimmers in cold water. Massive mediator release can result in hypotension and collapse, but these responses are rare. Cold urticaria is best treated with avoidance of exposure to cold, and its symptoms can be treated with antihistamines.
- Localized heat urticaria is rare; it occurs in response to local heat application and is difficult to treat. Antihistamines and cortisone have not been very effective in treating localized heat urticaria.
- Solar urticaria and aquagenic urticaria are rare conditions caused by exposure to light and water, respectively. In both cases, the treatment involves blocking the light or water by applying sunblocks and inert skin oils, respectively. Pharmacological treatment with antihistamines is also indicated.

Dermatographism

Dermatographism is an allergic reaction characterized by linear wheals that occur 1–3 minutes after the skin is stroked. Dermatographism has been described in football players wearing protective gear. Treatment with antihistamines is successful in most cases.

Angioedema

Angioedema (delayed pressure urticaria) is characterized by swelling or urticaria that occurs 4–6 hours after the application of pressure to the skin (footwear, tight clothing). It has been postulated that diet may have a role in causing angioedema. Treatments include avoiding skin pressure and using drugs such as H1-antagonists, as well as NSAIDs to control symptoms.

Exercise-induced anaphylaxis

Exercise-induced anaphylaxis (EIA) is not a localized allergic reaction affecting the skin. It is a rare, systemic, and serious allergic response to physical exercise. It is characterized by giant-sized urticaria (10–15 mm in diameter), URT obstruction, hypotension, angioedema, GIT colic, and headaches that last for up to 72 hours. Attacks of EIA are episodic, and the symptoms vary. EIA appears to be associated

178

with a family history of atopy and can be aggravated by certain foods and by menstruation.

Sun damage to the skin

Athletes participating in outdoor sports activity are exposed to the acute and chronic effects of sun exposure. Acute injury to the skin as a result of sun exposure is known as sunburn, whereas the long-term health risks of chronic exposure to the sun's radiation can result in premature aging of the skin and an increased incidence of skin cancer and melanoma.

The solar electromagnetic radiation spectrum includes wavelengths from 270 to 5,000 nm, but the main wavelengths causing skin effects are between 270 and 800 nm. Visible light (400–800 nm) is poorly absorbed by the ozone layer, and most of it reaches the earth's surface. Ultraviolet A (UVA) (320–400 nm) is poorly absorbed by the ozone layer and therefore also reaches the earth's surface. UVA is responsible for aging effects on the skin. Ultraviolet B (UVB (290–320 nm) is responsible for sunburn, carcinogenic effects on the skin, and vitamin D metabolism. It is moderately well absorbed by the ozone layer, but, depending on the ozone layer, significant amounts can reach the earth's surface and affect the skin. Ultraviolet C (UVC) (200–290 nm) is well absorbed by the ozone layer, and little reaches the earth's surface. This wavelength can cause sunburn, but also leads to protective thickening of the epidermis with chronic exposure. Infrared radiation (> 800 nm) is felt as heat on the skin. The water droplets in clouds absorb infrared radiation, but not UVA and UVB. Furthermore, wind, and the presence of light surfaces such as sand, snow, and water may aggravate sun damage.

Acute sun injury to the skin

Acute injury to the skin as a result of sun exposure is known as sunburn and is very common. Sun damage is caused mainly by the shorter-wavelength ultraviolet radiation (UVA and mainly UVB). There is a higher risk for sunburn when athletes are exposed to the sun when less filtering of UV radiation occurs, such as during

---

PRACTICAL CLINICAL POINT 26

Treatment of acute sunburn

- Cool tap-water compresses.
- Application of a topical corticosteroid cream (low-to-medium potency) (first 48 hours).
- Oral anti-histamines.
- Oral NSAIDs.

---

the middle of the day (10 a.m. to 2 p.m.), at high altitude, when there is reflection (snow, sand), increased humidity (reduced UV filtration), and at equatorial latitudes.

Shorter-wavelength radiation (UVB) is absorbed by the upper layers of the epidermis and can cause erythema, swelling, pain, blistering, and peeling owing to direct damage of the kartinocytes with the release of inflammatory mediators. UVA penetrates skin more, affecting the deeper layers (melanocytes, elastin, collagen).

Prevention of sunburn is the most important component of protection of the skin in athletes.

PRACTICAL CLINICAL POINT 27

Prevention of acute sun injury in athletes

- Avoid exposure to the effects of sunlight by exercising early in the morning or in the late afternoon.
- Cover exposed areas of skin with suitable clothing (fast-drying, tightly woven).
- Wear a wide-brimmed hat to cover ears, nose, and neck.
- Apply a sun-protection cream prophylactically at least 1 hour before sports to all exposed areas of the skin, choosing the correct sun protection factor (SPF) based on the skin type (lighter versus darker skins) (see Table 8.4).
- Re-apply sunscreen every 2 hours, particularly during activities such as swimming.
- Encourage the use of sunglasses with UVA and UVB filtering characteristics to avoid sun damage to the eyes.
- Use of oral photoprotective agents can be considered (Table 8.5).

Exposure to UV light results in an immediate and delayed protective response of the skin (commonly known as tanning). Immediate pigment darkening through oxidation of pre-existing melanin and redistribution of pre-existing melanosomes within melanocytes occurs immediately in response to sun exposure and fades a few minutes after exposure. The delayed-onset tanning effect starts 24–48 hours after exposure to UVA and UVB and consists of melanocyte division, increased synthesis of melanin, and redistribution of melanosomes to epidermal keratinocytes.

Table 8.4 Skin types and the use of sun-protection cream

Skin type	Sensitivity to UV radiation	History of exposure to sun	Suggested SPF*
I	Very sensitive	Always burns, never tans	10+
II	Very sensitive	Always burns, little tan	10+
III	Sensitive	Burns moderately, tans slowly	8–10
IV	Moderately sensitive	Burns little, tans well	6–8
V	Minimally sensitive	Rarely burns, tans dark brown	4
VI	Insensitive	Deeply pigmented, never burns	None

Note:

* The SPF is an area-specific factor and is a "time" measurement. Each geographical area has got a "safe sun time," which refers to the time that can be spent in the sun without damaging the skin. For example, in an area where the safe sun time is 10 minutes, this time gets multiplied with the SPF. An SPF of 10 gives 10 x protection, meaning 10 x 10 minutes = 100 minutes. Similarly an SPF of 30 gives protection for 300 minutes (5 hours), after which the sunscreen needs to be reapplied. Protection from exposure that lasts a full day would require the use of an SPF 60 = 10 hours.

Table 8.5 Oral photoprotective agents

Agent	Indication	Notes
Beta-carotene	Porphyria and other photosensitivity states, such as discoid lupus, polymorphous light eruption, and actinic reticuloid	– Protects against UVA – Becomes effective in 6 weeks – May be combined with a topical sunscreen – No serious adverse effects have been reported – Recommended adult dose is 120–80 mg per day
Chioroquine	Lupus, porphyria cutanea tarda, and other photosensitivity states	– Potentially toxic drug – Should never be used without careful supervision (regular visual-field checks) – Daily dose should not exceed 4 mg/kg
Psoralens	Enhances natural protective mechanism (keratin thickness and melanization of melano-somes)	– Used in combination with graded exposure to ultraviolet light – Should not be used without very careful monitoring by an experienced dermatologist

Conditions that are associated with photosensitivity

- Porphyria of various types (in particular, erythropoeitic protoporphyria).
- Lupus erythematosus (including chronic discoid, subacute, and systemic forms).
- Albinism (associated with the absence of melanin).
- Rare genetic disorders (xeroderma pigmentosum, Rothmund–Thomson syndrome, Bloom's syndrome, and Cockayne's syndrome).
- Polymorphous light eruption, actinic reticuloid, and solar urticaria (light-sensitive dermatoses of unknown cause).
- Medications (suphonamides, tetracyclines, oral hypoglycaemic agents, thiazide diuretics, and some anti-inflammatory drugs, e.g. naproxen sodium).
- Photosensitizing agents in soaps and cosmetics may also cause problems.

Chronic exposure to sun can result in a number of more serious skin conditions, including:

- damage to collagen and elastin manifesting as wrinkling, irregular pigmentation, epidermal thinning, and telangiectasia;
- pre-malignant skin lesions such as actinic keratosis;
- malignant skin conditions (basal cell carcinoma, squamous cell carcinoma, and malignant melanoma).

OTHER MEDICAL CONDITIONS IN ATHLETES

Jet lag

In recent years, there has been a large increase in the number of international sports competitions. This increase has been made possible in part through the development of an efficient, worldwide air-travel network. Athletes are required to travel to international competitions all over the globe. This can mean spending long hours of traveling overnight in a north–south direction, or to other destinations that involve crossing a number of time zones in the east–west or west–east direction. For example, during the Summer and Winter Olympic Games, many international teams travel across many time zones. Athletes are, nevertheless, expected to perform at peak level upon arrival.

It is understood that traveling across time zones is associated with a syndrome characterized by general malaise, together with a host of other non-specific symptoms. This syndrome, known as the "jet lag" syndrome, may have a detrimental effect on sports performance. It is important for any health professional who deals with the traveling athlete to be aware of the potential negative effects of inter-continental travel on sports performance.

Jet lag is a transient clinical syndrome that occurs in response to a disruption of normal biological rhythms and classically results in non-specific symptoms. The syndrome develops in most individuals when they travel across three or more time zones. The syndrome is characterized by two phases: (1) the development of circadian dysrhythmia (desynchronization), and (2) adaptation to the new time zone (resynchronization). An understanding of the basic physiology of these two phases is essential to give appropriate guidelines for the prevention of jet lag.

It is now fairly well established that jet lag is caused by circadian dysrhythmia. Circadian dysrhythmia refers to the disruption (desynchronization) of the normal biological clock (circadian rhythms) by external cues (light and dark cycles).

Circadian rhythms are characterized by an inherent periodicity of 24–26 hours and exist in a number of physiological systems in the body. These rhythms function as internal time indicators for the body and are important in the normal regulation of physical and psychological parameters, such as body temperature, blood cortisol levels, and alertness (sleep and wake cycle). These normal rhythms are influenced by external cues in the environment, in particular light and dark cycles.

When an athlete crosses several time zones, the circadian rhythms that are affected by the external cues of the previous time zone have to be adjusted to the new time zone. This adjustment is known as resynchronization and is correlated with the resolution of the symptoms of jet lag. A number of factors can influence the period required for resynchronization.

It is well established that, the more time zones crossed, the longer it takes to resynchronize the circadian rhythms. A rule of thumb is that it takes approximately 1 day per time zone crossed to resynchronize. The direction of the flight also has an important bearing on the time needed to adjust. A north–south flight that does not cross time zones requires no adjustment of circadian rhythms. Evidence shows that the time to adjust is 30–50% less if the flight is in an east–west direction (phase delay), compared with a west–east direction (phase advance). This difference is because the natural rhythm of the body is approximately 25 hours, which makes it easier to adjust to conditions that lengthen the day (east–west flights). Individual differences exist in the time needed for adjustment. "Night persons," usually extroverts, have their peaks in circadian rhythms later in the day, and therefore adjust more easily to west–east flight (phase advance). Conversely, "day people," usually introverts, will adjust easier to east–west flights (phase delay).

Age is associated with a change in the normal sleep pattern, usually involving going to bed and rising earlier. This change would therefore favor adjustment to west–east travel. The time to adjustment is also greatly influenced by how quickly the person is exposed to new environmental cues, in particular sunlight. Early exposure to the new day and night cycle results in a more rapid resynchronization. Minor factors that can influence the resynchronization time include the type and content of meals, as well as drugs known as chronobiotic drugs.

The effects of chronobiotic drugs on resynchronization require further discussion. Although none of the drugs discussed has been studied in actual flight experiments in humans, there may well be a future role for chronobiotic drugs in the prevention of jet lag. There are two basic mechanisms by which drugs can affect the resynchronization process.

184

First, drugs can act as external cues or synchronizers of biological rhythms. Examples of drugs that fall into this first category are adrenocorticotropin hormone (ACTH), levadopa, and parachlorophenylalanine. The timing of administration in the normal cycle is crucial in determining the effects of these drugs. If administered early in the cycle, they cause an advance in the normal cycle and thereby assist athletes who are traveling in a west–east direction (phase advance). Conversely, if administered later in the normal cycle, the drugs delay the cycle and assist athletes traveling in an east–west direction (phase delay).

The second mechanism by which chronobiotic drugs act is to intensify the effects of normal external cues. Drugs such as lithium and clorgyline facilitate resynchronization after east–west flights. Tricylic antidepressants, melatonin, and estradiol are drugs that are postulated to facilitate resynchronization after west–east flights.

The chronobiotic drug melatonin is commonly used by athletes to adapt to time-zone changes. Melatonin is secreted from the pineal gland between 9 p.m. and 7 a.m. and is regarded as a "dark pulse." Melatonin capsules taken in the evening for a few days before departing (at local time) and after arrival (at local time) may well facilitate resynchronization. When administrated under this schedule, melatonin has been shown to reduce the symptoms of jet lag in both men and women, and in both west–east and east–west travel directions. However, the exact mechanism by which melatonin facilitates resynchronization has not been established. A recent publication indicates that melatonin ingestion could alter the body clock. The use of melatonin in athletes, and in particular the effect of melatonin on exercise performance, needs further investigations.

Circadian rhythms of different bodily systems resynchronize at different rates. For example, body temperature, which varies from 36°C early in the morning to 38.5°C in the late afternoon, resynchronizes at a relatively rapid rate (40–50 minutes per day). The body temperature circadian rhythm is of particular importance in athletes, because it has been shown to be the most important rhythm determining athletic performance. Hormonal and renal function rhythms, on the other hand, can take longer to adjust to new time zones.

There is substantial anecdotal, but less scientific, evidence for the adverse effects of jet lag on sports performance. In one of the best-conducted scientific studies, it has been shown that west–east travel across six time zones results in a decrease in athletic performance of approximately 10%. In that study, decreases in athletic performance for specific events were 8–12% for a 270-m sprint, 8–9% for a 2.8-km run, 6–11% for isokinetic muscle strength, and 13% for isokinetic muscle endurance.

Practical guidelines to minimize the effects of jet lag in athletes or other patients who travel across time zones can be categorized according to the following two circumstances: (1) travel that involves small (less than three time zones) but consecutive time shifts; and (2) travel that involves one large (more than three time zones) time shift.

185

Guidelines to minimize the effects of jet lag in athletes

Small but consecutive time-zone shifts

- Schedule competitions in the morning after westward flights and in the evening after eastward flights.
- Travel in one direction when competing at different venues on an extended trip.
- Indulge in social and exercise activity (training sessions) immediately after arriving at the destination.
- Preset the sleep/wake cycles to that of the destination a few days before departing.
- Eat meals regularly after arriving at the destination.
- Avoid alcohol during the flight.

Single, large time-zone shift

- Arrive at the destination at least 1 day early for each time zone crossed (allow 14 days for resynchronization if the time-zone difference is greater than 6 hours).
- For flights crossing more than 10 time zones, it is better to take a west–east flight.
- Attempt to partially synchronize sleep/wake cycles and meals a few days before departing (for east–west flights, this means going to bed later).
- Indulge in social and exercise activity (training sessions) immediately after arriving at the destination.
- Maintain regular sleeping and eating times upon arrival.
- Alternate light/heavy meals for 3 days before the flight.
- Avoid alcohol during the flight.
- Chronobiotic drugs such as melatonin may be used.

Exercise and sexuality

The team physician is often the first or only contact point between health professionals and athletes. It is therefore quite common that the athlete will seek information from the team physician about aspects related to human sexuality and sport.

It must first be emphasized that human sexuality is complex and involves relationships between individuals, rather than just coitus (which, for purposes of this section, is defined as the physical act of "having sex"). The complex, intimate relationship between a man and a woman is referred to as sexual intercourse in

martin p. schwellnus and wayne derman

this section. Second, human sexuality is influenced by many factors, which can be physical, emotional, social, and psychological. The content of this section will deal with three questions that are commonly asked by athletes on the relationship between physical exercise and human sexual behavior.

It is important to point out that most of the research to date has focused only on the physiological aspects of the reproductive function, and to a lesser extent on aspects related to coitus. Very few data are available on the relationship between physical exercise and the emotional, social, and psychological aspects of sexual intercourse.

Effect of exercise on male fertility

Controversies exist on whether endurance training alters the reproductive physiology of men. The two aspects that have to be considered are the effects of endurance training on the hormonal profile (hypothalamic–pituitary–gonadal axis), and the effects of training on the semen profile. Some reports have indicated that training of high intensity or in large volumes can, in some men, be associated with a decrease in the concentration of circulating testosterone. The mechanism may be peripheral (enhanced hepatic clearance or increased tissue utilization) or central (a disturbance of the hypothalamic–pituitary–gonadal axis). Evidence for the central mechanism shows that some endurance-trained men have a decreased LH pulsatility, or a change in the pituitary response to hypothalamic stimulation by exogenous hormones such as GnRH, thyrotropin-releasing hormone, or corticotrophin-releasing hormone. However, the findings for decreased levels of circulating testosterone concentration in male athletes are not consistent, and the clinical significance is not known. In one study, excessive training in men was associated with a reduction in bone mineral density. Although firm scientific evidence is lacking, it has been suggested that this reduction may be related to decreases in circulating testosterone.

Quantitative and qualitative analyses of the semen ejaculate in male athletes has been conducted in four studies to date. In one of the best studies on the semen of high-mileage runners (> 100 km per week), compared with matched sedentary controls, the runner group showed a reduced total sperm count (but within normal limits), reduced sperm motility, a slight reduction in spermatozoa with normal morphology, a higher proportion of immature spermatozoa, and an increased leukocyte count in the semen.

The only study to date that has related hormonal changes and alterations in the semen ejaculate to reduced fertility capacity in highly trained male athletes is a report on an artificial insemination program. It is observed that donors with a high level of physical fitness have lower pregnancy rates compared with those with a normal level of physical activity. Although the interaction between male infertility and physical training requires further research, it appears that training of high intensity or in excessive volumes may reduce male fertility. Practical advice to highly trained athletes who are prospective fathers would be to reduce their training if there is a suggestion of male infertility.

Effect of exercise on female fertility

Female fertility can be influenced by factors that affect normal reproductive function. These factors fall into four broad categories – nutritional deprivation, physical illness, psychological stress, and an excessive or rapid increase in the amount of exercise. The common exercise-related changes in women are lack of ovulation (an obvious effect on fertility), shortening of the luteal phase, and oligomenorrhea.

Provided athletes are mature and well nourished, exercise is not associated with the development of amenorrhea. The proposed mechanism for the changes in female athletes caused by excessive training is an increase in the hypothalamic neurotransmitter corticotrophin-releasing hormone. Corticotrophin-releasing hormone can be affected by many factors (i.e., the four categories of factors).

Increased corticotrophin-releasing hormone results in a downward regulation of the pulsatile GnRH message to the pituitary hormones, LH, and FSH. Excessive exercise may lead to anovulatory cycles and cause female infertility. However, it is important to emphasize that other factors, such as emotional stress, nutrition, and physical illness, which are often present in high-level athletes, must be excluded first. Practical advice for the female athlete with possible infertility caused by excessive exercise is to: (1) decrease exercise intensity by 10–20%; (2) gain 1–2 kg weight; (3) monitor their basal body temperature for 3 months; and (4) seek psychological counseling to deal with any excessive emotional stress. Further investigations and the use of medication may be required, if ovulation has not returned to normal within 3–4 months.

Regular exercise and sexuality

Regular physical exercise is an integral component of a healthy lifestyle. Regular exercise is often a catalyst to other positive lifestyle elements, such as cessation of smoking, healthy nutritional habits, weight loss, stress management, and positive mood changes, including an improved self-image. Although not well studied, there appears to be a positive correlation between physical fitness and some aspects of human sexual activity. In a cross-sectional study, the sexual behavior of sedentary middle-aged men was compared with that of physically active men (exercising at moderate intensity for 3–4 hours per week). In that study, the physically active men reported the following: more frequent coitus, more frequent orgasms, lower prevalence of sexual abnormalities, and a higher percentage of satisfying orgasms. The postulated mechanisms for improved sexual function in moderately active males are less fatigue during coitus, improved cardiovascular function, possible increase in circulating testosterone (moderate-intensity exercise), and enhanced self-esteem.

188

In women, regular exercise and a healthy lifestyle will probably have similar effects. It has been shown that regular exercise enhances the self-esteem of women, reduces symptoms of premenstrual tension, and decreases some of the peri-menopausal symptoms. All these factors may improve female sexuality.

Sexual activity and athletic performance

A question commonly asked by athletes is whether coitus in the period immediately before competition (< 24 hours) affects athletic performance. Coitus does not result in excessive energy expenditure. It has been estimated that the total energy expenditure during one act of coitus is equivalent to a 100-m sprint. This energy expenditure will not adversely affect performance. However, two possible effects of coitus on exercise performance must be considered: the emotional effects, particularly if performed with an unfamiliar partner, and the sleep disturbance that results may adversely affect performance. Indeed, more energy may be expended in looking for a partner than during coitus!

Exercise and social drug use

Sports events are often associated with the use of alcohol and caffeine (in coffee, tea, and some commercial drinks). These associations stem from advertisements and sponsorships of major sports events, spectators and supporters who use these substances when watching sports events at home or at the venue, and, to a lesser extent, the use of these substances by athletes themselves. An intriguing question is whether these common "social drugs" affect sports performance and the health of the athlete. An ethical question is whether these drugs should be associated at all with sport, which is an activity that portrays health and vitality.

Alcohol

Alcohol use is almost synonymous with celebrating a win or reflecting on a loss in most sports circles. The question is whether this is good practice, or detrimental to performance, or indeed makes no difference. Perhaps the first question to answer is whether athletes do consume alcohol on a regular basis.

In studies from the United States, the reported use of alcohol in athletes attending institutions of higher education is 88%. This is significantly higher that the reported use of other social drugs such as caffeine (68%) and illegal drugs such as marijuana (36%). However, in the serious athlete, the reported use of alcohol is much lower, and there is considerable variability in alcohol use among different sports, as shown in Table 8.6. It therefore appears that alcohol use in athletes is common in the lower-level athlete, and consumption decreases as the level of performance increases.

It can be postulated that athletes have learned that alcohol is detrimental to sports performance, and therefore elite athletes avoid its use during training and competition. There is considerable scientific evidence to support this postulate.

Table 8.6	Reported use of alcohol among athletes participating in different sports	
Sport	**Alcohol use (% athletes)**	
Racket sports	12	
Golf	9	
Soccer	7	
Rugby	5	
Triathlon	2	
Hockey	0	

In a comprehensive analysis of scientific data, the American College of Sports Medicine came to the following conclusions:

- acute ingestion of alcohol has a deleterious effect on many psychomotor skills;
- alcohol ingestion does not improve muscular work capacity, and may decrease performance levels;
- alcohol consumption can impair temperature regulation during prolonged exercise in a cold environment; and
- alcohol consumption does not improve physiologic measures of sports performance, such as VO_2 max, respiratory variables, and cardiac parameters.

More recent studies have also shown that alcohol ingestion on the day before a sports event can decrease sports performance, in particular endurance performance. It is also noteworthy that a large percentage of fatal accidents in recreational sports activity, especially in aquatic sports, are related to excessive consumption of alcohol.

Caffeine

Caffeine is reported as being the most widely used drug in the Western world and possibly the world over. This means that it is also the most widely used social drug among sports participants. It is well documented that caffeine ingestion within 48 hours before sports participation can improve a number of sport performances, which include:

- work performed during a 2-hour cycle ride;
- running or cycling to exhaustion in laboratory studies;
- cycling time to exhaustion in repeated short-duration, high-intensity rides; and
- significant increases in maximal power output during a 6-second cycling bout at high intensity.

martin p. schwellnus and wayne derman

However, a number of variables can influence the outcome of performance tests when athletes consume caffeine. These include caffeine dose (mg/kg body weight), nutritional status, previous caffeine use, and individual variation in metabolism of caffeine (including urinary excretion).

SUGGESTED READING

Abarbanel J., Benet A.E., Lask D., Kimche D. Sports hematuria. *J. Urol.* 1990;143(5):887–90.

Adams B.B. Dermatologic disorders of the athlete. *Sports Med.* 2002;32(5):309–21.

Adams B.B. Skin infections in athletes. *Dermatol. Nurs.* 2008;20(1):39–44.

Adams B.B. Skin infections in sport. *ISMJ* 2003;4(3): www.ismj.com

Alonso J.M., Tscholl P.M., et al. Occurrence of injuries and illnesses during the 2009 IAAF World Athletics Championships. *Br. J. Sports Med.* 2010;44(15):1100–5.

Anderson S.D., Brannan J.D. Methods for "indirect" challenge tests including exercise, eucapnic voluntary hyperpnea, and hypertonic aerosols. *Clin. Rev. Allergy Immunol.* 2003;24(1):27–54.

Anderson S.D., Kippelen P. Exercise-induced bronchoconstriction: pathogenesis. *Curr. Allergy Asthma Rep.* 2005;5(2):116–22.

Arce J.C., De Souza M.J. Exercise and male factor infertility. *Sports Med.* 1993;15(3):146–69.

Beck C.K. Infectious diseases in sports. *Med. Sci. Sports Exerc.* 2000;32(7 Suppl.):S431–S8.

Bergstein J.M. A practical approach to proteinuria. *Pediatr. Nephrol.* 1999;13(8):697–700.

Bi L., Triadafilopoulos G. Exercise and gastrointestinal function and disease: an evidence-based review of risks and benefits. *Clin. Gastroenterol. Hepatol.* 2003;1(5):345–55.

Billen A., Dupont L. Exercise induced bronchoconstriction and sports. *Postgrad. Med. J.* 2008;84(996):512–17.

Bonini M., Braido F., et al. AQUA: Allergy Questionnaire for Athletes. Development and validation. *Med. Sci. Sports Exerc.* 2009;41(5):1034–41.

Cannavo S., Curto L., Trimarchi F. Exercise-related female reproductive dysfunction. *J. Endocrino.Invest.* 2001;24(10):823–32.

Carlsen K.H., Anderson S.D., et al. Exercise-induced asthma, respiratory and allergic disorders in elite athletes: epidemiology, mechanisms and diagnosis: part I of the report from the Joint Task Force of the European Respiratory Society (ERS) and the European Academy of Allergy and Clinical Immunology (EAACI) in cooperation with GA2LEN. *Allergy* 2008;63(4):387–403.

Chen E.C., Brzyski R.G. Exercise and reproductive dysfunction. *Fertil. Steri.* 1999;71(1):1–6.

Chipkin S.R., Klugh S.A., Chasan-Taber L. Exercise and diabetes. *Cardiol. Clin.* 2001;19(3):489–505.

Church T. Exercise in obesity, metabolic syndrome, and diabetes. *Prog. Cardiovasc. Dis.* 2011;53(6):412–18.

Constantinou D. Exercise-induced bronchoconstriction – Current update and implications for treating athletes. *Curr. Allergy Clin. Immunol.* 2010;23(10 (2)):64–70.

Cumming D.C., Wheeler G.D., Harber V.J. Physical activity, nutrition, and reproduction. *Ann. N. Y. Acad. Sci.* 1994;709:55–76.

Cunniffe B., Griffiths H., et al. Illness monitoring in team sports using a Web-based training diary. *Clin. J. Sport Med.* 2009;19(6):476–81.

Davis J.L. Sun and active patients. Preventing acute and cumulative skin damage. *Phys. Sports Med.* 2000;28(7):79–85.

Derman W. Medical care of the South African Olympic team – the Sydney 2000 experience. *SAJSM* 2003;Dec.:22–5.

Derman W. Profile of medical and injury consultations of Team South Africa during the XXVIIIth Olympiad, Athens 2004. *SAJSM* 2008;20(3):72–6.

Diagnosis and classification of diabetes mellitus. *Diabetes Care* 2009;32(Suppl. 1):S62–7.

Douglas R.M., Hemila H., et al. Vitamin C for preventing and treating the common cold. *Cochrane Database Syst. Rev.* 2004(4):CD000980.

Draznin M.B., Patel D.R. Diabetes mellitus and sports. *Adolesc. Med.* 1998;9(3):457–65.

Drust B., Waterhouse J., Atkinson G., Edwards B., Reilly T. Circadian rhythms in sports performance – an update. *Chronobiol. Int.* 2005;22(1):21–44.

Dryden D.M., Spooner C.H., et al. Exercise-induced bronchoconstriction and asthma. *Evid. Rep. Technol. Assess.* (Full Rep) 2010(189):1–154, v–vi.

Dubow J.S., Kelly J.P. Epilepsy in sports and recreation. *Sports Med.* 2003;33(7):499–516.

Dvorak J., Junge A., et al. Injuries and illnesses of football players during the 2010 FIFA World Cup. *Br. J. Sports Med.* 2011;45(8):626–30.

Engebretsen L., Steffen K., et al. Sports injuries and illnesses during the Winter Olympic Games 2010. *Br. J. Sports Med.* 2010;44(11):772–80.

Fitch K.D., Sue-Chu M., et al. Asthma and the elite athlete: summary of the International Olympic Committee's consensus conference, Lausanne, Switzerland, January 22–4, 2008. *J. Allergy Clin.Immunol.* 2008;122(2):254–60, 60.

Fountain N.B., May A.C. Epilepsy and athletics. *Clin. Sports Med.* 2003;22(3):605–6xi.

Friman G., Wesslen L. Special feature for the Olympics: effects of exercise on the immune system: infections and exercise in high-performance athletes. *Immunol. Cell Biol.* 2000;78(5):510–22.

Gambrell R.C., Blount B.W. Exercised-induced hematuria. *Am. Fam. Physician* 1996;53(3):905–11.

Ganio M.S., Casa D.J., et al. Evidence-based approach to lingering hydration questions. *Clin. Sports Med.* 2007;26(1):1–16.

Goodman L.R., Warren M.P. The female athlete and menstrual function. *Curr. Opin. Obstet. Gynecol.* 2005;17(5):466–70.

Harber V.J. Menstrual dysfunction in athletes: an energetic challenge. *Exerc. Sport Sci. Rev.* 2000;28(1):19–23.

Harrington D.W. Viral hepatitis and exercise. *Med. Sci. Sports Exerc.* 2000;32(7 Suppl.):S422–30.

Hawarden D., Baker S., et al. Aero-allergy in South African olympic athletes. *S. Afri. Med. J.* 2002;92(5):355–6.

Hayes C., Herbert M., Marrero D., Martins C.L., Muchnick S. Diabetes and exercise. *Diabetes Educ.* 2008;34(1):37–40.

Hayes C., Kriska A. Role of physical activity in diabetes management and prevention. *J. Am. Diet Assoc.* 2008;108(4 Suppl. 1):S19–23.

Heimer K.A., Hart A.M., et al. Examining the evidence for the use of vitamin C in the prophylaxis and treatment of the common cold. *J. Am. Acad. Nurse Pract.* 2009; 21(5):295–300.

Helenius I., Lumme A., Haahtela T. Asthma, airway inflammation and treatment in elite athletes. *Sports Med.* 2005;35(7):565–74.

Howard G.M., Radloff M., Sevier T.L. Epilepsy and sports participation. *Curr. Sports Med. Rep.* 2004;3(1):15–19.

Hull J.H., Hull P.J., et al. Approach to the diagnosis and management of suspected exercise-induced bronchoconstriction by primary care physicians. *BMC Pulm. Med.* 2009; 9:29.

Jeans A.K. Tropical infections in athletes: Malaria, schistosomiasis and African tick bite fever. *ISMJ* 2003;4 (3): http://www.ismj.com

Jones G.R., Newhouse I. Sport-related hematuria: a review. *Clin. J. Sport Med.* 1997; 7(2):119–25.

Katelaris C.H. Allergy and athletes. *Curr. Allergy Asthma Rep.* 2001;1(5):397–8.

Komarow H.D., Postolache T.T. Seasonal allergy and seasonal decrements in athletic performance. *Clin. Sports Med.* 2005;24(2):e35–50, xiii.

Kordi R., Wallace W.A. Blood borne infections in sport: risks of transmission, methods of prevention, and recommendations for hepatitis B vaccination. *Br. J. Sports Med.* 2004;38(6):678–84.

Lack L.C., Wright H.R. Chronobiology of sleep in humans. *Cell Mo. Life Sci.* 2007; 64(10):1205–15.

Lichaba M. Upper respiratory tract symptoms and allergies in Ironman triathletes. MPhil Sports Medicine dissertation, University of Cape Town 2006.

Luke A., d'Hemecourt P. Prevention of infectious diseases in athletes. *Clin. Sports Med.* 2007;26(3):321–44.

Martin S.A., Pence B.D., Woods J.A. Exercise and respiratory tract viral infections. *Exercise and Sport Sciences Reviews* 2009;37(4):157–64.

Mast E.E., Goodman R.A. Prevention of infectious disease transmission in sports. *Sports Med.* 1997;24(1):1–7.

Millward D.T., Tanner L.G., Brown M.A. Treatment options for the management of exercise-induced asthma and bronchoconstriction. *Physician Sportsmedicine* 2010;38(4):74–80.

Moehrle M. Outdoor sports and skin cancer. *Clin. Dermatol.* 2008;26(1):12–15.

Morris K.J. Management of exercise-induced bronchospasm in adolescents with asthma. *Nurse Pract.* 2010;35(12):18–26; quiz 27.

Morton A.R., Fitch K.D. Australian association for exercise and sports science position statement on exercise and asthma. *Journal of Science and Medicine in Sport/Sports Medicine Australia* 2011;14(4):312–16.

Mountjoy M., Junge A., et al. Sports injuries and illnesses in the 2009 FINA World Championships (Aquatics). *Br. J. Sports Med.* 2010;44(7):522–7.

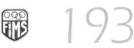

Nieman D.C. Current perspective on exercise immunology. *Curr. Sports Med. Rep.* 2003;2(5):239–42.

Nieman D.C. Immunonutrition support for athletes. *Nut. Rev.* 2008;66(6):310–20.

Page C.L., Diehl J.J. Upper respiratory tract infections in athletes. *Clin. Sports Med.* 2007;26(3):345–59.

Parsons J.P., Mastronarde J.G. Exercise-induced asthma. *Curr. Opin. Pulm. Med.* 2009; 15(1):25–8.

Parsons J.P., Mastronarde J.G. Exercise-induced bronchoconstriction in athletes. *Chest* 2005;128(6):3966–74.

Patel D.R., Torres A.D., Greydanus D.E. Kidneys and sports. *Adolesc. Med. Clin.* 2005; 16(1):111–9, xi.

Peirce N.S. Diabetes and exercise. *Br. J. Sports Med.* 1999;33(3):161–72.

Peters H.P., De Vries W.R. et al. Potential benefits and hazards of physical activity and exercise on the gastrointestinal tract. *Gut* 2001;48(3):435–9.

Pirozzolo J.J., LeMay D.C. Blood-borne infections. *Clin. Sports Med.* 2007;26(3):425–31.

Poortmans J.R., Vanderstraeten J. Kidney function during exercise in healthy and diseased humans. An update. *Sports Med.* 1994;18(6):419–37.

Poortmans J.R. Exercise and renal function. *Sports Med.* 1984;1(2):125–53.

Randolph C.C., Dreyfus D., et al. Prevalence of allergy and asthma symptoms in recreational road runners. *Med. Sci. Sports Exerc.* 2006;38(12):2053–7.

Rayner B., Schwellnus M.P. Exercise and the kidney. In: Schwellnus M.P. (ed), *The Olympic Textbook of Medicine in Sport*. Oxford: Wiley-Blackwell, 2008:375–89.

Reilly T., Atkinson G., Waterhouse J. Travel fatigue and jet-lag. *J. Sports Sci.* 1997; 15(3):365–9.

Reilly T., Waterhouse J., Edwards B. Jet lag and air travel: implications for performance. *Clin. Sports Med.* 2005;24(2):367–80, xii.

Roland P.S., Marple B.F. Disorders of the external auditory canal. *J. Am. Acad. Audiol.* 1997;8(6):367–78.

Romeo J., Warnberg J. Physical activity, immunity and infection. *Proc. Nutr. Soc.* 2010; 69(3):390–9.

Schwartz L.B., Delgado L., et al. Exercise-induced hypersensitivity syndromes in recreational and competitive athletes: a PRACTALL consensus report (what the general practitioner should know about sports and allergy). *Allergy* 2008;63(8):953–61.

Schwellnus M.P. Cause of exercise associated muscle cramps (EAMC) – altered neuro-muscular control, dehydration or electrolyte depletion? *Br. J. Sports Med.* 2009; 43(6):401–8.

Schwellnus M.P., Allie S., et al. Increased running speed and pre-race muscle damage as risk factors for exercise-associated muscle cramps in a 56 km ultra-marathon: a prospective cohort study. *Br. J. Sports Med.* 2011.

Schwellnus M.P., Derman E.W., Noakes T.D. Aetiology of skeletal muscle "cramps" during exercise: a novel hypothesis. *J. Sports Sci.* 1997;15(3):277–85.

Schwellnus M.P., Derman, E.W. Respiratory tract symptoms in endurance athletes – A review of causes and consequences. *Curr. Allergy Clin. Immunol.* 2010;23(2):52–7.

Schwellnus M.P., Drew N., Collins M. Increased running speed and previous cramps rather than dehydration or serum sodium changes predict exercise-associated muscle cramping: a prospective cohort study in 210 Ironman triathletes. *Br. J. Sports Med.* 2011;45(8):650–6.

Schwellnus M.P., Drew N., Collins M. Muscle cramping in athletes – risk factors, clinical assessment, and management. *Clin. Sports Med.* 2008;27(1):183–94.

Schwellnus M.P., Dvorak J., et al. Medical conditions and illness in elite football players during international competition: a pilot study (unpublished data in preparation).

Schwellnus M.P., Jeans A., et al. Exercise and infections. In: Schwellnus M.P. (ed), *The Olympic Textbook of Medicine in Sport*. Oxford: Wiley-Blackwell, 2008:344–64.

Schwellnus M.P., Nicol J., et al. Serum electrolyte concentrations and hydration status are not associated with exercise associated muscle cramping (EAMC) in distance runners. *Br. J. Sports Med.* 2004;38(4):488–92.

Schwellnus M.P., Patel D.N., et al. Healthy lifestyle interventions in general practice. Part 4: Lifestyle and diabetes mellitus. *S. Afr. Fam. Pract.* 2009;51(1).

Schwellnus M.P., Tune M., et al. Post ultra-marathon upper respiratory tract symptoms are not caused by an infection. *Med. Sci. Sports Exerc.* 2002;34(5 (Suppl.)):S168.

Shang G., Collins M., Schwellnus M.P. Factors associated with a self-reported history of exercise-associated muscle cramps in ironman triathletes: a case-control study. *Clin. J. Sport Med.: Official J. Canadian Academy of Sport Medicine* 2011;21(3):204–10.

Sharpe R.M. Lifestyle and environmental contribution to male infertility. *Br. Med. Bull.* 2000;56(3):630–42.

Simons S.M., Kennedy R.G. Gastrointestinal problems in runners. *Curr. Sports Med. Rep.* 2004;3(2):112–16.

Smoot M.K., Hosey R.G. Pulmonary infections in the athlete. *Curr. Sports Med. Rep.* 2009;8(2):71–5.

Speed C. Exercise and menstrual function. *BMJ* 2007;334(7586):164–5.

Spence L., Brown W.J., et al. Incidence, etiology, and symptomatology of upper respiratory illness in elite athletes. *Med. Sci. Sports Exerc.* 2007;39(4):577–86.

Stacey A., Atkins B. Infectious diseases in rugby players: incidence, treatment and prevention. *Sports Med.* 2000;29(3):211–20.

Standards of medical care in diabetes – 2009. *Diabetes Care* 2009;32(Suppl. 1):S13–61.

Sulzer N.U., Schwellnus M.P., Noakes T.D. Serum electrolytes in ironman triathletes with exercise-associated muscle cramping. *Med. Sci. Sports Exerc.* 2005;37(7):1081–5.

Turbeville S.D., Cowan L.D., Greenfield R.A. Infectious disease outbreaks in competitive sports: a review of the literature. *Am. J. Sports Med.* 2006;34(11):1860–5.

Walsh N.P., Gleeson M., et al. Position statement. Part one: Immune function and exercise. *Exerc. Immunol. Rev.* 2011;17:6–63.

Walsh N.P., Gleeson M., et al. Position statement. Part two: Maintaining immune health. *Exerc. Immunol. Rev.* 2011;17:64–103.

West N.P., Pyne D.B., et al. Probiotics, immunity and exercise: a review. *Exerc. Immunol. Rev.* 2009;15:107–26.

Wright H., Collins M. Are splanchnic hemodynamics related to the development of gastrointestinal symptoms in ironman triathletes? A prospective cohort study. *Clin. J. Sport Med.: Official J. Canadian Academy of Sport Medicine* 2011;21(4):337–43.

Wright H., Collins M., Schwellnus M. Gastrointestinal (GIT) symptoms in athletes: a review of risk factors associated with the development of GIT symptoms during exercise. *ISMJ* 2009;10(3):116–23.

CHAPTER 9

YOUNG ATHLETES

Michelle Burke, Angela D. Smith,
and Keith J. Loud

INTRODUCTION

Adult males still comprise the majority of members of athletic teams, and it is this population that has been the focus of most sports medicine research. Children and adolescents demonstrate significant differences from the adult male, and so, while most of the principles in the rest of this volume also apply to young athletes, this chapter will emphasize issues specific to this group. Team physicians caring for young athletes should be aware of differences, not only in injury patterns and management, but also in training response, training safety, and therefore injury prevention.

HEALTHY CHILDREN AND ADOLESCENTS

Injury patterns

Pre-pubertal children

Pre-pubertal children have more joint laxity and often more musculotendinous flexibility than adolescents and adults. They rarely sustain musculotendinous strains. However, Achilles and patellar tendon pain are common among jumping athletes, and patellar tendon pain is seen in kicking athletes. It is now clear that pre-pubertal children may tear ligaments, including the anterior cruciate ligament. In the ankle and the elbow, however, the weakest link in this age group is more frequently the growth plate rather than the ligament.

The physis (growth plate) can be three to five times weaker than adjacent connective tissue structures, depending on the rate and phase of growth. Both Salter–Harris types I and V physeal fractures can be difficult to recognize on plain X-rays, and so a careful clinical examination is needed to rule out these diagnoses before allowing return to play, and appropriate immobilization should be provided until healing is complete. Remember to rule out the presence of a fracture, at least clinically, before performing stress tests on an injured joint in a skeletally immature athlete. Also, acute avulsion fractures and chronic apophyseal traction injuries must be considered in the differential diagnosis of joint complaints. For example, the commonest cause of heel pain in 6–10-year-old athletes is calcaneal apophysitis.

Temporary or repetitive interruptions of normal circulation may involve the epiphysis and cause bone collapse, leading to softening, deformity, or fragmentation and loss of the overlying articular cartilage. Legg–Calve–Perthes disease involves the proximal femoral epiphysis and typically causes groin or anteromedial thigh pain. Kohler's disease affects the tarsal navicular bone in the foot and may be asymptomatic. Both of these conditions usually occur in the pre-pubertal age group but may first be diagnosed during adolescence. Osteochondritis dissecans of the femoral condyles of the knee, talar dome in the ankle, or humeral capitellum in the elbow may heal with activity restriction – that is, allowing the young athlete to do only those activities that cause no pain or swelling. Surgical intervention may be necessary in adolescent athletes, those who do not heal with non-operative care, or those whose lesions are partially or completely detached.

Fortunately, head and neck injuries occur relatively infrequently among prepubertal children playing sports, with the exception of participants in cycling and equestrian sports and contact sports such as American football and ice hockey. The use of helmets for these sports has been shown to reduce the risk and severity of head injury. However, adolescents seem more susceptible to the effects of recurrent concussion, recovering more slowly than adults. The dreaded second-impact syndrome has only been observed to occur in younger adolescent males. For these reasons, any child or adolescent athlete who sustains a head injury should not be allowed to return to competition that day and should be evaluated by a clinician skilled in concussion management before returning to strenuous activities.

All sport injury rates increase with age throughout childhood. Increasing sport specialization at younger ages seems to be related to increased rate of injury, particularly overuse injury, among pre-pubertal athletes. Greater volume and intensity of training appear to increase the risk of injury among all children and adolescents.

Adolescents

Adolescence is a time of rapid growth. Longitudinal growth occurs through the articular cartilage, epiphysis, and primarily the physis. Long bones increase in width by appositional growth of the shaft, and by physeal and appositional growth at the apophyses (where muscles attach). Bony growth often outpaces muscle and tendon lengthening during the adolescent growth spurt, rendering these regions particularly vulnerable to injury.

Acute injuries to the apophyses are maximal in mid to late adolescence, as physeal closure approaches. The mechanism of avulsion injury is most often a sudden violent muscular contraction, often occurring when unexpected resistance is encountered, such as with a blocked kick. The youth may have pre-existing pain

197

Table 9.1 Sites of avulsion fractures and muscles involved

Anterior superior iliac spine	Sartorius muscle
Anterior inferior iliac spine	Rectus femoris muscle
Ischial tuberosity	Hamstring muscle group
Iliac crest	Hip abductor muscle group; abdominal muscle, lumbar muscles
Lesser trochanter	Iliopsoas tendon
Tibial tubercle	Patellar tendon (patellar ligament)
Medial epicondyle	Common flexor–pronator origin

in the region of the apophysis from repetitive or chronic injury before the avulsion injury occurs. The most usual sites for avulsion fractures and muscles involved are shown in Table 9.1. The muscles most frequently involved are those that cross more than one joint.

Apophysitis is a repetitive traction injury of an apophysis associated with rapid growth, tight tendons, and increased activity during the growth spurt. Any of the apophyses in Table 9.1 may be involved. Some of these injuries are often well known by their famous eponyms. Their locations are shown in Table 9.2. Iliac apophysitis may affect any portion of the iliac crest, even causing back pain. Treatment includes determining and removing the cause of the injury (tight muscle, biomechanical abnormality, incorrect technique, too much intensity or repetition for the tissues to adapt), active rest, and appropriate rehabilitation.

In addition to traction injuries to apophyseal growth plates, repetitive stress may also injure a growth plate that is responsible for longitudinal growth. The locations where this type of injury is most often observed are in the upper extremity – the distal radial physis in gymnasts and the proximal humeral physis in pitchers. Treatment of these injuries focuses on removing the overload by decreasing the frequency or intensity of the activities causing the injury. Occasionally, complete rest from weight bearing on the hands (for the distal radius) or throwing (for the proximal humerus) is necessary for the physis to heal.

Acute fractures of the physis and epiphysis are sometimes missed, being diagnosed as sprains. Careful physical examination that shows tenderness of the injured bone

Table 9.2 Injuries and their locations

Sever's disease	Calcaneal tuberosity
Osgood–Schlatter's	Tibial tubercle
Sinding–Larsen–Johansson	Inferior pole of the patella
"Little league elbow"	Medial epicondyle of the humerus

m. burke, a.d. smith, and k.j. loud

provides good evidence for fracture, even if the X-ray appears normal. Wrist sprains are very unusual in adolescence, and so a significant wrist injury should be considered a fracture or dislocation until proven otherwise. Particularly in the situation of a badly swollen knee, radiographic and clinical findings must be correlated, as all Salter–Harris physeal fracture types may not be apparent on the acute injury films, and immobilization may prevent displacement of the fracture fragments.

Always included in the differential diagnosis of an adolescent with knee, thigh, or groin pain is acute or chronic slipped capital femoral epiphysis. The diagnosis is usually suspected by the finding of decreased medial rotation of the affected hip and pain with hip motion, especially rotation.

General guidelines for evaluation of musculoskeletal injuries in children and adolescents:

1. Palpate the growth plates carefully; do no stress tests of the joint if you suspect a fracture until you have plain X-rays of the suspicious area, or do the stress test carefully, under fluoroscopic control.
2. Always obtain X-rays if there is bone tenderness; X-ray the joints proximal and distal to the known injury – an unsuspected distal radius fracture may accompany a supracondylar humerus fracture, for example.
    (a) Perform a minimum of two orthogonal views on X-ray; additional oblique or special views may be indicated, depending on the particular bone and situation.
    (b) Comparison views of the uninjured side can help clarify questions of developmental variations and ossification centers.

Other considerations: pre-pubertal children

Pre-pubertal children have specific psychological, medical, and training needs. Increasingly, pre-pubertal children participate in organized sports. Children who participate in multiple different sports throughout the week and throughout the year may have injury patterns that differ little from children participating in free play. However, children who begin to specialize into one sport – or a few sports – are at risk for increased incidence of injury without appropriate preparation.

Psychological issues

Children play. From the infant beginning to roll, to the toddler taking the first steps, to the pre-school child learning to hop, skip, and jump, children derive pleasure from physical activity. Children in this age group want more to have fun than to win. Coaches need to understand this and need to allow for potential variations in competitive drive among children. A sense of play should definitely be encouraged, and participation should be emphasized over competition.

Starting sports

There are numerous guidelines about when and how children should begin participating in sport and fitness activities. Unfortunately, evidence is lacking to support most guidelines, which are often based on adult physical activity guidelines that are designed to improve fitness parameters and decrease risk factors for disease. There is no solid evidence to support the assumption that childhood activity translates into improved childhood health, adult activity, or adult health and fitness.

Musculoskeletal overuse injuries typically occur more frequently among children who intensively train in one sport compared with those who participate in several different activities. Surprisingly, though, one group found elite pre-pubertal athletes to have a lower injury rate than their sub-elite counterparts, suggesting that the former may be genetically endowed for such intensive training in their chosen sports.

Based on available reports and expert opinions, it would seem prudent that pre-pubertal children who choose to participate in organized sport activity should be advised to engage in a variety of activities that they enjoy, and delay sport specialization until adolescence. However, team physicians should recognize that participants in sports such as gymnastics, diving, figure skating, and more recently even soccer football generally specialize in their sports at very early ages in order to learn the required skills. This is particularly true for girls, who usually must learn to complete rotational maneuvers while they are small and lean. Even athletes in these sports, however, have been shown to benefit from participation in other activities, known as cross-training.

Training response: strength training effective

Numerous well-conducted scientific studies now indicate that strength training is both effective and safe for pre-pubertal children. In fact, strength training may make a critical difference in preventing injuries for those children who specialize in a few sports at an early age. Strength training is particularly important for the child who has previously been relatively inactive and then begins intensive sport activity. All of the musculoskeletal structures – the bones, musculotendinous units, and ligaments – must gradually and progressively adapt by gaining strength and size to support the demands that the sport may be placing on the child's body.

Most of the principles of strength training for children are the same as those for adults. The training must be gradual, and the resistance and intensity must increase slowly and progressively. The percentage increase of strength is similar in both children and adults who do a similar strength-training program. The strength increase appears to be mainly from neuromuscular adaptation, as little hypertrophy of the skeletal muscles occurs. There is no evidence of gender difference in trainability of pre-pubertal children.

m. burke, a.d. smith, and k.j. loud

A strength-training program for children must be well supervised. All equipment must be adjusted to be appropriate for the child's size. Exercises may be done with either appropriately adjusted equipment, with free weights, or with equipment such as a stability ball. If free weights are used, the amount of weight should be relatively small, the child's form and technique must be correct, and close supervision is extremely important. The increases in resistance should be gradual and progressive. The resistance used should always be submaximal, typically 60–80% of the maximum that the child can lift. The child must be able to complete each repetition of the exercise with good form. Practically speaking, the child should always use a resistance that allows the young athlete to complete 8–15 repetitions with correct technique. Competitive weight lifting and comparison of maximum resistance should be prohibited. We encourage exercises that use the child's own weight, such as push-ups and pull-ups, or exercises using large balls to balance on, which add increasing challenge related to the factor of instability.

It is best if the strength-training program is part of a periodized conditioning program. The components of the conditioning program should vary in intensity and in volume during the year. Other components of the conditioning program typically include flexibility and aerobic and anaerobic training. Flexibility exercises should be incorporated into the strength training so that the muscles are maintained at an adequate length as they gain in strength. It appears likely that many children's sport injuries are prevented by a program that combines strength training with flexibility increases. In addition to improved performance, the goals of a youth strength-training program are learning safe strength-training principles, improving balance and proprioception, and injury reduction.

STRENGTH TRAINING FOR YOUTH

- Strength training can be effective and safe and help prevent injuries.
- It is mainly for neuromuscular adaptation.
- Its goals are: learn safe strength-training principles, improve balance and proprioception, decrease injury incidence/severity.
- For safety, it must be well supervised, and equipment must be adjusted for size; there should be a gradual, progressive increase in submaximal resistance.

Training safety: exercise in heat or cold

Those who coach or provide medical care for pre-pubertal children who exercise in hot or cold conditions must always be aware of how the child's response to these environments differs from that of the adult. Children have greater skin surface area relative to total body mass than adults. Therefore, they are more susceptible to developing hypothermia and hyperthermia. Young children also do not have fully mature thermal regulatory mechanisms and may have sweat rate and sweat composition that are different from adults', depending on age and acclimatization. In addition, children often do not feel thirsty until they are quite dehydrated, and so that they must be encouraged to drink during exercise long before they begin to feel thirsty.

Furthermore, children generate more thermal energy, proportionally, than adults, owing to relative physiologic and metabolic inefficiency. Children have higher heart and respiratory rates than adults do and therefore use more oxygen per kilogram of body weight at baseline. Stroke volume does not increase greatly, and so increases in cardiac output with endurance exercise require increases in heart rate, with concomitant metabolic expenditure. Their gait mechanics are not yet mature, and so they typically expend more energy for a given amount of running work compared with adults.

The best treatment for illness or injury caused by, or exacerbated by, heat is prevention. Adequate hydration is key. An average 40-kg child should have approximately 150 ml of fluid to drink every 20–30 minutes while exercising. This translates to roughly 7.5 ml/kg/hour of exercise; a more easily remembered conversion is to replace every kilogram of weight loss during an exercise session with 1 l of fluid. For exercise in heat for less than 1 hour, plain water is generally the replacement liquid of choice. For exercise lasting longer than 1 hour, sports drinks that are flavored and contain electrolytes and carbohydrates are recommended, as their palatable taste may prompt greater intake.

Those who care for young athletes should also be prepared to modify, postpone, or even cancel events when environmental conditions make them unsafe. Extra care with regard to exercise in hot conditions must be taken for children with cystic fibrosis, diabetes, developmental delay, chronic renal disease, or other conditions that impair thermoregulation, thirst, or fluid balance.

Injury prevention

Potential mechanisms for reducing injuries in all youth sports include improving the sports environment. A properly conducted pre-participation medical evaluation identifies medical conditions that place the young athlete at risk and musculoskeletal conditions that should be rehabilitated before competing. The four principles of musculoskeletal rehabilitation are: (1) limit additional injury and control pain and swelling; (2) regain normal range of motion; (3) progressively increase strength, flexibility, proprioception, and aerobic and anaerobic endurance to the levels needed for the sport; and (4) resume sport-specific skills and return to activity symptom-free.

The team physician should make appropriate recommendations to the coach concerning good practice conditions. At sporting events, the team physician's roles include ensuring adequate hydration of the players and proper coaching, officiating, equipment, and field/surface playing conditions. The team physician

m. burke, a.d. smith, and k.j. loud

should be aware of potentially risky situations on the field and observe all play carefully. Of course, the physician provides medical care as needed.

Other considerations: adolescents

Many of the preceding principles continue to apply to younger adolescents, whereas older adolescents may be considered similar to the adults described throughout this text. The difficulty in caring for adolescents is that the process of moving from early to late adolescence is marked by substantial changes, not all of which proceed at consistent, predictable, or uniform rates.

Growth and development

Growth and development occur rapidly during adolescence. Ongoing body changes alter balance, height-to-strength ratio, and flexibility. Whereas boys gain muscle mass owing to the effects of testosterone, girls gain both lean body mass and fat. As a consequence, from age 6 to age 18, the "average" (50th percentile for age) boy increases his body fat percentage from 10 to 13%, whereas the average girl increases from 14 to 25%. Athletic adolescent males are typically 5–12% body fat, whereas most athletic adolescent females are 16–18%.

As the onset and pace of pubertal development is variable, there may be wide differences in maturity level within a team, or on opposing teams. Smaller athletes would seem to be at greater risk of injury compared with larger, more muscular opponents. Although some competitive groups are determined by weight class, others are simply determined by chronologic age. Matching participants of similar developmental stage rather than chronologic age in order to minimize competitive disparity and reduce risk of injury is intuitively attractive. Physiologic parameters such as Tanner classification, bone age, and grip strength have been proposed, but are impractical for the vast majority of organized athletic endeavors. Weight classification is used in some settings but has a major limitation in that differences in body composition (e.g., muscle vs. fat) render weight a poor measure of athletic fitness. Additionally, the pressure to "make weight" has potential adverse health outcomes of its own. Finally, there is no evidence at this time to substantiate the hypothesis that having athletes of differing developmental or physiological levels directly competing against one another increases risk of injury.

These issues pose a challenge to the physician advising adolescent athletes concerning the type and level of sport to play during a particular stage of development. Unfortunately, there is little evidence that can be used to guide the level and intensity of participation. The higher injury rates reported among athletes with more mature Tanner stages may reflect their greater body masses colliding, greater speed, or greater intensity of effort. Another factor is the decreased strength of growth plates and adjacent metaphyseal bone at periods of fastest growth (near peak height velocity).

Some coaches of athletes and dancers, particularly in Eastern Europe, have long monitored athletes' growth rates and decreased intensity of training during growth spurts in an effort to decrease injury incidence. As the bones rapidly grow longitudinally, the lengthening of adjacent muscles may lag behind. This "mismatch" is particularly notable with muscles that cross two joints, such as the hamstrings, rectus femoris, iliotibial band, and gastrocnemius. Among growing children and adolescents, flexibility deficits have been associated with calcaneal apophysitis and anterior knee overuse syndromes. Among older adolescents, poor muscle flexibility is often described in those most prone to developing injury.

Weight control

In adolescence, weight control often becomes a significant issue for athletes. For boys, this is mainly a concern for those involved in the sports of wrestling and rowing – those in which the competitive class is determined by weight. For girls, there are also concerns in sports that have classes determined by weight. However, among adolescent girls, there are also major concerns with regard to aesthetics. Being thin is a particular concern for girls involved in sports that are judged subjectively, such as gymnastics, diving, and figure skating. In addition, many coaches stress the necessity of low weight in other sports, such as running and swimming, even though there is evidence that weight (within a typical range for athletes) makes no difference at all in performance of these sports. Attempting to control weight does, however, increase the risk of dehydration, heat illness, disordered eating, malnutrition, frank eating disorders, and, in females, amenorrhea, contributing to impaired bone-mass acquisition. Many of the above abnormalities can directly or indirectly lead to severe morbidity or even mortality.

Psychological issues

Just as they grow physically and physiologically, adolescents must progress through several psychological stages. The major developmental tasks of adolescence are separation from their parents and families and individuation into adults. Peer relationships and opinions gain primacy in middle adolescence. Advice from friends, inaccurate as it may be, can be given greater credence than that from coaches, teachers, parents, or even physicians! Because participation in the peer group holds so much importance, the adolescent who does not make a team or is removed owing to injury can consider the loss as emotionally difficult as parental separation or divorce, or a friend's death.

Early-maturing athletes may have experienced early success, but then become "average," as their peers mature physically and catch up in size and strength, causing additional psychological stress. On the positive side, adolescents also increasingly develop the ability for more complex and abstract thought, which may facilitate interactions with the team physician and improve the description, diagnosis, and rehabilitation of injuries. Participation in sports helps to foster a positive self-image in the developing adolescent.

Substance abuse

In the process of separation and individuation, adolescents may experiment with substances such as tobacco, alcohol, and drugs. Fortunately, there is evidence that participation in sports reduces these risk-taking behaviors. Young athletes may use anabolic steroids for performance enhancement or for cosmetic reasons. They may also use nutritional supplements as ergogenic aids. These are, as a rule, poorly controlled and poorly studied, particularly with regard to adolescents. Nonetheless, many supplements are legal, non-prescription, and readily available. The majority of adolescent users of anabolic steroids and nutritional supplements have cited non-medical sources of information, taken higher than recommended dosages, and continued to use the substance despite experiencing adverse effects. Perhaps the best general advice regarding these substances is that they are often ineffective, unsafe, impure, expensive, and banned by sports organizations.

ADOLESCENTS

- Pubertal development is variable; growth is rapid; body composition changes.
- There is decreased strength of bone at physis (growth plate) and metaphysis near peak height velocity; fractures are more likely than sprains at wrist and ankle.
- Muscles may be "short" relative to adjacent long bones, especially muscles that cross two joints.
- Weight control is an issue for sport weight class, or for psychosocial reasons.
- There can be substance experimentation/abuse.

Gender differences during development

Motor skill acquisition

In general, there are very few gender differences in the pre-pubertal age range. The vast majority of motor skills are acquired at similar ages for both girls and boys. However, there is a definite difference in throwing ability before approximately 6 years of age, the boys becoming more accomplished in this skill than the girls at an earlier age.

Skeletal muscle strength

There is no significant difference in absolute strength gain between pre-pubertal boys and girls. Both groups have a linear increase in strength from about 5 years of age through puberty. Following puberty, there is a marked acceleration in the strength gain of boys, coinciding with the boys' serum testosterone increase. This accelerated strength gain in boys continues through their late teens. There are no similar post-pubertal strength gains among girls.

Similar differences are found when comparing the ratio of strength to body mass. For both boys and girls aged 5–17 years, absolute strength increases more than the ratio of strength to body mass. However, by the time the girls are approximately 10–12 years old, the decreased upper body strength relative to body mass ratio for the girls begins to be apparent. By age 14 years, boys are noticeably stronger than girls.

There is only a small difference in muscle cross-sectional area until about age 14 years. However, by age 20 years, the difference in muscle cross-sectional area between young men and young women is 30–50%. The differences are greater in the upper than the lower extremities. By adulthood, women have 50% of the upper-body muscle size, but about 65–70% of the lower-extremity muscle size of men. Similar differences are seen in the size of the bones as well.

Strength training

By adolescence, the gender differences in strength-training results are greater than they were in the pre-pubertal years. After puberty, adolescent boys doing strength-training exercises increase their upper body strength more than adolescent girls do with the same training. With similar strength training, the boys' lower body strength also increases to a greater extent than the girls', but the gender difference is less than it is for upper body strength.

Aerobic capacity

Before 12 years of age, the VO_2max of girls is typically 85–90% that of boys. This is consistent with the 70% lower relative muscle mass of girls compared with boys. By late adolescence, the VO_2max of girls is only 70% that of boys. However, if the VO_2max of boys versus girls is compared relative to their fat-free mass, the VO_2max of the boys is only 10% greater than the girls.

For submaximal work, at the same absolute workload, pre-adolescent and adolescent girls have higher heart rates than boys. In childhood, the more rapid heart rate is probably best explained by the relatively lower stroke volume of girls.

Endurance activities

In endurance running, the gender difference widens between the performance of 11–12 year olds and that of 15–16 year olds. This finding is probably related to the development of greater muscle mass in boys. The muscle mass in turn affects both running economy and endurance, or maximal aerobic power.

Implications

Although pre-pubertal boys and girls can likely participate together in sports safely, it seems reasonable – in light of these physiologic differences found during adolescence – to recommend generally that adolescent boys and girls do not compete head-to-head in contact or collision sports. Nonetheless, there are no data available from mixed-gender sports to support this concern for possibly increased rates of injury. In fact, there may be situations where the perceived or theoretical risks are minimal, particularly if a physically strong, mature, well-conditioned, skilled female athlete wants to play a contact sport for which only male teams are fielded.

GENDER DIFFERENCES

- *Pre-pubertal*: almost all motor skills are acquired at similar ages; there is a similar linear increase in muscle strength; VO_2max of girls is 85–90% that of boys; there is no difference in endurance running performance.
- *Adolescence*: there is a marked acceleration of boys' strength gain, and gender differences are greatest for upper extremities; boys gain more strength than girls with the same training program; girls' VO_2max decreases to 70% that of boys, but is still approximately 90% when expressed relative to fat-free mass; there is greater gender difference in endurance running performance by mid teens.

ADDITIONAL CONSIDERATIONS FOR FEMALE ADOLESCENTS AND YOUNG ADULTS

Injury patterns

Young adult women (and skeletally mature female adolescents more than two years after menarche) in organized athletics sustain the same injuries as their male counterparts and are injured at the same overall rate. However, the distribution of injuries among young women is different, owing in part to their differing participation rates. For example, American-rules football is largely unavailable to women, rendering them less susceptible to traumatic shoulder dislocations. In other cases, such as the anterior cruciate ligament (ACL) discussed later, intrinsic differences cause a much higher risk of injury for female adolescents and young adults engaged in similar activities, such as basketball and soccer. Thus, we use the term "injury patterns" to describe the differences between males and females.

Musculoskeletal differences

There are numerous musculoskeletal differences between men and women that may contribute to differing injury patterns, including decreased strength among women (discussed later). The woman's wider pelvis and greater knee valgus angulation make patellofemoral dysfunction more common among female than male athletes. The vast majority of cases of patellofemoral dysfunction in athletes can be controlled with exercise programs that stretch any tight muscles that cross the knee joint and strengthen the quadriceps (particularly the vastusmedialis), combined with correction of other biomechanical problems – such as excessive pronation – when present.

In general, women have greater ligamentous laxity than men, which may lead to knee pain and shoulder instability. Most symptoms related to joint laxity can be controlled by increasing the strength and endurance of the muscles that control the painful, lax joint.

There is a markedly increased incidence of ACL injury among women compared with men, particularly for non-contact mechanisms. The causes of this are not yet fully determined, but are hypothesized to include body composition, the effects of estrogen, anatomic considerations including the thickness of the ACL and the width of the intercondylar notch, as well as conditioning and technique differences. For example, recent research showed that male basketball players typically land with greater knee flexion than female players, with their weight on the balls of their feet and the center of gravity well balanced over the toes. In contrast, the female basketball players studied more often land with straighter knees, more flat footed, with the center of gravity behind the toes. The quadriceps force pulling the tibia forward was therefore greater. Other research has indicated relative weakness of the hamstrings among women athletes compared with men, so that the effective quadriceps/hamstrings force mismatch was sufficient to cause ACL tears in this situation. Early studies of female basketball players who have altered their technique to include greater knee flexion, softer jump landings, and keeping their weight over their toes with sudden decelerations and with jump landings have found a decrease in their incidence of ACL injury.

Women have higher incidence of scoliosis, but symptoms should limit sports participation very rarely. Young athletes undergoing brace treatment for scoliosis may have specific limitations on sport participations, but generally there are none, and many athletes are allowed to train and compete a few hours per day without the brace.

Other issues

Cultural issues

For a young adult woman, sports opportunities vary markedly depending on her region and her culture. Some cultures require women to wear appropriate garb that covers much of the body and interferes with peripheral vision. Dissipation of heat may become a problem with the greater amount of clothing in these situations. As the team physician makes advance plans for medical treatment in such a cultural situation, an appropriate treatment venue and an appropriate provider, often female, are usually required.

Performance differences

Among women, like men, running performance is closely related to maximal aerobic power. The slower running times reported for elite female athletes are mainly attributed to their lower VO_2max. The gender differences in VO_2max are probably mainly related to body composition and to hemoglobin concentration. Typically, no difference in VO_2max is found between similarly trained men and women when VO_2max is expressed relative to fat-free mass. In addition, iron deficiency is common among women because of iron loss during menses. This further decreases the oxygen-carrying capacity of the blood and decreases performance.

Training response: strength and endurance training

As mentioned above, by age 20 years, the difference in muscle cross-sectional area between young men and young women is 30–50%, with differences greater in the upper than the lower extremities. However, men and women have little difference in response to strength training, if the parameters examined are relative increase in strength and muscle size. Women can show muscle hypertrophy with strength training, although the maximum hypertrophy is typically less than that for men, without the use of exogenous anabolic steroids. Nonetheless, some studies have shown that the amount of training-induced muscle hypertrophy is similar among men and women who are involved in similar training regimens. It is not yet known if there are gender differences in the optimal training intensity or optimal training frequency for strength training. With regard to endurance training, the trainability of women has been found to be equal to that of men.

Menstrual cycle

Although there have been many studies of athletic performance throughout the menstrual cycle, no change in aerobic capacity has been found related to the menstrual phase. Although study findings vary, the best-controlled studies seem to indicate that there is also no change in anaerobic capacity with regard to the menstrual phase. There is also no consistent evidence that menstrual phase significantly affects athletic performance or injury occurrence, so there is no rationale to restrict a woman's sport participation at any phase of the menstrual cycle.

Disordered eating and the female athlete triad

Although amenorrhea associated with athletic participation has been appreciated for decades, greater attention was focused on its connections with disordered eating and osteoporosis by the American College of Sports Medicine in describing the "female athlete triad" in 1992. More recently (2007), the triad has been refined to describe the interrelationships between energy availability, menstrual cycle, and bone mineral density, emphasizing that the spectrum can be either beneficial or deleterious. The concern for menstrual irregularity is that it is thought by many to be related to inadequate nutrition relative to the energy that the athlete is expending, causing a significant negative energy balance. With prolonged decreased estrogen exposure, impaired bone mineral density may follow.

No study has shown a direct relationship between athletic performance and being overweight. In fact, several studies have shown that there is no such relationship. However, aesthetic issues are often paramount for the athlete, judge, and coach involved. It is clear that severe dieting can decrease performance and can especially affect aerobic capacity. Impaired bone mineral density may lead to stress fractures that severely limit training. The bone loss may be permanent. Finally, although menstrual irregularity by itself does not affect thermoregulation, those with anorexia nervosa do typically have abnormal thermoregulation.

Overall, the benefits of sport for women far outweigh the risks of the triad. In fact, athletes such as gymnasts and figure skaters, even when having irregular menstrual cycles, have been found to have greater bone mass in the bones that are impact-loaded than sedentary controls, or even other athletes such as runners and swimmers. Amenorrheic and eumenorrheic gymnasts have stronger upper-extremity bones than controls or other athletes, and figure skaters have stronger lower-extremity bones and pelvis, even skaters not menstruating regularly.

Other nutritional differences

Women who restrict their caloric intake often have inadequate intake of protein, vitamins, and minerals. They may require supplementation, particularly of B vitamins, folate, and iron. They should be encouraged to eat breakfast and consume snacks throughout the day, in order better to balance their energy intake and output on an hourly basis throughout the day. Female athletes who eat throughout the day between exercise bouts have been shown, in small studies, to have improved performance, increased lean body mass, and decreased body fat.

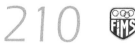

m. burke, a.d. smith, and k.j. loud

In an interesting nutritional difference between men and women, the benefits of a high carbohydrate diet and carbohydrate loading seem to be less pronounced among trained female endurance athletes than among males. This finding is probably related to the lower daily energy intake for the female athletes.

Training safety: thermoregulation

There appear to be significant differences in thermoregulation between men and women. First, women have cyclical changes in core body temperature. During the luteal phase of the menstrual cycle, core body temperature at rest increases by 0.3–0.6°C. Heart rate and rating of perceived exertion are also higher during prolonged exercise during the luteal phase.

Compared with men, women have a larger ratio of skin surface area to body mass. The increased body fat of women adversely affects their response to heat, but it is advantageous in cold environments. In equal heat, women's core body temperature increases more than men's, both at rest and with exercise. Women sweat less, and they have a higher sweating threshold. However, among women and men of similar aerobic capacity, these previous two differences are not apparent. Women are at a disadvantage when exercising in dry heat, compared with men. However, they are at less of a disadvantage when exercising in humid heat, as continued sweating in humid exposure has a greater likelihood of leading to dehydration.

Training safety: pregnancy

A great deal of work has been done in the last decade with regard to physical activity and sport participation during pregnancy. It now appears that regular exercise during pregnancy actually enhances maternal fitness, without apparent risk to either the mother or the fetus. Regular exercise before and during pregnancy seems to enhance a pregnant woman's physiologic reserve. Premature labor occurs with equal frequency in women who do and do not exercise.

Special attention needs to be paid to certain safety principles during exercise in pregnancy. In particular, the pregnant woman needs to pay special attention to appropriate nutrition, hydration, and rest. It is recommended that exercise bouts not occur until at least 3 hours after eating, and that the exercise be followed with a snack. As a reflection of hydration status, weight loss during a single exercise session should be no more than 1 kg.

The pregnant woman should avoid exercising in extremely hot and humid environments. She should avoid high-intensity activities that may lead to hyperthermia, which is a significant concern during pregnancy. First-trimester hyperthermia may be teratogenic. Clapp suggests that a pregnant woman's rectal temperature should not rise by more than 1.5–1.8°C and should not exceed 38.7°C on a regular basis or for a prolonged period of time. According to him, the commonly accepted teratogenic level is 39.2°C. Exercising in water may help thermoregulation by dissipating heat.

During pregnancy, a woman who is participating in sports or an exercise program should modify her training program if she has musculoskeletal discomfort or other uncomfortable symptoms. She should also consider modifying or avoiding exercise with risk of blunt abdominal trauma. She should avoid activities done at high altitude (such as mountain climbing) or in deep water (such as scuba diving). Additional modifications are indicated in the situation of multiple fetuses, bleeding, poor fetal growth, or evidence of premature change in the cervix.

Finally, the exercising pregnant woman should monitor her training intensity carefully. She may do this by monitoring her rating of perceived exertion. In addition, fatigue or poor performance may indicate that she is overtraining.

Other gynecologic issues

Team physicians caring for women athletes must consider gynecologic concerns such as ovarian cysts, endometriosis, and more urgent problems such as pelvic inflammatory disease and ectopic pregnancy in their differential diagnosis of pelvic, hip, and low-back pain. Days of persistent nausea may be caused by pregnancy rather than representing post-concussive symptoms or labyrinthitis, and so pregnancy should always be in the diffential diagnosis of persistent nausea of the female athlete. Also, the differential diagnosis of amenorrhea in an athlete of course includes pregnancy.

WOMEN: YOUNG ADULT

- There are wide cultural variations in sport activities available to women; required clothing may increase hyperthermia risk or interfere with vision.
- Compared with young adult men, young adult women have lower VO_2max (but the same VO_2max when expressed relative to fat-free mass); decreased muscle cross-sectional area and bone size; and less muscle hypertrophy with strength training (unless using exogenous anabolic steroids).
- Compared with young adult men, young adult women show no difference in strength trainability expressed as percentage increase.
- There are special musculoskeletal considerations: more frequent patellofemoral dysfunction, anterior cruciate ligament rupture, and idiopathic scoliosis.
- There are special medical considerations: iron deficiency, disordered eating/female athlete triad, and thermoregulation differences.
- Pregnancy: regular exercise is good for mother and fetus. The mother should eat, rest, and hydrate appropriately; avoid exercise in heat/humidity, especially exercise of high intensity; and monitor intensity carefully.

---

m. burke, a.d. smith, and k.j. loud

Breast protection

Many women with larger breasts prefer to wear a sports bra that decreases breast motion, for comfort. For some contact and collision sports, breast padding is appropriate to prevent trauma to the breast. The nipple is the most prominent and most commonly injured part of the breast. For both women and men, repetitive vigorous abrasion or cold-induced thermal injury of the nipple may lead to bloody discharge and concern about possible breast cancer. Prophylactic measures include application of plastic bandages and/or petroleum jelly over the nipples before exercise.

YOUNG ATHLETES WITH SPECIAL CHALLENGES

General principles

Physically and cognitively challenged youth find many benefits from participating in sports. However, they may have certain risks that are not commonly found among able-bodied populations. Each individual must weigh the risks and benefits of participation. The vast majority of physically challenged youth can participate in at least some type of sport. Special Olympics Games have been developed for athletes with mental disabilities. The Paralympics provides athletic venues for those who have limited or no use of their lower extremities.

Medical challenges

Specific medical challenges are discussed in previous chapters. These include exercise-induced bronchospasm, diabetes mellitus, and seizure disorders. For those with hemophilia, in addition to medical management, injury prevention is important. The team physician can emphasize the importance of good muscle strength to provide better control about a joint, the use of appropriate protective equipment, and avoidance of contact and collision sports.

Obese youth may have altered response to heat, feeling less cold when exercising in cold environments, but overheating when exercising in warm environments. In addition, they may need to pay greater attention to pre-participation conditioning.

Athletes with cystic fibrosis can have surprising exercise endurance, and affected athletes have actually completed marathon runs. Most studies have shown that exercise tolerance and peak oxygen consumption VO_2 increase in regularly exercising patients. In addition, exercising cystic fibrosis patients have decreased dyspnea.

Athletes with congenital heart disease should tailor their activities to their cardiopulmonary abilities as advised by their cardiologists. The American College of Cardiology has devised and published detailed guidelines on cardiovascular disease and athletic participation (Bethesda Guidelines). The American Academy of Pediatrics Council on Sports Medicine and Fitness has similarly published guidelines for participation in sports by children and adolescents with systemic hypertension and an extensive list of medical conditions (see page 24).

Neuromuscular disabilities

Progressive

People with progressive neuromuscular disorders such as Duchenne muscular dystrophy may find that participation in sports improves their self-image. There is some evidence that physical activity such as weight lifting prolongs maintenance of muscle strength. Athletes with mild, progressive neuromuscular disorders, such as some forms of Charcot–Marie–Tooth disease, may be able to participate even in running sports using only an ankle–foot orthosis.

Non-progressive

Individuals with non-progressive neuromuscular disorders, such as cerebral palsy, may have intellectual as well as physical disabilities. Those with the diagnosis of cerebral palsy may have a very wide range of abilities, from nearly normal to profoundly involved. It is important that the training be adjusted to the level of the individual's ability.

Other non-progressive neuromuscular disorders include spina bifida and spinal cord injury. Here, also, the athlete's ability is related to the functional level and whether the intellect is impaired. Athletes with distal involvement, such as those with sacral-level spina bifida, may participate in a regular sports program using only ankle–foot orthoses. Wheelchair sports are excellent for lower-level quadriplegics and for paraplegics. They may also participate in many sports on ice and snow.

Amputees

Athletes with lower-extremity amputations often put forth remarkable performances. Champion athletes range from a world champion figure skater who had a partial foot amputation to ultra-distance runners with high above-knee amputations. Modern prostheses may be highly engineered for sophisticated mobility and shock absorption. Indeed, the most recently developed lower-extremity prostheses may outperform the human leg, causing some controversy. Upper-extremity amputees may also participate in sports that require upper-extremity use, with appropriate prosthetic devices.

Down syndrome

Down syndrome (trisomy 21) patients often find great joy in sports participation. They should be checked for cervical spine stability, particularly if they choose to participate in sports where contact or collision occurs. Although recurrent patellar dislocation is not uncommon in Down syndrome, it rarely interferes with the athlete's ability to participate in sports. Evaluation guidelines for athletic participation with Down syndrome have also been published by the American Academy of Pediatrics (see page 24).

SUMMARY

Sports and exercise are beneficial for virtually all populations. The physical, mental, and sociological benefits are all significant. However, physicians caring for the athletes described in this chapter need to be aware of their special needs and must be prepared to provide appropriate care.

SUGGESTED READING

Agostini R. (Ed.) *Medical and Orthopedic Issues of Active and Athletic Women*, Hanley & Belfus, Philadelphia, PA, 1994.

Bar-Or O. (Ed.) *The Child and Adolescent Athlete, The Encyclopedia of Sports Medicine*, International Olympic Committee Medical Commission Publication, in collaboration with the International Federation of Sports Medicine, Blackwell Science, Oxford, England, 1996.

Bar-or O., Lamb D.R., and Clarkson P.M. (Eds.) *Exercise and the Female, a Life Span Approach, Perspectives in Exercise Science and Sports Medicine*, vol. 9, Cooper Publishing Group, Carmel, IN, 1996.

Clapp, J. *Exercising Through Your Pregnancy*, Champaign, IL, Human Kinetics, 2002.

Drinkwater B.L. (Ed.) *Women in Sport*, International Olympic Committee Medical Commission Publication, in collaboration with the International Federation of Sports Medicine, Blackwell Science, Oxford, England, 2000.

Dyment P. (Ed.) *Sports Medicine: Health Care for Young Athletes*, 2nd edition, Committee on Sports Medicine and Fitness of the American Academy of Pediatrics, American Academy of Pediatrics, Elk Growth Village, Illinois, 1991.

Goldberg B. (Ed.) *Sports in Exercise for Children with Chronic Health Conditions*, Human Kinetics Publishers, Champaign, Illinois, 1995.

Gordon S.L., Gonzalez-Mestre X.G., and Garrett W.E. (Eds.) *Sports and Exercise In Midlife*, American Academy of Orthopaedic Surgeons, Rosemont, Illinois, 1993.

IOC Consensus Statement: The Female Athlete Triad. *Med. Sci. Sports Exercise* 11(1), 2006.

Micheli L.J. (Ed.) The young athlete, *Clin. Sports Med.* 14(3), 1995.

Micheli L.J. (Ed.) Pediatric and adolescent sports injuries, diagnosis, management, and prevention. *Clin. Sports Med.* 19(4), 2000.

Micheli L.J. (Guest Ed.), Cannon W.D., and DeHaven K.E. (Eds.) Adolescent sports medicine, *Sports Medicine and Arthroscopy Review* 4(2), 1996.

Nicholas J.A. and Hershman E.B. (Eds.) *The Lower Extremity and Spine in Sports Medicine*, Mosby, St. Louis, MO, 1995.

Reider B. Sports medicine, *The School-Age Athlete*, Philadelphia, PA: Saunders Press, 1991.

Rippe J.M. (Ed.) *Lifestyle Medicine*, Blackwell Science, Oxford, England, 1999.

Stanitski C.L., DeLee J.C., and Drez D. (Eds.) *Pediatric and Adolescent Sports Medicine*, W.B. Saunders, Philadelphia, PA, 1994.

CHAPTER 10

SPORTS MEDICINE AND PHYSICAL CHALLENGE

Peter Van de Vliet, Pia Pit-Grosheide, and Oriol
Martinez Ferrer

INTRODUCTION

Although sport has value in everyone's life, it is even more important in the life
of a person with a disability. This is because of the rehabilitative influence sport
can have, not only rehabilitating the physical body, but also rehabilitating people
with a disability into society. Furthermore, sport teaches independence.

Although sport for people with a physical disability is of all times, it was more or
less systematically introduced after World War II to assist the medical and
psychological needs of the large number of injured ex-servicemen, -women, and
civilians. In the search for new methods to minimize the consequences of their
immobility, it provided a new and great possibility for reviving the idea of sport
as a means of treatment and rehabilitation. As a result, nowadays, people with a
disability participate in high-performance, as well as competitive and recreational,
sport across the world, and sports and physical activity also found their way into
rehabilitation. The impact of such programs in early phases of rehabilitation are
well documented in the literature, including higher employment rates, increased
psychological stability and life satisfaction, reduced medical aftercare, and
increased independent living. Sport programs and opportunities worldwide have
increased in scope and number, and sport has become a viable option for
individuals with a disability.

Sports medicine has evolved in similar fashion. Although commonly established
for many years, it is only since the early twenty-first century that sports medicine
has emerged as a distinct entity in disability sport. This went hand in hand with
the increased sport participation of individuals with a disability and the increased
professionalism in disability sport. Despite the growing awareness, there remains
a relative paucity of published research on sports medicine specifically for this
athletic population.

YOUR AUDIENCE: IMPAIRMENT GROUPS

Disabled athletes can be categorized in different groups, each requiring a particular approach with regard to medical care: athletes with loss of limb or limb deficiency (e.g. amputation); athletes with loss of muscle power (e.g., spinal cord injury, post-poliomyelitis, spina bifida); athletes with coordination problems (e.g., hypertonia, ataxia, or athetosis as clinically manifested in, e.g., cerebral palsy (CP)); athletes with visual impairment; athletes with auditive impairment; athletes with intellectual impairment; and athletes with loss of body function of the cardiovascular, haemato-logical, immunological, or respiratory system.

This chapter limits itself to describing sports medicine applications for athletes with physical impairments (loss of limb, limb deficiency, loss of muscle power, coordination problems).

Athletes with loss of limb or limb deficiency either suffer from congenital disorders, acquired amputations, or limb deformity. Common causes are traumatic or disease-related (bone cancer, bone infection, diabetes). Occasionally, amputee athletes experience phantom sensation, painful cramping feelings, and hypersensitivity. Amputee athletes may compete with or without orthotic or prosthetic devices, depending on the sport in which they participate. The use of such assistive devices brings an additional component of medical care, e.g., soft-tissue problems and skin breakdown (see below).

The group of athletes with loss of muscle power typically includes: spinal cord injury, spina bifida, and post-polio paralysis. Spinal cord injury is an acquired condition involving the motor, sensory, and autonomic nervous systems and due to spinal (bone) fracture or infection. The neurological level of injury corresponds with the lowest level of the spinal cord that exhibits intact motor and sensory function. Associated conditions can include spasms and spasticity, urinary tract infections, thermoregulation disorders, skin breakdown, pressure sores and decubitus ulcers, autonomic hyperreflexia, osteoporosis and heterotopic ossification, and joint contractures. Athletes with spina bifida or myelomeningocele experience muscle weakness, sensory loss, and bowel and bladder dysfunction similar to the issues experienced with a spinal cord injury. Particular attention should be given to orthopedic complications of the spine and legs and the enhanced risk of development of hydrocephalus. Poliomyelitis is an infectious impairment caused by a virus that destroys motor nerve cells and causes permanent muscle weakness and paralysis. Unlike with spinal cord injury and spina bifida, post-polio paralysis results in problems with movement but not with sensation or autonomic nervous system function. Depending on the extent of the paralysis, the athlete may experience joint contractures and osteoporosis. Asymmetrical muscle function often results in the development of muscle tightness and restriction around limb joints, and spine curvatures.

The group of athletes with coordination problems includes a wide range vulnerable to problems with control of voluntary movement or coordination. CP, as an example, usually results from a complication in the pre-, peri- or postnatal period that leads to an injury to the areas of the brain that control movement, speech, muscle tone, and coordination. Associated conditions often include seizures and perceptual, speech, and swallowing disorders.

SPORTS INJURIES AND ILLNESSES

With participation in sport comes an associated risk of injury. Despite the growing awareness and popularity of disability sport, there continues to be a relative paucity of understanding of the injury patterns and risk factors for injury among these athletes. Although athletes with physical disabilities can experience the same spectrum of medical conditions as athletes without disabilities, furthering understanding through longitudinal and systematic investigation of injuries and illnesses in elite athletes, e.g., as initiated in 2002 by the International Paralympic Committee Sports Injury Survey, is extremely helpful in this regard. The few studies that have been published comparing sport participation in both able-bodied and disabled individuals suggest that the latter do not have a significantly greater overall risk of injury than their able-bodied counterparts, although the functional consequences of injury to an athlete with an underlying impairment can be considerably greater than for an able-bodied athlete. For example, a comparatively "routine" shoulder overuse injury that might be a mere "nuisance" for an able-bodied athlete could compromise the ability of a C6-lesion tetraplegic athlete (athlete with high neck lesion, impacting the function of both lower and upper limbs) to remain independently mobile, to say nothing about dramatically interfering with his or her participation in sport.

A better understanding of common disabilities and injuries will assist athletes and their coaches, therapists, and trainers, as well as all event (medical) staff, in identifying possible medical problems and activities that may lead to injuries or medical complications. This enables all involved to take the steps necessary to ensure safe and effective training techniques and maximize competitive performance on the one hand, and optimize sports medicine and event-related medical services on the other hand.

MANAGEMENT OF COMMON MEDICAL PROBLEMS

Generally, the same safety and medical considerations apply to both disabled and able-bodied athletes. Precautions should be taken in order to prevent accidents from happening and to make the sporting environment a safe and positive one. However, precautions should not be so extreme as to take away the "sense of achievement" that is inherent to sports participation. One of the greatest "handicaps" that people with a disability, in general, have had to confront has

218

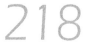
p. van de vliet, p. pit-grosheide, and o. martinez ferrer

been to deal with the overbearing concerns of caregivers and society in general. Although these types of concern have been well intended, they have often stifled the independence and hampered the freedom of disabled athletes.

As with able-bodied athletes, athletes with a disability should be "cleared" for sport and checked for medical complications that may limit or prohibit involvement in (competitive) sport. Team physicians should have a medical history report on all athletes with them at all times. Athletes themselves have the responsibility to pass on appropriate medical (and technical) information to coaches, event organizers, and the like upon request.

An awareness of the risks of common medical problems experienced by Paralympic athletes is essential to prevent unfortunate condition(s), and it is important for care staff to identify in advance the possible medical problems the athletes might face. Issues such as the extent of muscle and joint involvement, muscle tone and coordination, sensory loss, heat/cold intolerance, susceptibility to fractures, dangers of exacerbation, or the likelihood of progression of disease symptoms are all important considerations in anticipation of sports participation.

Although it is expected that Paralympic athletes should practice routine preventive measures to achieve and maintain optimal health to achieve maximal performance, research has shown that Paralympic athletes often do not seek medical consultation for problems they consider inherent to their impairment. Consequently, they too often try to "work through" an illness or disease. Unfortunately, this "self-manage-ment" sometimes prevents proper assessment of the problem and appropriate medical care at an early stage.

COMMON MEDICAL PROBLEMS AND INJURIES

The medical care in athletes with a disability should be related to the sport-specific risks and demands, as well as to the nature of the impairment. Although relatively few studies are available, wheelchair track and road racing, para-cycling, alpine skiing, wheelchair basketball, and wheelchair rugby are among the higher-risk sports. More importantly, however, medical problems and injuries are positively correlated with frequency and intensity of training and competition.

Analysis of medical encounters reported at major events shows that athletes with a disability present to medical stations more often for the same medical problems as the general population than they do for medical problems usually related specifically to their impairment.

The following are the commonest injuries occurring in athletes with a disability.

Soft-tissue injuries

Soft-tissue injuries (abrasions, contusions, strains, and sprains) typically result from repetitive stress on joints and muscles. Shoulder and elbow joints are particularly

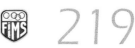

vulnerable to repetitive motions, as well as contact surfaces between amputee stump and socket. Particular attention should be given to carpal tunnel syndrome: the repetitive trauma of wheelchair propulsion creates additional forces on the nerves that run from the forearm to the palm of the hand. The carpal tunnel compresses these nerves. This results in pain, tingling, and loss of strength and/or hand sensation.

Muscles are often strained when in a stretched position and contracting with great force against strong resistance, which commonly occurs in sports performance. Weaker, smaller muscles are particularly prone to such strain in disabled athletes, e.g., the shoulder rotator cuff. The result is an impingement syndrome or painful condition caused by continued compression of a tendon that then inflames. As soft-tissue injuries are related to direct and repetitive trauma, it is essential to schedule adequate rest and recovery between practice times and competitions.

In addition to soft-tissue problems, degeneration of bony surface coverings (cartilage), tears in the fibrous tissue surrounding the joint, and loss of bone circulation may occur over time. Extensive forces imposed by weight-bearing and continuous overhead activity decrease circulation to the structures of, in particular, the shoulder (e.g., wheelchair users) and hip (e.g., lower-limb amputees) joints. Surgical decompression is sometimes the only action left to relieve chronic shoulder pain resulting from repetitive strains.

Often reported are scrapes, cuts, bruises, blisters, and floor and wheel burns. Disabled athletes are particularly at risk for accidental injury from incidental contact with the wheelchair, prosthesis, or ground after a fall. Occasionally, friction burns occur owing to inappropriate fitting of the device (wheelchair too wide, prosthesis too small) (see below). If a prosthesis is not fitted correctly and it rubs on the stump, or if the stump sock moves against the stump, then friction occurs. This can cause blistering of the stump and result in several days' loss of training and competition. Particular attention should be given to the problems occurring when the skin is wet (e.g., swimming, rowing, sailing). Athletes sensitive to abrasions and lacerations often wear protective long sleeves or gloves, or strap themselves into their chairs to minimize injuries during falls (e.g., wheelchair-rugby players).

Sensory disorders and skin breakdown

Spinal cord injury, spina bifida, and other nervous-system-related impairments interfere with the normal protection that pressure, temperature, and pain sensations provide. This often goes together with excessive friction related to repetitive movements. The result is pressure sores due to shearing of the superficial tissue over bone, in particular in tissue areas over bony prominences (especially on the buttocks and hips). The blood supply to the skin and underlying tissues is cut off. Athletes vulnerable to pressure sores should (visually) inspect insensitive skin very regularly. Persistent redness, hardening of the skin, or a raised area are first signs of pressure sores and should immediately result in relief of all pressure from sitting, restrictive clothes, or prosthesis fitting until the redness resolves and normal skin color returns. If not treated appropriately, skin breakdown (decubitus ulcer) may progress to serious deep infection in muscle and bone. Caretakers should also be sensitive to any redness or hardened or raised area that has been subjected to sustained pressure. If pressure is not relieved immediately, the area can progress to an open sore (ulcerate decubitus) and result in a serious infection involving skin, muscle, and bone. Customized seating may alleviate pressure, but horizontal rest, mostly lying on the stomach or side, is recommended.

Temperature-regulation disorders

Thermal injuries are common in all Paralympic athletes. Paralysis affects the body's ability to perspire below the site of the lesion, most severely in athletes with high-level lesions. Similarly, owing to the loss of a limb, the ratio of surface area to body volume in amputee athletes is different. Consequently, both paralyzed, as well as amputee, athletes may suffer from overheating.

Athletes with higher lesions (C5 and higher) often also have problems with core body-temperature regulation owing to the loss of normal blood-flow regulation via the central nervous system. This may be compounded by their inability to sweat or shiver below the level of the spinal cord injury. Typically, these athletes wet their own t-shirts or moisten themselves with plant sprinklers. Fans are also a common aid alongside the field of play (e.g., in wheelchair rugby).

Muscle paralysis induces impaired circulation. In addition, blood flow to the skin and deep tissues is relatively low. A sensory deficit also often causes lack of pain sensation, which normally serves as a warning mechanism. As a result, it is easier to sustain both burns and cold injuries (frostbite). In addition, the same circulatory problems slow down and complicate the healing of the wounds afterwards.

Although sunscreens may be a first-hand aid, athletes with more severe dysfunction may have difficulties applying their own protective cream or clothing. And, although sunscreen helps to prevent sunburn, it can also make the athlete susceptible to heat intolerance, as the sunscreen may inhibit and impair cooling, especially in athletes who do not sweat normally.

High temperatures and humidity intensify heat intolerance. Initial symptoms include muscle cramps, whereas more severe heat illness results in heat exhaustion, with similar symptoms as in able-bodied athletes.

Dehydration is underestimated as an important cause of thermoregulatory disorders. Athletes, in particular CP athletes, easily become dehydrated, because the athletes start breathing rapidly and lose water from perspiration. Athletes with high support needs are less able to take fluids during sports participation without assistance, owing to their severe mobility problems. Some athletes may also restrict water intake because of bladder problems (see under 'Bladder dysfunction and urinary tract infections').

Bladder dysfunction and urinary tract infections

Athletes with neurological disorders often have neurogenic bladders, causing inadequate or incomplete bladder emptying. Indwelling catheters or intermittent catheterization may be necessary and, consequently, increase vulnerability to bladder infections, kidney stones, and urinary tract obstruction. Bladder infections often cause pain and increased muscle spasticity, as well as blood-pressure disturbances (see 'Blood-pressure and blood-flow problems'). In a worst-case scenario, i.e., with continued physical activity or sport participation, bladder infection extends to kidney and blood-stream infections, causing severe illness or worse. Many athletes take preventive medication. In case of an acute infection, antibiotic treatment should be initiated, and the athlete should refrain from any activity before body temperature has normalized.

Although infections can be treated, they are best prevented by simple measures. By far the simplest one is to ensure adequate fluid intake to regularly flush out the bladder. Additionally, athletes require clean areas in order to avoid contamination during handling and use of catheters, connecting tubes, and bags.

Blood-pressure and blood-flow problems

Some muscle and joint diseases have associated problems with blood circulation. This can be caused by artery spasm of the hands or feet and may be induced by lower temperatures. Athletes with paralyzed muscles may lack blood return owing to impairment of the muscular pumping action. Edema in the paralyzed limbs is likely to occur, in particular when blood flow is obstructed by tight clothing or straps around the legs or trunk.

Disabled athletes often also experience low blood pressure in hot or humid environments, especially when they are already dehydrated (see also under 'Bladder dysfunction and urinary tract infections'). Athletes are very vulnerable to this hypotension during long opening and closing ceremonies or when they watch peer sports while exposed to full sunshine.

Blood-flow problems also occur when athletes rapidly change position, in particular from lying to sitting or standing. In particular, wheelchair-bound athletes may lack rapid response from the heart and blood vessels to changes in position or movement. Those athletes often may be exposed to orthostatic hypotension, owing to the inability of the sympathetic nervous system to accommodate a rapidly shifting blood volume.

Autonomic dysreflexia

A particular case of high blood pressure in athletes with a disability is autonomic dysreflexia, a reflex syndrome that is unique to individuals with spinal cord injury at lesion levels above T6. This reflex can occur spontaneously, resulting in a

p. van de vliet, p. pit-grosheide, and o. martinez ferrer

sympathetic discharge that elevates the arterial blood pressure and associated cardiovascular responses, which can enhance physical performance. The stimulus usually occurs in an area without sensation and triggers a series of reflexes resulting in abnormally high blood pressure, sweating, goose bumps, and/or flushing of the face and neck. The symptoms mostly go along with headache. Athletes with spinal cord injury who compete in wheelchair sports can also voluntarily induce autonomic dysreflexia prior to, or during, the event in order to enhance their performance. Research has demonstrated that this practice, which is commonly referred to as "boosting" in athletic circles, improves middle-distance wheelchair-racing performance by approximately 10% in elite athletes with quadriplegia. However, autonomic dysreflexia is a medical emergency, as stroke due to elevated blood pressure can occur. As the situation is triggered by a stimulus from a bladder or bowel obstruction, immediate action to empty the bladder or evacuate the bowels is to be taken, together with moving the athlete to a sitting position to reduce blood pressure. A recent study has indicated the need to strengthen awareness and education in this area, as close to 20% of athletes vulnerable to autonomic dysreflexia used the mechanism to voluntarily enhance performance, whereas 40% were not aware of the mechanism at all. Both conditions, however, carry significant risk.

Osteoporosis and fractures

Although fractures are not a common problem and only occur in a few sports (e.g., Alpine skiing), bones in, for example, paralyzed athletes are often thin (osteoporosis) and may fracture from minor injuries. As many disabled athletes lack the sensation that accompanies a bone fracture, any evidence of an abnormal body position, swelling, redness, bruising, or grinding sensations should be further examined through imaging, with the bone stabilized or splinted in the meantime.

Fractures are also likely to occur owing to falls as a consequence of reduced balance. This can be the result of loss of sensation (e.g., incomplete lesions), coordination problems (e.g., CP athletes), loss of proprioception (e.g., prosthesis running), or unforeseen obstacles (e.g., visually impaired athletes).

Other

In the case of tetraplegic athletes, the diaphragm muscle is generally the only respiratory muscle that remains functional. The respiratory function of the muscles of the chest wall is usually paralyzed below the level of the injury. This loss of function affects the ability to cough and thereby clear the respiratory passage. Consequently, respiratory infections are more likely to occur, particularly when the sports activities are performed under less favorable environmental conditions.

Athletes with CP are more likely to have convulsive disorders than their able-bodied peers. Not only is fatigue a major inductor, but CP athletes, similar to athletes with intellectual disability, may induce epilepsy when they become overly distressed. Team physicians, however, should have this status reported on the individual athlete's medical files and should monitor athletes with epilepsy more closely in cool-down periods, as seizures are more likely to occur in this period rather than during the activity itself.

There is some evidence to suggest that there may be an increase in intraocular pressure during activities that can cause pressure increases (e.g., powerlifting, rowing, judo, shot put), in particular in athletes with glaucoma (eye disorder).

PHARMACOLOGY

Whereas team physicians should emphasize injury prevention techniques, pharmacological management of athletes with a disability should not be forgotten. Disabled athletes, in the first instance, are *athletes* and thus bound by the same rules, regulations, and responsibilities as any other athlete under the World Anti-Doping Code. Team physicians in turn have a similar responsibility toward these athletes as they do have toward any other athlete. Disabled athletes often have to be treated with medications owing to their impairment or intensive sports participation, or owing to secondary health problems affiliated with the impairment. This may vary from exercise-induced bronchospasm, through hypo- or hypertension, urinary tract infections, and muscle spasticity, to diabetes mellitus and seizure disorders. Pharmacological literature unfortunately does not offer much relevant information concerning the effects of medication on exercise performance in disabled athletes, and data on medication use in this athlete group are not systematically available.

The personal and financial rewards of modern-day sport can create an unhealthy desire to win at all costs and that also exists in the Paralympic Movement. To gain a competitive advantage, some athletes find their way to so-called ergogenic aids, which enhance sporting performance beyond that attainable through genetic ability and sustained effective training. Ergogenic aids, including pharmacological (e.g., performance-enhancing drugs) and physiological (e.g., blood-doping) supplies, are commonly referred to as "doping." A discussion on pharmacology and medication use in athletes with a disability therefore cannot go without consideration of prohibited substances and prohibited methods and, thus, the need to apply – where relevant – for a therapeutic use exemption (TUE). As with any medical treatment, it is recommended that individuals who may benefit from these medications be treated by a specialist with extensive knowledge of the individual's condition. Periodic review of the individual's status is necessary to ensure that the correct treatments are being administered in the correct doses. It is recognized that, although some of the medications listed can substantially enhance an individual's ability to function on a daily basis with everyday activities, they may simultaneously affect an individual's ability to participate in sports. There is no

p. van de vliet, p. pit-grosheide, and o. martinez ferrer

clear or objective distinction between obtaining an improvement in activities of daily living and obtaining enhanced sports performance. Therefore, it is imperative that the individual and the healthcare provider proceed with the spirit of sport in mind.

Athletes have an increased awareness of the rules and regulations and the particular provisions put in place for disabled athletes with regard to sample collection (WADC International Standard for Testing, Appendix B). This awareness occasionally contrasts with the support these athletes get from coaches and, more importantly and of greater concern, the support from professional support staff. In recent years, the Paralympic Movement has dealt with cases in anti-doping rule-violation management in which, in particular, team or athlete physicians played an important – though unfortunate – role. Ultimately, the athlete is bound by strict liability for any substance found in his/her body, but the above indicates that many cases could have been avoided if proper advice and follow-up had been considered by professionally qualified individuals, whose role it is to support athletes to excel in performance. The most recent WADA production, "Toolkit for physicians," is no doubt a welcome addition to a successful series in this regard.

TRAVEL MANAGEMENT

With the growth of the Paralympic Movement, athletes with exceptionally diverse categories of disability are more frequently traveling great distances to compete on the world stage. In addition to sport-specific training, preparation for travel and maximizing one's ability to arrive at a competition refreshed and ready to perform are essential components of an athlete's success.

Prior to travel, athletes should discuss with the team physician how best to prepare. This includes discussing current medication prescriptions, need for extra prescriptions to bring along in case travel is unexpectedly prolonged or medication is unavailable on site, medications or supplies that may necessitate special arrangements with airline staff (such as medications that will need refrigeration, or insulin syringes that need to be taken on board the plane), medical supplies such as catheters, gloves, and necessary immunizations for the region to which the athlete is traveling. Athletes should also address the level of accessibility of the destination: bed and bathroom, training and competition venues, transportation, etc. This may impact on the need to bring, for example, a slide board or a shower chair. Boarding an aircraft can be stressful and also a potential source of injury for athletes if lifting and handling are performed carelessly. This will require handling agencies to be informed how athletes like to be lifted and to ensure that the athlete controls the procedure.

Team physicians should advise athletes on sleep–wake cycles and adjustment to changes in time zone, maintaining adequate hydration at all times (circulated air inside planes is extremely dry and can cause dehydration in and of itself), medication intake during (long-haul) flights over different time zones, and climate conditions of the place where the next competition takes place (pollution, air quality, temperature).

Upon arrival at the destination, team physicians should assist athletes in conducting a primary health check, including hydration status, leg swelling (increased risk for edema), pressure areas, and skin control.

Often forgotten, but crucial from a health-care perspective, is the fact that all the above also apply for the return journey. Athletes (and support staff) are eager to get home, particularly after long competition periods. Sometimes, in this eagerness, athletes forget about all the good things they did to keep healthy on the return.

EQUIPMENT

Equipment such as prostheses and wheelchairs are fundamental in allowing some people with a disability to carry out the tasks of daily living, as well as to participate in sport. Advances in technology underpin such assistive devices. For example, the development of an energy-storing prosthetic foot can make a lower-limb amputee's gait more efficient and ambulation faster. The application of such technology in a sport environment, however, can be controversial, as demonstrated by the Oscar Pistorius or "Blade Runner" case. With the evolvement of Paralympic sport, athletes have found that standard devices inhibit their sporting performance, and significant new technological developments in, for example, sport-specific wheelchair design and protheses, seated throwing chairs, and adaptive sit skis have revolutionized sports medicine thinking. Ambulatory amputee runners, for instance, have benefited considerably from advances in prosthetic technology, but, besides a question that some of these aids could be considered performance enhancing, no consideration so far has been given to the influence on the stump–socket interface of the prosthesis and the body. This is particularly important owing to the far greater loads on the body in high-intensity sport. As a biological structure, the anatomical stump is influenced by factors such as changes in altitude and local climatic conditions (e.g., humidity), which may impact on the volume of the stump and alter the stump–socket contact points. Also, not-so-obvious compensatory factors require further attention. Amputation in the lower leg alters the orientation of the pelvis, in turn altering the orientation of the vertebral column. This may have far-reaching consequences on the functional ability of the athlete and requires the evaluation of technology in a holistic manner. Similar reasoning applies for wheelchair or sit-ski use. The increase in the mechanical performance of any sports assistive device must always be considered together with the compensatory consequences of disability within the athlete, and it always will remain a challenge to effectively "match" the technology with the athlete's requirements.

226

PSYCHOLOGY

Besides the medical care, team physicians should not forget about the psychological component of disability sport. Research on athletic identity has demonstrated that, although many athletes with a disability view themselves as committed and serious athletes, they typically feel that the public does not view them as legitimate athletes. Limited, or no, access to excellent coaching (too often still an issue in disability sport) means that many athletes still overtrain, train inconsistently in non-sport-specific ways, fail to taper for major competitions, and fail to rest after major performance efforts. The ramifications of an inadequate coaching support system are that athletes may need extra support and (medical) care. This certainly applies when an athlete leaves the sport and transitions back to being an "individual in daily life." Intense commitment to sport, the lack of coaching, and issues of overtraining raise questions as to how the quality of (further) life may be affected in, for example, athletes with chronic pain due to overuse injuries. Knowledge of the disability paradox, coping with a disability, disability stereotypes, and disability culture are just a few salient considerations of value, and physicians may play a major role in facilitating the understanding of the subtle differences between disability and non-disability sports.

COORDINATING MEDICAL SERVICES AT EVENTS

Despite the best planning, accidents do occur. It is, therefore, important that organizers solicit experienced medical personnel and carefully determine emergency contingencies. Prior to the event, medical staff should have information about the common disability-related problems of the competing athletes and orientation regarding the medical services, facilities, policies, and procedures. Nearby hospitals with comprehensive emergency services should be identified and contracted, and consultation with a specialized rehabilitation care centre is advisable. Prosthetists, orthotists, and wheelchair repair specialists should be at hand. Accessible (medical) services will largely facilitate the work for all involved.

It is recommended that the emergency medical teams have experience in extricating athletes from adaptive equipment (e.g., mono-ski shells, ice sledges, racing chairs, hand cycles), or at least familiarize themselves with the adaptive equipment that is in use.

Health-care professionals should hold malpractice and professional-liability insurance coverage and be licensed to practice in the area where the competition is being held. Additionally, the organizers should have adequate liability insurance to cover participants. It is important to note, at this stage, that this insurance policy should not exclude the occurrence of injuries on previously existing injuries or impairments.

Owing to the variety of disability sports, event medical services need to be "tailored" to reflect the needs and demands of a particular sport or discipline.

227

Based on the above, considerations of the particularities of disability sports and athletes with a disability will facilitate the planning and ensure appropriate provisions are put in place. The following should be considered:

- who participates (impairment groups: wheelchair users vs. amputees vs. visual-impaired athletes);
- which (adaptive) equipment will be used;
- where does the activity take place (outdoor vs. sports hall vs. water);
- what are the environmental conditions (winter vs. summer; altitude vs. air quality).

It is recommended that key medical staff attend disability-sport events in preparation for their own event.

ACKNOWLEDGMENT

This chapter could not have been compiled without the expert input provided by the members of the IPC Medical Committee and additional experts on medical care with Paralympic athletes/athletes with a disability.

SUGGESTED READING

Australian Sports Commission (2005). Coaching athletes with disabilities. An Australian resource. www.ausport.gov.au/publications/catalogue/index.asp

Burkett, B. (2010). Technology in paralympic sport: Performance enhancement or essential for performance? *British Journal of Sports Medicine*, 44, 215–20.

Curtis, K.A. (1996). Health smarts: Strategies and solutions for wheelchair athletes. *Sports 'n Spokes*, Sept, 63–68.

Emery, C. and Thompson, W.R. (2012). Paralympic sports medicine – current evidence in winter sport. Thematic issue, *Canadian Journal of Sports Medicine*, in press.

Ferrara, M.S. and Peterson, C.L. (2000). Injuries to athletes with disabilities: Identifying injury patterns. *Sports Medicine*, 30, 137–43.

Krassioukov, A. (2009). Autonomic function following cervical spinal cord injury. *Respiratory Physiology & Neurobiology*, 169: 157–64.

Van de Vliet, P. (2011). Event Medical Care for Paralympic Athletes. In D.O. McDonagh, L.J. Micheli, W.R. Frontera, F. Pigozzi, K. Grimm, C.F. Butler, A.D. Smith, R. Budgett, C. Parisis, and I. Lereim (Eds.), *FIMS Sports Medicine Manual: Event Planning and Emergency Care*. Lippincot Williams & Wilkins.

Vanlandewijck, Y.C. and Thompson, W.R. (2011). *The Paralympic Athlete. Handbook of Sports Medicine and Science*. Wiley-Blackwell.

Webborn, A.D.J. (1999). "Boosting" performance in disability sport. *British Journal of Sports Medicine*, 74–5.

Webborn, A.D.J. (2010). Paralympic Sports. In D.J. Caine, P.A. Harmer, and M.A. Shiff (Eds.), *Epidemiology of Injury in Olympic Sports. The Encyclopedia of Sports Medicine* (475–88). Wiley-Blackwell.

Webborn, N., Willick, S., and Reeser, J.C. (2006). Injuries among disabled athletes during the 2002 winter Paralympic Games. *Medicine and Science in Sports and Exercise*, 38, 811–15.

Williams, R. (2006). *First Aid: A Guide for Adapted Sports Coaches*. Atlanta: The American Association of Adapted Sports Programs.

World Anti-Doping Agency (2011). WADA Sport Physician's Toolkit. www.wada-ama.org/en/Education-Awareness/Tools/For-Sport-Physicians/

CHAPTER 11

FEMALE ATHLETES

S. Talia Alenabi and Angela D. Smith

For a young adult woman, sports opportunities vary markedly, depending on her region, her culture, and the sport. There are still some barriers for women's participation in competitions in some areas and sports, but, despite all these barriers, the number of female participants in athletic events is increasing. For instance, 42% of the athletes in the 2008 Beijing Olympic Games were female. By 2010, only three countries had never sent female athletes to the Olympic Games, and boxing was the only sport that did not include events for women. Considering the increased participation of girls and women in different types of sport and competition, the subject of the "female athlete" has been receiving more attention from the sports medicine community. This chapter will review some findings in this vast area.

ANATOMICAL AND PHYSIOLOGICAL CONSIDERATIONS IN FEMALE ATHLETES

Anatomical considerations

Generally, women are shorter than men, with shorter limbs and smaller articular surfaces. In the lower limb, the proportion of leg length to total height is less than in men. Combining this characteristic with a broader pelvis, women have a lower center of gravity. The greater pelvic width contributes to a greater Q angle in women than in men. The static Q angle is determined by measuring the acute angle produced by the intersection of two lines, the first drawn from the anterior superior iliac spine to the midpoint of the patella and the second line from the midpoint of the patella to the tibial tubercle (Figure 11.1). The volume of the femoral intercondylar notch has been found to be smaller in women compared with in men, and studies have shown that subjects with smaller notches also had smaller anterior cruciate ligaments. These structural differences may relate to the increased likelihood of knee injuries in female athletes compared with men.

In the upper limbs, narrower shoulders and a smaller forearm-to-arm ratio are seen in women, and they may have a larger carrying angle (cubitus valgus).

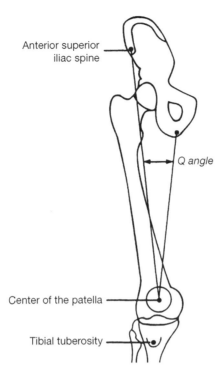

Anterior superior
iliac spine

Q angle

Center of the patella

Tibial tuberosity

Figure 11.1 Q angle
Source: Dr. Micheli, Chapter 23

Idiopathic scoliosis is more prevalent in girls, but it very rarely limits sports participation. Young athletes undergoing brace treatment for scoliosis are generally allowed to train and compete a few hours per day without the brace.

Physiological considerations

Aerobic and anaerobic capacities

The changes of puberty affect the body-fat percentage of females, resulting in an average body-fat percentage in adult women of 23–27%, versus a range of 13–15% in adult men. With intensive training and/or dietary manipulation, female athletes can reduce their body fat to lower levels (for example, 10–12%) but rarely as low as the level in an elite male athlete. After puberty, there is a relatively little muscle mass increase compared with a greater body-fat increase.

The gender differences in VO_2 max are probably mainly related to these body composition differences and to hemoglobin concentration, which is lower in an adult woman. Among women, as with men, running performance is closely related to maximal aerobic power. The slower running times reported for elite female athletes are mainly attributed to their lower VO_2 max. Typically, no difference in VO_2 max is found between similarly trained men and women when VO_2 max is expressed relative to fat-free mass. Iron deficiency is common among women because of iron loss during menses. This further decreases the oxygen-carrying capacity of the blood and decreases performance.

The Wingate test and short repeated sprints have been used to test gender differences in anaerobic performance characterized by peak and mean power outputs. Although previous studies found women achieved approximately 60% of the peak power output of men, more recent studies have shown that, when matched for VO_2 max relative to fat-free mass, the results are very similar. Lower lactate accumulation has been reported by a single Wingate test in one study, but others have shown similar lactate thresholds in male and female endurance athletes.

Strength and endurance training

By age 20 years, the difference in muscle cross-sectional area between young men and young women is considerable. The differences are greater in the upper than the lower extremities. By adulthood, women have 50% of the upper-body muscle size, but about 65–70% of the lower-extremity muscle size of men. When lean body mass and muscle group are taken into consideration, women's upper-body strength is less than men's, regardless of how they are compared, but women's lower-body strength is comparable with that of their male counterparts.

Men and women have little difference in training response to strength training, if the parameters examined are relative increase in strength and muscle size. Women can show muscle hypertrophy with strength training, but the maximum hypertrophy is typically less than for men, without the use of exogenous anabolic steroids. Nonetheless, some studies have shown that the amount of training-induced muscle hypertrophy is similar among men and women who are involved in similar training regimens. It is not yet known if there are gender differences in the optimal training intensity or optimal training frequency for strength training. With regard to endurance training, the trainability of women has been found to be equal to men's.

Thermoregulation

There appear to be significant differences in thermoregulation between men and women. First, women have cyclical changes in core body temperature. During the luteal phase of the menstrual cycle, core body temperature at rest increases by 0.3–0.6°C. Heart rate (HR) and rating of perceived exertion are also higher during prolonged exercise during the luteal phase.

Compared with men, women have a larger ratio of skin surface area to body mass. The increased body fat of women adversely affects their response to heat, but it is advantageous in cold environments. In equal heat, women's core body temperature increases more than men's, both at rest and with exercise. Women sweat less, and they have a higher sweating threshold. However, among women and men of similar

s. talia alenabi and angela d. smith

aerobic capacity, these previous two differences are not apparent. Women are at a disadvantage when exercising in dry heat, compared with men. However, they are at less of a disadvantage when exercising in humid heat, as continued sweating in humid exposure has a greater likelihood of leading to dehydration.

Some cultures require women to wear appropriate garb that covers much of the body during competitions when male spectators are present. Dissipation of heat may become a problem with the greater amount of clothing in these situations. As the team physician makes advance plans for medical treatment in such a cultural situation, an appropriate treatment plan is needed.

SEXUAL MATURATION AND MENSTRUAL CONSIDERATIONS

Limited longitudinal data suggest that young female athletes have similar patterns of timing and progression of development of secondary sex characteristics. Most samples of adolescent athletes have mean ages of menarche within the normal range, but some studies of gymnasts and ballet dancers showed a mean age older than 15. It has been suggested that the delay in menarche may be 5 months for each year of intense training before the onset of puberty. Nonetheless, a strong predictor of age at menarche is the menarcheal age of the athlete's mother and sisters. Low energy availability relative to training energy demands likely plays a part in delayed menarche in these young athletes and performers.

Adult athletes' menstrual dysfunction includes oligomenorrhea (intervals longer than 35 days), secondary amenorrhea (no menstrual cycle in 3 months or more), and luteal phase dysfunction. Secondary amenorrhea is reported frequently among female ballet dancers, gymnasts, distance runners, and cyclists. The percentage of all menstrual irregularities is much higher in these athletes, as well as swimmers, triathletes, and vigorous exercisers, compared with sedentary women. The relationship between athletics and delay in menarche or amenorrhea is confounded by other factors such as genetics, percentage body fat, exercise intensity, age, weight, nutritional deficits, and stress. A widely accepted theory suggests that menstrual irregularity in athletes results from low energy availability due to an imbalance between caloric intake and the energy requirements of intense exercise. A history of previous menstrual problems, positive family history, and chronic illnesses can be additional factors of menstrual dysfunction.

Exercise during menstruation

Although there have been many studies of athletic performance throughout the menstrual cycle, no change in aerobic capacity has been found related to the menstrual phase. Although study findings vary, the best-controlled studies seem to indicate that there is also no change in anaerobic capacity with regard to the menstrual phase. There is not consistent evidence that menstrual phase significantly affects athletic performance or injury occurrence, and so there is no scientific reason to restrict a woman's sport participation at any phase of the menstrual cycle. Studies have also suggested fewer menstrual symptoms such as pain, bleeding, and premenstrual syndrome in regular exercisers.

FEMALE ATHLETE TRIAD

The term "female athlete triad" was first introduced in 1992 to describe an association of amenorrhea, osteoporosis, and disordered eating among female athletes such as gymnasts, ballet dancers, and distance runners. Ongoing research showed that a more appropriate model of this disorder is a spectrum of wellness-to-disease within the three components of the triad: energy availability, menstrual function, and bone mineral density (BMD). Energy availability is the remaining amount of energy relative to lean body mass when exercise-energy expenditure is subtracted from dietary-energy intake. It can be reduced by low caloric intake (restricted diet or bulimic condition) or very-high-energy expenditure (for example, increasing running without a compensatory change in diet). The second component – menstrual dysfunction – includes a spectrum from normal menstrual cycles and oligomenorrhea to amenorrhea. Bone health can range from healthy bones to low BMD or osteoporosis. Because of this wide spectrum of symptoms, it is difficult to estimate the prevalence of the female athlete triad.

No study has shown a direct relationship between athletic performance and fatness. In fact, several studies have shown that there is no such relationship. However, aesthetic issues are often paramount for the athlete, judge, and coach involved. It is clear that severe dieting can decrease performance and can especially affect aerobic capacity. Bone loss may lead to stress fractures that severely limit training. The bone loss may be permanent. Some studies have shown that irreversible bone loss can occur after only 3 years of amenorrhea. Finally, although amenorrhea by itself does not affect thermoregulation, those with anorexia nervosa do typically have abnormal thermoregulation.

We recommend that female athletes, especially those who compete in aesthetic and weight-dependent sports, be routinely screened for disordered eating. For the detection of eating disorders and disordered eating, several validated screening tools exist: the Eating Disorder Examination Questionnaire (EDE-Q), the SCOFF Questionnaire, the Eating Disorder Screen for Primary Care (ESP), or the Eating Attitude Test. Referral and treatment are necessary for those who have disordered eating. For all athletes, even those with apparently normal diets, their energy availability should be evaluated. Detailed assessment of an athlete's calorie intake and daily energy expenditure can prevent the triad's complications. If the athlete is diagnosed with an eating disorder (Table 11.1), then psychologist referral is indicated.

Any athlete with abnormal menses should receive a comprehensive evaluation. History and physical examination are very important, and the evaluation should investigate the positive findings of congenital anomalies, short stature, galactorrhea,

Table 11.1 DSM IV-TR criteria for eating disorders

Anorexia nervosa	• Refusal to maintain body weight at or above minimally normal weight for age and height (e.g. < 85% of that expected) • Intense fear of gaining weight or becoming fat • Disturbance in the way in which one's body weight or shape is experienced • The absence of at least 3 consecutive menstrual cycles

Bulimia nervosa	• Recurrent episodes of binge eating:
	  – eating in a discrete period of time (2-hour period)
	  – a sense of lack of control over eating during the episode
	• Recurrent inappropriate compensatory behavior
	• Binge eating and compensatory behavior occur at least twice a week for 3 months
	• Self-evaluation is unduly influenced by body shape and weight
	• The disturbance does not occur during episodes of anorexia nervosa

Eating disorder not otherwise specified (EDNOS)	• All of the criteria for anorexia nervosa except:
	  – amenorrhea
	  – despite significant weight loss, the individual's weight is in the normal range
	• All of the criteria for bulimia nervosa except:
	  – binge eating and inappropriate compensatory behaviors occur less than twice a week or for a duration of less than 3 months
	  – inappropriate compensatory behaviors may occur after eating small amounts of food

virilization, and hypoestrogenemia, in young athletes, and other endocrine findings or disorders in adult female athletes. A pregnancy test should be the first laboratory evaluation. Characteristically, patients with functional hypothalamic amenorrhea related to the female athlete triad will demonstrate a low FSH level and very low LH and estradiol levels and may not have a withdrawal bleed to a progesterone challenge. However, they also could have normal FSH and LH levels and may indeed have a withdrawal bleed to hormones.

A DEXA scan has been used as a diagnostic tool for the evaluation of bone health and particularly low BMD. In adolescents and premenopausal women, a Z-score, or a comparison with age-matched controls, is commonly reported. The estrogen-deficient state has a detrimental effect on BMD, but the effect varies at different stages of a woman's development and is compounded by the nutritional compromise seen in the triad. A Z-score below −2.0 in premenopausal women is reported as "low bone density," but a Z-score less than −1.0 in an athlete requires evaluation. Athletes with recurrent stress fractures, prolonged amenorrhea

(> 6 months), and frequent phases of oligomenorrhea should be screened with at least a baseline DEXA, keeping in mind that normal athletes, particularly those participating in weight-bearing sports, generally have BMD measurements 12–15% higher than those of sedentary women.

The best treatment is prevention, or at least early detection before these disorders become chronic. Screening for disordered eating can be conducted at the pre-participation physical evaluation, along with evaluation for stress fractures, recurrent illness or injury, menstrual changes, cardiac arrhythmias, and depression. The history and physical examination of the female athlete should address each component of the female athlete triad. If one component of the triad is present, it is essential to look further for the others. After careful evaluation, if the menstrual dysfunction of an athlete is related to her intense exercise patterns and low energy availability, advice should be given to decrease exercise intensity and increase nutritional intake. Increases in BMD occurring with return of menses and weight gain are often more significant than those achieved by pharmacologic means. It appears that more than 45 kcal/kg of lean body mass per day may be required to actually increase BMD. Women who restrict their caloric intake often have inadequate intake of protein, vitamins, and minerals. They may require supplementation, particularly of B vitamins, folate, and iron, for general health purposes. Protein intake of at least 1 g/kg of body weight, calcium at 1,000–1,500 mg/day, and vitamin D at 400–800 IU/day are all recommended.

Overall, the benefits of sport for women far outweigh the risks of the triad. In fact, athletes such as gymnasts and figure skaters, even when amenorrheic, have been found to have greater bone mass in the bones that are impact-loaded than sedentary controls or even other athletes, such as runners and swimmers. Amenorrheic and eumenorrheic gymnasts have stronger upper-extremity bones than controls or other athletes, and figure skaters have stronger lower-extremity bones and pelvis, even skaters not menstruating regularly. Educational programs for athletes and coaches focused on prevention of the female athlete triad are recommended to decrease the incidence of health concerns, to maximize athletic performance, and to ensure that female athletes enjoy the benefits of sport participation.

GENDER VERIFICATION

Sex testing was officially mandated by the IOC in 1968 and continued until 1999, when the IOC announced the ending of the process of gender verification during the Olympic Games. The right to test individual cases is still held by this organization. The reason was to prevent masquerading males and women with "unfair, male-like" physical advantage from competing in female-only events. However, gender verification has long been criticized by geneticists, endo-crinologists, and others in the medical community, owing to the combination of invalid screening tests, failure to understand the problem of intersex individuals, and discrimination and emotional trauma to female athletes. Disorders of sexual development may be chromosomal, gonadal, or phenotypic in origin. We just mention a few causes in this chapter.

Androgen insensitivity (testicular feminization) is one of the causes of sex-verification problems, especially when the verification is based on sex chromosome or androgen level. These individuals are genetically male 46 XY, with a complete lack of androgen receptor function and, hence, female phenotype. The external genitalia develop in a female direction, the uterus is absent, and they present with primary amenorrhea. They may have little or no pubic hair, but normal breast development owing to secretion of estrogen from their testes. These XY females are taller than average women. Normal-sized testes are usually found in the pelvis or at the inguinal ring. Most commonly, androgen insensitivity is complete, but partial sensitivity may be present in about 10% of patients. The testosterone levels are those of a normal male. These women's testes should be removed at the age of 20 because of a high risk of testicular cancer.

Female pseudohermaphroditism occurs in 46 XX women who have bilateral ovaries but variable virilization of the urogenital tract because of androgen excess during fetal life. This usually is associated with congenital adrenal hyperplasia (CAH; most commonly 21-hydroxylase deficiency), developmental disorders of müllerian ducts, or other non-adrenal enzymatic deficiencies. In mixed gonadal dysgenesis, affected individuals usually have a testis on one side and a streak gonad on the other. The phenotype varies depending on the proportion of XY cells and their distribution. Most of these individuals are raised as females. Despite hyperandro-genism (non-pharmacologic), according to the new recommendations, a legally eligible female athlete can compete in female competitions, provided that she has androgen levels below the male range (as shown by the serum concentration of testosterone), or, if within the male range, she has an androgen resistance such that she derives no competitive advantage from such levels.

New rules also permit transsexual athletes to compete in the Olympic Games after having completed sex reassignment surgery, being legally recognized as a member of the sex they wish to compete as, and having undergone 2 years of hormonal therapy (unless they transitioned before puberty).

IRON DEFICIENCY IN FEMALE ATHLETES

Several studies found greater prevalence of iron deficiency anemia in female athletes than the general population. Compared with male athletes, fertile female athletes have a disadvantage of blood loss due to menstruation, and have lower dietary intake of iron. Moreover, intense physical activity has the potential to worsen their hematologic profile. Therefore, it is reasonable to consider performing routine hematological assessment during a pre-participation examination for female athletes. Low-dose iron supplements under medical and dietary supervision may sometimes help to prevent a decline in iron status during training.

INJURY PATTERNS

Although many of the sports injuries faced by the female athlete affect the male athlete as well, some occur exclusively, or more commonly, in women. Sports injuries are discussed in other chapters, and in this chapter a few injuries that typically affect female athletes disproportionately are reviewed.

Patellofemoral pain syndrome

According to some reports, adolescent females and young adult women are affected 2–10 times more often with patellofemoral pain (PFP) than their male counterparts. Their wider pelvis and greater knee valgus may cause more patellofemoral dysfunction (Figure 11.2). Shortened quadriceps muscles, an altered vastus medialis obliquus muscle reflex response time, decreased explosive strength and jumping power, and a hypermobile patella have been shown to be significantly related to the incidence of PFP. A recent study found that high-school cross-country runners with abnormal frontal plane static alignments (Q-angle measurements of 20° or more) were more likely to miss practice or competition because of knee problems. PFP often limits participation in recreational and sports activities. The vast majority of cases of patellofemoral dysfunction in athletes can be controlled with exercise programs that stretch any tight muscles that cross the knee joint and strengthen the quadriceps (particularly the vastus medialis), combined with correction of other biomechanical problems – such as excessive pronation and weak hip abductors and external rotators – when present.

Non-contact ACL injuries

There is a greater incidence of ACL injury among female athletes than male. This may be a result of anatomical, biomechanical, strength, and/or hormonal differences. Although studies have found anatomical differences of bone contour between male and female knees, these differences probably contribute little to the increased rate of ACL injuries in female athletes. Studies of hormone levels have found varying results related to the likelihood of ACL injury. Female athletes have a decreased quadriceps-to-hamstring-strength ratio and a shorter time to peak hamstring torque than male athletes. The effective quadriceps–hamstrings force mismatch has been showed to contribute to ACL tears. Female basketball athletes tend to land with knees less flexed than male athletes, more flat-footed, and less on the balls of their feet. Early studies of female basketball players who altered their technique, to include greater knee flexion, softer jump landings, and keeping their weight over their toes with sudden decelerations and with jump landings, found decreased incidence of ACL injury. More recent training programs designed to improve proprioception and balance and alter landing and deceleration positions and patterns may decrease ACL injury among female athletes, but more studies of larger athlete populations are needed to test this hypothesis further.

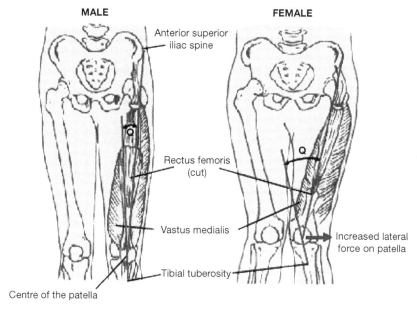

MALE   FEMALE

Anterior superior iliac spine

Rectus femoris (cut)

Q

Vastus medialis

Increased lateral force on patella

Tibial tuberosity

Centre of the patella

Figure 11.2 Patellofemoral position
Source: Google image

Stress fractures

Multiple studies in both male and female athletes have found that females sustain a higher incidence of stress fractures. Male and female stress-fracture distributions are typically similar for similar activities, such as long-distance running or military activities, with common sites at the tibia, metatarsals, femur, and calcaneus, but pelvis fractures occur more often among females. The etiology of stress fractures is multifactorial. A higher injury rate In female athletes has been attributed to lower aerobic capacity, reduced muscle mass, lower BMD, narrow tibia, wide pelvis, low BMI, and inadequate energy, calcium, and vitamin D intake. Female athletes with normal weight and bone health are less likely to develop stress fractures, showing that gender itself might be less important than overall physical conditioning.

Forefoot disorders

Hallux valgus is a common disorder of the forefoot that results from medial deviation of the first metatarsal and lateral deviation and/or rotation of the great toe, with or without medial soft-tissue enlargement of the first metatarsal head (bunion). The female–male ratio has been reported as 9:1, which is likely due to both biomechanics (joint laxity/instability) and types of shoe wear. The presence of an asymptomatic hallux valgus deformity in the athlete does not warrant treatment.

Morton's neuroma is a mechanical entrapment neuropathy of the interdigital nerve. Related pain occurs during the toe-off phase of running or during repetitive positions of toe rise. Like bunions, this problem is nine times more common in females. Symptoms are exacerbated by poorly fitting, narrow shoes that compress the forefoot. Poor shoe selection for training and sport may increase the impact forces on the forefoot and contribute to neuroma symptoms. High-heeled shoes increase forefoot pressure and will also exacerbate symptoms of interdigital neuroma (see Chapter 20).

Breast trauma

Many women with larger breasts prefer to wear a sports bra that decreases breast motion, or even two or more supportive/compressive bras, layered, for comfort. For some contact and collision sports, breast padding is appropriate to prevent trauma to the breast. The nipple is the most prominent and most commonly injured part of the breast. For both women and men, repetitive vigorous abrasion or cold-induced thermal injury of the nipple may lead to bloody discharge and concern about possible breast cancer. Prophylactic measures include application of plastic bandages and/or petroleum jelly over the nipples before exercise.

PREGNANCY AND EXERCISE

A great deal of work has been done in the past decade with regard to physical activity and sport participation during pregnancy. Many of the concerns related to exercise during pregnancy focus on the safety of the fetus rather than the athlete herself. It now appears that regular exercise during pregnancy actually enhances maternal fitness, without apparent risk to either the mother or the fetus. Regular exercise before and during pregnancy seems to enhance a pregnant woman's physiologic reserve. Premature labor occurs equally frequently in women who do and do not exercise.

Special attention needs to be paid to certain safety principles during exercise in pregnancy. In particular, the pregnant woman needs to pay special attention to appropriate nutrition, hydration, and rest. It is recommended that exercise bouts not occur until at least 3 hours after eating, and that the exercise be followed with a snack. As a reflection of hydration status, weight loss during a single exercise session should be no more than 1 kg.

The pregnant woman should avoid exercising in extremely hot and humid environments. She should avoid high-intensity activities that may lead to hyperthermia, which is a significant concern during pregnancy. First-trimester hyperthermia may be teratogenic. Clapp suggests that a pregnant woman's rectal temperature should not rise by more than 1.5–1.8°C and should not exceed 38.7°C on a regular basis or for a prolonged period of time. According to Clapp, the commonly accepted teratogenic level is 39.2°C. Exercising in water may help thermoregulation by dissipating heat.

Some elite athletes want to maintain a high level of performance throughout pregnancy. One of the concerns of a pregnant female athlete is that, by reducing her training during pregnancy, she will lose a significant amount of aerobic fitness and her VO_2max will decline. However, most studies do not support this concern. More vigorous exercise is regarded as safe for women who are well trained before the pregnancy. Actually, a woman's aerobic fitness will decline very little if she continues to exercise as her pregnancy-related symptoms permit. Regarding strenuous exercise, it has been suggested that exercise intensity should not exceed 90% of maximal maternal HR, as there may be simultaneous reduction in uterine blood flow. There is little research on the interaction between pregnancy and physiologic responses to resistance training. One study noticed fetal HR accelerations during resistance training performed in the seated position, but occasional, brief HR decelerations in the supine position. Therefore, pregnant athletes should be prudent and avoid supine exercises during their workouts and choose alternate positions that work the same muscle groups.

During pregnancy, a woman who is participating in sports or an exercise program should modify her training program if she has musculoskeletal discomfort or other uncomfortable symptoms. Musculoskeletal problems in the physically active pregnant woman are related to weight gain, ligamentous relaxation, lumbar lordosis, and change in the center of gravity. The pregnant woman should also consider modifying or avoiding exercise with risk of blunt abdominal trauma. She should avoid activities done at high altitude (such as mountain climbing) or in deep water (such as scuba diving). Although athletes can perform many activities safely and effectively during pregnancy, this is not the time to focus on "extreme sports" competitions. Finally, the exercising pregnant woman should monitor her training intensity carefully. She may do this by monitoring her rating of perceived exertion. In addition, fatigue or poor performance may indicate that she is overtraining.

CONCLUSION

As more girls and women take advantage of greater sports opportunities, researchers have increasingly investigated their physiology, training, and injury patterns. Despite earlier concerns that sports participation might harm women's health and reproductive capacity, sports and physical activity have been shown to enhance a woman's overall health. As long as she practices moderation in training, a sportswoman's pregnancy and fetal health are not endangered, and delivery may even be enhanced.

Not surprisingly, differences have been found between athletic men and women. Women's body proportions, body composition, upper-body strength, flexibility, and injury patterns differ from those of men. However, despite their very different hormonal profiles, women can increase aerobic capacity, strength, and physical performance through training (though generally to a lesser extent than similarly trained men). Trained women typically find marked improvements in strength, for

241

example, even when muscle hypertrophy is considerably less than a similarly strength-trained man would gain.

The greater incidence of patellofemoral pain among girls and women is likely related to anatomic differences from men, but optimized hip and leg strength and flexibility can treat, and may prevent, patellofemoral pain. The markedly increased incidence of ACL injuries – especially among women in jumping/pivoting sports – may be multifactorial, but strength and neuromuscular training programs that alter landing, pivoting, and deceleration patterns show promise in preventing these injuries. The increased incidence of stress fractures found among female military recruits compared with their male counterparts may be caused by less adequate previous training. In sports, stress fractures among girls and women have been related to inadequate nutrition and/or abnormal hormonal profile, as in the female athlete triad. This is one area of greater study of women than of men, even though male athletes have been found to have similar problems of interrelated inadequate energy intake, abnormal hormonal profile, and poor bone health.

Especially at this time of increasing obesity incidence throughout much of the world, girls and women should be encouraged to be physically active. Sports provide many opportunities for physical activity for the twenty-first-century woman. For women as for men, the potential benefits far outweigh the risks discussed here.

ACKNOWLEDGMENT

The editors acknowledge the assistance of Wendy Holdan, MSPT, of Boston Children's Hospital, for contributing to, and reviewing, this chapter.

SUGGESTED READING

Alleyne J.K., Exercise and pregnancy. Position Stand of Canadian Association of Sport Medicine, 2008; www.sirc.ca/newsletters/may08/documents/PregnancyPositionPaper.pdf
Clapp J., Exercising Through Your Pregnancy. Champaign, IL: Human Kinetics, 2002.
Loud K., Micheli L., Common athletic injuries in adolescent girls, Current Opinion in Pediatrics Issue 2001; 13(4) (August): 317–22.
Renström P., et. al., Non-contact ACL injuries in female athletes: An International Olympic Committee current concepts statement, Br. J. Sports Med. 2008; 42: 394–41.
Witkop C., Warren M., Understanding the spectrum of the female athlete triad, Obstetrics & Gynecology 2010; 116(6) (December): 1444–8.

 s. talia alenabi and angela d. smith

CHAPTER 12

THE MASTERS, OLDER, AND SENIOR ATHLETES

Julia Alleyne and Neil Dilworth

INTRODUCTION

Over the last decade of sport science research, we have witnessed the emergence of evidence that challenges our traditional perception of aging and exercise. We have often assumed that, with age, our bodies will lose strength, our energy will be reduced, and new-skill acquisition will be difficult. Yet, we are actually finding that active seniors can participate in training and sport well into their ninth decade and compete in the seventh and eighth decades. The limits to strength, stamina, and skill are being tested continually, and the boundaries reset by experience, training, and research.

The World Health Organization estimates that the number of people over 65 years of age will reach 1 billion by 2030 and comprise 15% of the population. This is a significant sector of our patients with imperative needs for exercise as treatment for chronic disease, maintenance of function, and increasing recreational purpose. It is hard to define the older athlete in strict terms of age, hours of exercise, or level of competition. The "masters" athlete is often defined as an athlete who maintains a high level of training and participates in competition, although the initial entry categories vary from 35 to 50 years of age, and competition can carry on to any age, as long as function is maintained as competitive. The emphasis is on the stage of the athlete versus the age of the athlete. The "senior" athlete is often defined by age, with 55 or 65 years being the commonest entry levels, and 10-year categories separate the age groups. The "older" athlete is a more recent term, used to define the athletic stage as being one that is associated with age-related changes that require training and/or competition modifications, but where there is no imposed limit on participation due to age.

As a team physician, it is important to understand older athletes in the context of their physiological changes related to aging, such as cardiovascular capacity, their musculoskeletal system changes, including strength and flexibility, and degenerative conditions, as well as the effect that exercise may have on concurrent medical conditions.

MEDICAL CONDITIONS AND TRAINING

It is important to understand that with age comes the increased incidence of medical conditions that affect circulation, endurance, joint mobility, and strength.

Atherosclerotic disease increases with age, and it is well known that exercise can trigger sudden death and myocardial infarction (MI). The incidence of an exercise-related cardiac event in those with coronary artery disease (CAD) is approximately 10 times higher than that of a healthy adult. As an example, it has been estimated that 1 in 15,000 joggers will die from sudden cardiac causes yearly (Maron et al., 2001). With this in mind, it is recommended that all masters competitions have automatic external defibrillators (AEDs) and persons present who are trained to perform CPR and use AEDs. Finally, it is important that physicians use the opportunity to educate masters and senior athletes on the signs and symptoms of angina and myocardial infarction. Cardiovascular diseases can be impacted by metabolic disease such as diabetes mellitus, which can lead to dysfunction in neuromuscular physiology, compromised renal function, and increased lipid profiles, adding to the barriers to exercise.

Degenerative joint disease is common with aging and can lead to reduced joint mobility and increased instability, secondary to recurrent effusions and inactivity. It is important for exercise regimes to be modified so that the quality of streng-thening and stretching is preserved, without an excessive quantity of repetition that might exacerbate joint irritation. When a joint is swollen, painful at night, or warm to touch, it is advised that exercise should be reduced or avoided. Degen-erative joint disease most commonly affects the knee, hip, spine, and shoulders. Cross-training in water or with low-impact machines such as bicycles can be beneficial to avoid exacerbation.

Respiratory conditions can impact exercise tolerance if there is a restrictive pattern, as seen with emphysema or chronic obstructive pulmonary disease. Exercise toler-ance needs to be reduced to ensure that overload to the lungs and heart is not experienced. However, a low, progressive level of exercise, such as walking and cycling, can be beneficial treatment. Warning symptoms may include difficulty with resuming normal breathing after exercise, painful or prolonged shortness of breath, or inability to speak a phrase during exercise.

SCREENING FOR PARTICIPATION

The major concern in pre-participation screening of older athletes involves cardiovascular disease and the risk of death. The cardiovascular system affects the health of many body systems, and a focus on both primary and secondary factors provides the best approach to screening. Therefore, pre-participation screening should include a thorough history, physical examination, and pertinent investigations.

Table 12.1 Summary of pre-participation evaluation

System	History	Examination	Investigations
Cardiovascular	Fatigue Exertional dyspnea Exertional chest pain Smoking Positive family history of sudden death	Murmurs Hypertension Jugular venous pressure (JVP) Decreased peripheral capillary filling Femoral pulses	Lipid profile EKG Exercise test
Metabolic	Presence of diabetes	Weight Body mass index Waist–hip ratio	Fasting blood glucose Hemoglobin A1C Insulin sensitivity
Respiratory	Smoking Persistent cough Exertional dyspnea Exertional wheeze	Breath sounds Chest expansion Rapid exhalation time	VO_2 max test Optional chest X-ray

Table 12.2 Summary of exercise stress testing with ECG recommendations

Masters athletes (sex and age)	Without CAD risk factors	CAD risk factors
Males > 40	No	Yes
Females > 50	No	Yes
Both > 65	Yes	Yes

CONTRAINDICATIONS TO MASTERS ATHLETES PARTICIPATING IN HIGH-INTENSITY SPORTS

High-intensity sports are defined as those requiring a VO_2 max greater than 70%, moderate-intensity sports require 40–70% of VO_2 max, and low-intensity sports require less than 40% of VO_2 max.

The following conditions are contraindications to masters athletes participating in high-intensity sports:

1. CAD with greater than 50% blockage (may compete in low-intensity sports such as bowling, curling, golf, etc.);
2. left ventricular ejection fraction less than 50%;

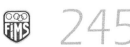

3. evidence of exercise-induced MI;
4. evidence of exercise-induced frequent or complex supraventricular or ventricular arrhythmias;
5. exercise-induced systolic hypotension;
6. moderate-to-severe systemic hypertension (systolic > 160 mmHg; diastolic > 100 mmHg); these athletes should be restricted from highly static competitive sports, such as weight lifting, until BP is controlled;
7. unequivocal diagnosis of hypertrophic cardiomyopathy (HCM).

Athletes with known mitral valve prolapse (MVP) who have no complicating factors may participate in sports. However, if a masters athlete has known MVP, participation may be contraindicated if it is associated with a history of syncope, a family history of sudden death secondary to MVP, repetitive supraventricular tachycardia (SVT) or complex ventricular tachyarrythmias, moderate-to-severe mitral regurgitation, and/or a prior embolic event.

Another cardiac condition that may be encountered by the team physician is myocarditis. Masters athletes may return to competition when there is no longer evidence of active infection, and they have had normal Holter or exercise tests.

Finally, a mention should be made of Chagas disease, common in South America. It is estimated that 5% of Brazilians are infected. If chronic myocarditis or an apical aneurysm is present, intense competition is contraindicated. However, if there is no evidence of cardiac involvement, participation may be unrestricted.

AGING AND THE MUSCULOSKELETAL SYSTEM

After age 35, we lose 1.25% of our muscle mass per year, and, after age 70, this decline often accelerates. This loss is primarily due to a decrease in the fast-twitch (Type II) fibers, in both quantity and quality. The cross-sectional ratio is decreased between Type I and Type II fibers, from 1:1 to 1:2. In addition to a volume change, the remaining Type II fibers are not as quick to reach their contractile peak strength with effort. This age-associated loss of muscle mass is characterized by muscle fibers being replaced by fat and fibrosis, a process called sacropenia. This process may be compounded by medical conditions that affect glucose metabolism (diabetes), cardiovascular circulation (peripheral vascular disease), and neuromuscular disorders affecting balance and strength.

A decrease in joint mobility, along with muscular and tendon flexibility, also contributes to the decline in performances in masters athletes. For example, compared with their younger counterparts aged 19–40, sprinters aged between 60 and 85 years had an approximately 40% shorter stride (Forsberg et al., 1991), which means that they have to take more steps to reach the same distance. There is low-level evidence that range-of-motion exercises can be beneficial. Therefore, the key to the success of a masters athlete is minimizing these physiological changes that occur

julia alleyne and neil dilworth

with age. When motivated, and with regular training, they can potentiate their cardiovascular performance, muscular strength, and range of motion.

TRAINING PRINCIPLES

The declines in VO_2 max, maximum HR, muscle mass, bone density, and flexibility all affect the overall performance of the masters athlete. Although it is impossible to stop these changes altogether, it has been shown through various studies that regular training can actually attenuate these decreases. Maximum aerobic capacity is estimated to decline by approximately 10% per decade after the age of 25. Studies following men over 20 years have shown a total decline to be 12% over a 20-year period and a decrease to 5.5% per decade compared with the predicted decline with high-intensity training. The same 20-year prospective study of masters athletes showed a maximum HR decrease with high-intensity training of 13 beats per minute (bpm) v. 20 bpm in the predicted population, and also showed 11 bpm higher maximum HR than predicted at age 65.

It has been postulated that muscle loss is more consistent with disuse and training type rather than an age-related decline. Several studies have shown an increase in Type II fibers, with intense exercise and endurance training maintaining muscle mass. Therefore, the decline in muscle loss appears to be related to a decline in training intensity. Muscular decline is accompanied with a decrease in bone mineral density (BMD). An estimated 0.5% loss of bone density per year occurs after the age of 40 in men, with a 3–5% loss in post-menopausal women. A study of male endurance runners showed an attenuation of BMD scores over a 5-year period. Among senior athletes surveyed and tested at a national seniors games, those involved in high-impact sports versus those involved in other sports demonstrated a positive 3% variance in BMD.

Table 12.3 Summary of physiological changes with average population aging

Physiological factor	Decrease
VO_2 max	10% per decade
Maximum heart rate	1.0 bpm/year
Muscular power	3.8% per year (Tanaka and Seals, 2003)
Bone loss (BMD)	0.5% per year in men after 40 years of age
	3–5% per year in post menopausal women
Flexibility	40% reduction in stride

Exercise prescription

Training regimens should be personalized and tailored to the individual athletes to meet their needs and goals and should include endurance, resistance, and flexibility regimes.

Endurance training

High-intensity interval training has been shown to result in up to a 25% increase in VO$_2$ max. To help improve VO$_2$ max and maximum HR, as well as to provide high-impact exercise to promote positive bone effects, endurance training is recommended. Athletes should be endurance training 3–5 days per week. The intensity of this training should range from 40 to 80% of maximum oxygen uptake reserve, or 55 to 90% of maximum HR, depending on the duration and type of exercise. The time and duration depend on the athlete's level of training, but should range from a minimum of 20 minutes to more than 60 minutes and can be continuous or in intervals. Generally speaking, the types of exercise for endurance training should be using as many large muscle groups as possible. Examples include running, walking, swimming, and elliptical training.

Table 12.4 Summary of training principles (Chodzko-Zajko et al., 2009)

Endurance training	
Frequency	3–5 days per week
Intensity	40–85% of maximum oxygen uptake reserve 55–90% of maximum HR
Time/duration	20–60 minutes continuous or intervals/intermittent
Type	Running, elliptical, swimming, walking
Resistance training	
Frequency	2–3 days per week
Intensity	Multiple sets, 8–12 repetitions (reps) to volitional fatigue If > 50–60 years of age, 10–15 reps

Time/duration	Sets:
	    One for high intensity (< 6 reps)
	    Two for moderate intensity (8–15 reps)
	    Three for low intensity (> 15 reps)

Type	Generally 8–10 exercises that work the main muscle groups in upper and lower body
Flexibility training	
Frequency	2–3 days per week
Intensity	Stretching sensation without pain
Time/duration	15–30 seconds static stretching
Type	Major muscle and tendon groups

Resistance training

Resistance training is recommended to help maintain muscular strength and Type II muscle fibers. Masters athletes should be doing weight-resistance exercises two to three times per week for best results. The athlete is aiming to use resistance that results in the muscles reaching volitional fatigue at between 8 and 12 repetitions (moderate intensity). For greater gains, or maintenance of muscle strength, an athlete may increase the resistance where muscle fatigue occurs after only 6 repetitions. In athletes over the age of 50–60, lower-intensity exercises are recommended with higher repetitions (e.g., 15). Generally, between 8 and 10 weight-resistance exercises can be used by the athlete to target the large muscle groups in the upper and lower body.

Flexibility

There is low-level evidence that flexibility could also have beneficial effects for the aging athlete. The recommendations are that athletes partake in flexibility training 2 or 3 days per week. The large muscle and tendon groups are targeted once again, with static exercises for four repetitions of approximately 15–30 seconds with breathing.

Finally, motivation for continual training is essential for the compliance of a masters athlete with a training regime. Motivational factors include the personal-health benefits of training, the effect on longevity of life, and quality of life. Other motivational factors involve setting specific goals for training, as well as competition and signing up for competitions so as to have a timeline.

PERFORMANCE AND COMPETITION PREPARATION

Masters and senior athletes also differ from their younger counterparts in their dietary requirements for training and competing. The effects of age on human physiology involve changes in energy requirements and decreases in lean body mass and training volume. The Institute of Medicine's Food and Nutrition board has the following dietary reference intake (DRI) values for diet: 45–60% carbohydrates, 10–35% protein, and 20–35% fat.

Carbohydrates

For competitors in training, carbohydrate intake should be in the range 5–7 g/kg/day for moderate-intensity exercise of less than1 hour per day. Athletes with higher training loads should aim for 7–10g/kg/day of carbohydrates. Regular activity has been demonstrated to maintain the body's ability to store carbohydrates as glycogen in the liver and muscles of the aging athlete. Whole grains are an ideal source of carbohydrate and should be taken with water or fluids for optimal glycogen storage. There is evidence for using energy drinks containing 6–8% carbohydrates during competition lasting less than an hour, and this is ideally consumed every 15–20 minutes during the competition.

Fat

Fat intake should consist of healthier monounsaturated and polyunsaturated sources. Fat sources should include 14 g/day of Omega-6 fatty acids for older men and 11 g/day for older women. Omega-3 fatty acid intakes of 1.6 g and 1.1 g/day are recommended for men and women, respectively.

Protein

Protein intake should be 1.2 g/kg/day, which is greater than the usual recommended adult intake of 0.8 g/kg/day. Proteins can be in the form of lean meat, dairy, soy, eggs, or nuts.

Fluids

There are some general recommendations regarding hydration prior to competition or training, and the first involves using the athlete's urine as a guide. The two aspects of urine that can be easily assessed are the amount and color. Athletes should try to hydrate prior to events or training to pale-colored urine. However, if they notice their urine is dark and/or they aren't producing urine, they should hydrate more. Older athletes with reduced renal function must be particularly careful about their hydration balance.

Table 12.5 Summary of performance and competition preparation

Intake	Recommended amounts	When
Carbohydrate		
– Low–moderate intensity	5–7 g/kg/day	Through day up until 2–4 hours prior to competition
– High intensity	7–10 g/kg/day	
– In competition < 1 hour	6–8% carb energy drink	At leisure through event
– In competition > 1 hour	30–60 g/hour*	Every 15–20 min during exercise
Fat		
– Omega 6	11(♀)–14 g(♂)/day	Through day up until 2–4 hours prior to competition
– Omega 3	1.1(♀)–1.6 g(♂)/day	
Protein	1.0–1.2 g/kg/day	Through day up until 2–4 hours prior to competition
Fluids		
– Pretraining/competition	5–7 ml/kg	2–4 hours prior to training
– During training	4–800 ml/hour at leisure	Per hour during training

Note: * May obtain from an energy drink containing 6–8% carbohydrate.

julia alleyne and neil dilworth

During training and competition, fluid replacement during exercise is more complicated, as it is highly dependent on the event/training type, equivalent sweat rates, temperature at event, and, finally, the individual athlete. For longer-duration events of greater than 1 hour, it is recommended that individual athletes drink, at their leisure, between 400 and 800 ml/hour.

RECOVERY STRATEGIES

The focus for recovery strategies is on recommended nutrition and fluids. The timing of nutrient and fluid intake post exercise is essential to the athlete's recovery and maintenance of muscle gains from training, as well as to any potential gains. There are several changes that occur during exercise, including depletion of muscle glycogen stores, an increase in oxidative stress markers, and fat and protein losses. The best results are seen when the nutrients and fluids are taken as close to the conclusion of training as possible. The post-exercise meal should include carbohydrate for glycogen resynthesis. One study showed results with a mixture of 10 g protein, 7 g carbohydrate, and 3 g fat. Other studies have shown no further benefit with protein intake in relation to glycogen resynthesis, when post-exercise carbohydrate intake has been sufficient. However post-training protein intake may aid body-protein repair (Rodriguez et al., 2009). When taken by elderly adults participating in resistance training immediately after exercise, compared with after a 2-hour delay, the results were greater muscle mass and strength changes. As well as energy losses, there have been marked increases in antioxidant defense-system markers post-endurance competitions for up to 48 hours after competition.

Similar to younger competitors, masters athletes are competing to find the edge either to give them that extra gain or maintain their performance in competition. Striegel et al. (2006) conducted a survey of 598 participants in the 2004 World Masters Athletics Championships Indoors on supplement consumption. The commonest supplements used were vitamins, at 35.4%, followed by minerals, 29.9%, then proteins, 10.6%, and creatine, 6.5%.

In general, vitamin supplements are not required if athletes are eating adequately; however, if they are restricting certain food types, they may indeed need to supplement with the diet-deficient vitamins. There has been some evidence to recommend creatine monohydrate (CM), mainly for sports requiring higher maximal voluntary contractions, such as weight lifting. High-level evidence from three large, randomized control trials showed that there is an increase in fat-free mass and strength when using CM in conjunction with resistance training. The recommended amount of CM is 5 g/day. There may be no further benefit outside of 6 months or with endurance sports. There is little evidence to support the adverse effects of CM on the kidneys; however, it should probably be avoided in patients with reduced renal function until further studies are conducted. If the athlete has demonstrated deficiencies in iron, selenium, vitamins B12, D, and E, they should be treated, as they are connected with myopathy and neuropathy. Vitamin D deficiency should be suspected in athletes training in northern latitudes or mostly indoors. As for iron deficiencies, even in the absence of anemia, athletes may benefit from iron supplementation with ferrous sulphate, 100 mg daily for 4–6 weeks.

Masters and senior athletes have a decreased thirst sensation, compared with their younger counterparts. There is, thus, a higher risk of dehydration in the older athlete, compared with younger athletes. The wide variation in training amounts, sweat rates and totals, diets, training environments, and age between athletes requires that an individual have a customized fluid loading and replacement plan. For example, water polo athletes' average sweat rate is just under 0.3 l/hour, compared with tennis players whose rates are 2.6 l/hour (Sawka et al., 2007). This method may simplify the issue, as different medications, vitamins, and diets may affect the colour of the urine and lead to hyperhydration and, possibly, hyponatremia. The risk of hyponatremia with hyperhydration becomes more likely with events over 3 hours, in larger athletes who hyperhydrate throughout the competition. A more customized method is for the athlete to weigh him/herself prior to the event and afterwards. There is good-quality evidence that body weight (BW) can be used accurately to determine individual fluid losses and fluid replacement requirements (Sawka et al., 2007). It is important, however, that the pre-event weight be based on a nude BW first thing in the morning, after urinating. This will negate the dependency of BW on numerous factors, including food and fluid intake and bowel movements, as well as provide a less than 1% deviation from subsequent measurements. The post-race BW should discount the mass of the fluid intake during the race. Post-training fluid intake should ideally occur with meals and snacks containing sodium to enhance fluid replacement. Athletes should aim for 1.5 l per kg BW lost during event (Shirreffs and Maughan, 1998).

Table 12.6 Summary of recovery recommendations

Intake	Recommended amounts	When
Macronutrients	Carbs: 1–1.5 g/kg	< 30 min post exercise
Supplements		
– Vitamins	Obtain from diet Replace if deficient	Throughout day
– Creatine monohydrate	5 g/day if in high MVC sports	Throughout day
Fluids	1.5 l per kg BW lost	After training/competition

Note: MVC = maximal voluntary contraction.

INJURY PREVENTION

The key elements of injury prevention in the senior athlete include:

- equipment size and fit;
- appropriate dynamic warm-up for muscle responsiveness;
- skill acquisition for complex or new learning;
- recovery strategies embedded in training regime.

The time required to increase muscle temperature and circulation is about 10–15 minutes in adults under 50 years of age, but the older adult may require 30–50% of their exercise time to provide adequate warm-up. This translates into 20–30 minutes of dynamic warm-up time for most activities of 1-hour duration. This warm-up can include simulating the sport or doing repetitions of sport-specific tasks and skills.

The older athlete needs to include balance and proprioception training into their regime as a key preventive measure for falls and joint instability. This will reduce avoidance injuries and enhance training. A balance program should be progressive and challenging, and yet have the safety net of railings, supports, or spotters. Balance should include dynamic standing positions on one or both legs, requiring quick-response reactions. This can be achieved with activities, such as yoga and tai chi, that promote multiple changes of positions using arms and legs, while balance and stability are maintained.

Equipment modifications may be required to tailor the weight, grip, or mobility of equipment to the older athlete's strength and body shape. An example of this is finding the right tennis racquet weight, handgrip, and length to accommodate for joint-mobility and strength changes. There are advancements in equipment that may be beneficial to the senior athlete which are new to the marketplace since they bought equipment, and, therefore, they may not be aware of these advancements. For example, ski boots, curved parabolic skis, and light-weight snow shoes have all made winter-sport participants less injury prone.

CONCLUSION

There is encouraging evidence that older athletes who continue to be active, with a well-balanced program of strength and aerobic training, can achieve optimal levels of performance for sport, and this may reduce the effects of decline that often accompany aging. The athlete should have a screening physical prior to starting intense regular exercise and with any health changes. Recovery strategies are important, particularly in the areas of nutrition and hydration.

ABBREVIATIONS

AED   artificial external defibrillator
BMD   bone mineral density
bpm   beats per minute
BW   bodyweight
CAD   coronary artery disease
Carbs   carbohydrates
CM   creatine monohydrate
DRI   dietary reference intake
ECGs   electrocardiograms
Max HR   maximum heart rate = (220 − age)
MI   myocardial infarction
MVC   maximal voluntary contraction

ACKNOWLEDGMENT

The editors acknowledge the assistance of Wendy Holdan, MSPT, of Boston Children's Hospital, for contributing to, and reviewing, this chapter.

SUGGESTED READING

Chodzko-Zajko W.J., Proctor D.N., Fiatarone Singh M.A., Minson C.T., Nigg C.R., Salem G.J., Skinner J.S. Exercise and physical activity for older adults. *Medicine & Science in Sports & Exercise.* July 2009; 41(7):1510–30; Special Communications: Position Stand.

Esmarck B., Andersen J.L., Olsen S., et al. Timing of postexercise protein intake is important for muscle hypertrophy with resistance training in eldery humans. *J. Physiol.* 2001; 535:301–11.

Forsberg A.M., Nilsson E., Werneman J., Bergström J., Hultman E. Muscle composition in relation to age and sex. *Clin. Sci. (Lond).* Aug 1991; 81(2):249–56.

Franklin B.A., Fern A., Voytas J. Training principles of elite senior athletes. *Current Sports Medicine Reports.* 2004; 3:173–9.

Hecht H.S. Recommendations for pre-participation screening and the assessment of cardiovascular disease in masters athletes. *Circulation.* 2001; 104(11):E58.

Kasch F., Wallace J., Van Kamp S. A longitudinal study of cardiovascular stability in active men aged 45–65 years. *Physician Sports Med.* 1988; 64:1038–44.

Leigey D., Irrgang J., Francis K., Cohen P., Wright V. Participation in high-impact sports predicts bone mineral density in senior olympic athletes. *Sports Health: A Multi-disciplinary Approach.* 2009; 1:508.

Maron B.J., Araujo C.G., Thompson P.D., Fletcher G.F., de Luna A.B., Fleg J.L., Pelliccia A., Balady G.J., Furanello F., Van Camp S.P., Elosua R., Chaitman B.R., Bazzarre T.L., World Heart Federation, International Federation of Sports Medicine, American Heart Association Committee on Exercise, Cardiac Rehabilitation, and Prevention. Recommendations for pre-participation screening and the assessment of cardiovascular disease in masters athletes. *Circulation.* 2001; 103(2):327–34.

Melanson K.J. Exercise nutrition for adults older than 40 years. *American Journal of Lifestyle Medicine.* 2008; 2:285–9.

Mitchell J.H., Haskell W., Snell P., Van Camp S.P. Task Force 8: Classification of sports. 36th Bethesda Conference. *J. Am. Coll. Cardiol*. 2005; 45:1364–7.

Nisevich P. Nutritional needs of senior athletes. *Fitness Journal*. September 2009.

Pollock M.L., Meglelkoch, L.J., Graves J.E., et al. Twenty year follow up of aerobic power and body composition of older athletes. *J. Appl. Physiol*. 1997; 82:1508–16.

Powell A.P. Issues unique to the masters athlete. *Current Sports Medicine Reports*. 2005; 4(6):335.

Rodriguez N.R., DiMarco N.M., Langley S. Nutrition and athletic perfomance. *Medicine & Science in Sports & Exercise*. 2009; 41:3, 709–31.

Rogers M., Hagbery J., Martin III W., et al. Decline in VO_2max in master athletes and sedentary men. *J. Appl. Phyiol*. 1990; 68:2195–9.

Rosenbloom, C.A. Nutrition recommendations for masters athletes. *Clin. Sports Med.*. 2007.

Sawka M., Burke L.M., Eichner E.R., Maughan R.J., Montain S.J., Stachenfeld N.S. Exercise and fluid replacement. *Medicine & Science in Sports & Exercise*. 2007; 39(2):377–90.

Shirreffs S.M., Maughan R.J. Volume repletion after exercise-induced volume depletion in humans: Replacement of water and sodium losses. *American Journal of Physiology*. 1998; 274:F868–75.

Striegel H., Simon P., Wurster C., Niess A.M., Ulrich R. The use of nutritional supplements among master athletes. *International Journal of Sports Medicine*. 2006; 27(3):236–41.

Tanaka H., Seals D.R. Invited review: Dynamic exercise performance in Masters athletes: insight into the effects of primary human aging on physiological functional capacity. *J. Appl. Physiol*. Nov. 2003; 95(5):2152–62.

Tarnopolsky M.A. Nutritional consideration in the aging athlete. *Clin. J. Sport Med*. 2008; 18:531–8.

Tarnopolsky M., Zimmer A., Paikin J., Safdar A., Aboud A., Pearce E., Roy B., Doherty T. Creatine monohydrate and conjugated linoleic acid improve strength and body composition following resistance exercise in older adults. *PLoS ONE*. 2007; 2(10):e991.

Volpe S.L. Physiological changes and nutrition for masters athletes. *ACMS Health and Fitness Journal*. 2010; 14(1):36–8.

Whiteson J.H., Bartels M.N., Kim H., Abla A.S. Coronary artery disease in masters-level athletes. *Archives of Phys. Med. Rehabil*. 2006; 87(3 Suppl. 1):S79–81.

Wright V.J., Perricelli B.C. Age-related rates of decline in performance among elite senior athletes. *Am. J. Sports Med*. Mar. 2008; 36(3):443–50. Epub Nov. 30, 2007.

CHAPTER 13

ENVIRONMENTAL PROBLEMS

S. Talia Alenabi and Farzin Halabchi

HEAT-RELATED PROBLEMS

Introduction

Each team physician should be familiar with the prevention and management of heat-associated illnesses, as many sports events occur in hot, humid conditions. Heat is produced by endogenous sources, including metabolism associated with muscle activity, and exogenous sources, which include heat transfer to the body when the environmental temperature is higher than body temperature. Thermally, the body can be divided into two zones: the core and the shell. The core consists of the deeper tissues, including all the vital organs such as the heart and brain; the shell comprises the remainder, including the skin, subcutaneous tissue, and muscles. The core temperature is stable over a remarkable range of environmental thermal stressors. On the other hand, the temperature of the shell differs significantly with the environment, the degree of protection, and the activity of the individual.

Heat loss occurs by conduction, convection, radiation and/or evaporation. During exercise, 15–20 times more heat is produced compared with resting conditions. This internal heat, in addition to the heat from the external environment, must be offset to avoid hyperthermia. In convection and conduction, heat is transferred from a warm object to a cooler object. The amount lost by conduction depends on the temperature difference between two surfaces in direct contact. It accounts for less than 2% of heat loss in most situations, including during exercise. Convection is the exchange of heat between a solid medium and one that moves, such as air or body fluids. When a person is at rest in a moderate environmental temperature, thermoregulation is performed by convection of heat to the body surface and radiation to the environment, but, during exercise, evaporation through sweating is more important, especially when the environmental temperature is equal to, or higher than, the body temperature. Radiation and evaporation are maximized by increasing skin blood flow and diaphoresis. Heat loss by radiation occurs when the air temperature is lower than the body temperature.

Relative Humidity

Air Temperature	40	45	50	55	60	65	70	75	80	85	90	95	100
80°	80	80	81	81	82	82	83	84	84	85	86	86	87
82°	81	82	83	84	84	85	86	88	89	90	91	93	95
84°	83	84	85	86	88	89	90	92	94	96	98	100	103
86°	85	87	88	89	91	93	95	97	100	102	105	108	112
88°	88	89	91	93	95	98	100	103	106	110	113	117	121
90°	91	93	95	97	100	103	105	109	113	117	122	127	132
92°	94	96	99	101	105	108	112	116	121	126	131		
94°	97	100	103	106	110	114	119	124	129	135			
96°	101	104	108	112	116	121	126	132					
98°	105	109	113	117	123	128	134						
100°	109	114	118	124	129	136							
102°	114	119	124	130	137								
104°	119	124	131	137									
106°	124	130	137										
108°	130	137											
110°	136												

The heat index chart is designed to provide general guidelines for assessing the potential severity of heat stress. Individual reactions to heat will vary. In addition, studies indicate that the susceptibility to heat disorders tends to increase with age. **Exposure to full sunshine can increase Heat Index values by up to 15° F.**

How to use Heat Index:
1. Locate on the chart above the current Air Temperature down the left side
2. Locate the current Relative Humidity across the top
3. Follow across and down to find apparent Temperature (what it feels like to the body)
4. Determine heat stress risk on **chart below**

Heat Illness Risk

Apparent Temperature	Heat Stress Risk with Physical Activity and/or Prolonged Exposure
80° to 90°	Exercise caution: dehydration likely if athlete fails to drink adequate fluids
91° to 103°	Exercise extreme caution: Heat cramps or heat exhaustion possible
104° to 124°	Danger: Exertion heat cramps or heat exhaustion likely, heatstroke possible
125° and up	Extreme danger: Exertional heatstroke highly likely

Figure 13.1 Heat index chart
Source: National Oceanic and Atmospheric Administration (NOAA)

When the air temperature is above the body temperature, the athlete absorbs heat from the environment and depends entirely on evaporation for heat loss. When the environmental temperature is higher than 35°C (95°F), evaporation is the main mechanism for heat dissipation. In hot, dry conditions, evaporation can dissipate more than 98% of heat, but, normally, 30% of the cooling effect is related to evaporation, because this process is dependent on the humidity level. When the environmental humidity is high (greater than 75%), the evaporation of sweat is limited, and then its cooling effect is limited (Figure 13.1).

Dehydration can also limit the evaporation effect. Solar and ground radiation, air temperature, barometric pressure, wind speed, and clothing insulation are all important in this regard.

Monitoring of the environmental temperature

The relative risk of heat illness can be calculated using the wet-bulb and globe temperature (WBGT) index. The WBGT index for the outdoor environment is computed from readings of a natural wet bulb (TWB), which accounts for humidity-related heat stress, a black globe (TBG), which accounts for radiant heat stress, and a dry bulb (TDB), for ambient temperature, according to the following formula (WBGT = 0.7TWB + 0.2TBG + 0.1TDB). It was developed to minimize the occur-rence of heat casualties, first among military trainees and then in occupational environments and athletic events (See Table 13.1). Several recommendations have been published for distance running, which may not be allowed when the WBGT index exceeds 28°C.

Table 13.1 Prediction of heat-illness risk

Risk	WBGT temperature (°C)
Low	< 18
Moderate	18–23
High	23–8
Extreme	> 28

Risk factors

Obese and unconditioned people, children and prepubescent athletes, the elderly and disabled are all at higher risk of heat illnesses. Dehydration may also increase the rate. Those who are unacclimatized to heat and people with a prior history of heat illness are more prone to heat problems. Users of some medications, such as antidepressants, diuretics, antihypertensives, antihistamines, and stimulants, and alcohol consumers are all at higher risk. Some researchers believe that consumption of ephedrine and related alkaloids, which are used for weight loss, can cause thermoregulatory dysfunction. Athletic equipment and rubber or plastic suits do not allow water vapor to pass through and, like helmets, also limit heat dissipation. Any condition that can enhance dehydration, such as gastroenteritis, upper respiratory illness, sweat-gland dysfunction, and viral infections with fever, should be taken into consideration when the risk of heat illness is evaluated. People with chronic medical illness are at a greater risk of developing an exertional heat-related illness. Prolonged sun exposure and wearing heavy or excessive clothing are also important risk factors.

Heat-associated illnesses

In this section, five common types of heat illness and exertional hyponatremia are introduced. The milder heat illnesses include heat edema, heat cramps, heat syncope, and heat exhaustion. Heat stroke is a medical emergency.

Heat edema
Heat edema occurs more commonly in persons in a very hot situation. The edema results from peripheral vasodilatation and is more evident in the lower extremities.

RISK FACTORS OF HEAT ILLNESSES

- Extremes of age.
- Obesity.
- Lack of fitness.
- Unacclimatization to heat.
- Dehydration.
- Previous history of heat illness.
- Alcoholism
- Medications and drugs: diuretics, beta blockers, alcohol, ephedrine, amphetamines, and cocaine.
- Skin-altering conditions (sunburn, psoriasis, eczema, burns).
- Prolonged exposure to heat (occupational or exertional).
- Acute gastroenteritis.
- Upper respiratory illness.
- Chronic medical illnesses.
- Sweat-gland dysfunction (cystic fibrosis, scleroderma).
- Sickle-cell trait.
- Sleep deprivation.
- Lack of proper air conditioning.
- Wearing heavy or excessive clothing.
- Barriers to evaporation such as helmets, rubber, or plastic suits.

It resolves spontaneously as acclimatization takes place, but can be treated symptomatically with rest and elevation of the lower limbs. Diuretics should be avoided.

Heat cramps

This problem presents with annoying pain and spasm in different skeletal muscles. The muscles employed in the exercise are usually affected, especially the leg and abdominal muscles. It was believed that severe dehydration and sodium loss causes heat cramps, but recent research showed that cramps can occur in any environmental conditions and result from alterations in neural activity. In fact, fatigue can change the spinal neural activity in some susceptible individuals, resulting in cramps. However, cramps are more common in unacclimatized persons and diuretic users.

Heat cramps are treated with rest, ice therapy, mild stretching, and massage, along with rehydration using a sport drink. Intravenous fluids may be required if nausea or vomiting limits oral intake.

MILD HEAT ILLNESSES

Heat edema
- Presentation: peripheral edema.
- Treatment: rest, elevation of limbs, acclimatization.

Heat cramp
- Presentation: painful muscle cramp, palpable muscle spasm.
- Treatment: fluid intake, massage, stretching, ice therapy.

Heat syncope
- Presentation: loss of consciousness.
- Treatment: rest, Trendelenberg position, fluid intake.

Heat exhaustion
- Presentation: inability to continue exercise, fatigue, nausea, vomiting, chills, hypotension, syncope, elevated core temperature.
- Treatment: ABC, cooling therapy, rehydration.

Heat syncope

Syncope results from orthostatic hypotension due to inadequate cardiac output. Usually, it occurs after completing an endurance event in the heat. After exercise, the athlete develops hypotension, general weakness and fatigue, and a brief loss of consciousness. It is a benign situation, and the patient usually recovers immediately when supine. Most cases have a rectal temperature lower than 40°C. In this situation, a team physician should also consider other causes of collapse. Treatment includes supine positioning of the patient, with the pelvis and legs elevated (Trendelenberg position), cooling, and fluid-replacement therapy. Usually, sports drinks containing glucose and electrolytes are appropriate, provided the patient can drink. In case of severe dehydration, intravenous fluid replacement may be indicated.

Heat exhaustion

This is the commonest form of heat illness. The athlete is unable to continue exercising and sweats profusely. He/she may be confused or irritated, suffering from fatigue, nausea, vomiting, headache, vertigo, weakness, heat cramps, heat sensations in the head and neck, chills, tachycardia, and hypotension. Hyperventilation, muscle incoordination, agitation, and impaired judgment may occasionally be present. Cognitive changes are usually minimal, but the function of the central nervous system should be assessed. This problem results when the cardiovascular response to exercise is not sufficient, especially when the athlete is dehydrated, and the external temperature is high. In this situation, the skin blood vessels are so dilated that blood flow to vital organs is reduced. Usually, the core body temperature is between 38 and 40.5°C. Rectal temperature is the most accurate method of monitoring core temperature in the field. The patient should be removed from the heat, cooled as soon as possible, and rehydrated orally or intravenously.

Heat stroke

This is the most serious condition of heat-related illness and the third commonest cause of death in high-school athletes. Heat stroke is a medical emergency that needs special attention and does not reverse spontaneously. This problem, which is sometimes irreversible and life threatening, is characterized by impairment of thermoregulatory mechanisms. Heat stroke can be exertional or non-exertional. In both situations, body temperature is high enough to deteriorate the function of multiple organs.

HEAT STROKE

- *Symptoms*: Changes in mental status, fatigue, dizziness, nausea, vomiting, uncoordinated movements, hot and dry skin, irritation or drowsiness, syncope.
- *Signs*: Core temperature > 40.5°C, hypotension, tachycardia, possible cessation of sweating, coma, disseminated intravascular coagulation (DIC), ATN, liver damage.
- *Treatment*: ABC, cooling therapy, monitoring, hospitalization.

Clinical presentation

The rectal temperature increases to more than 40.5°C. The athlete may have failings of sweating or complete cessation of sweating, but, in general, the presence or absence of sweating does not influence the diagnosis. Key points for diagnosis of heat stroke include a rise of the core body temperature to greater than 40.5°C and moderate-to-severe mental status impairment or central-nervous-system dysfunction. Decreased level of consciousness, delirium, and frank coma are the severe manifestations, but patients may present with impaired judgment or inappropriate behavior. Some believe that the neurologic dysfunction is a clinical hallmark of this problem, but other authors think that an elevated body temperature and neural dysfunction are necessary, but not sufficient, to diagnose heat stroke. Some other clinical signs and symptoms, such as fatigue, dizziness, weakness, nausea and vomiting, headache, confusion, disorientation to place, person and time, irritation or drowsiness, uncoordinated movement, hot and dry skin, and reddened face, are frequently observed.

Owing to peripheral vasodilatation and reduction in afterload, the patient has tachycardia, widened pulse pressure, and warm skin at first, but, in a severe hypovolemic state, the late finding of hypotension and circulatory collapse may occur. The compensatory vasoconstriction of internal organs can result in multi-organ damage. Acute tubular necrosis due to decreased renal perfusion, elevated liver enzymes as a result of liver-cell damage, and gastrointestinal signs and symptoms due to reduced mesenteric perfusion are some of the examples. As the problem progresses, encephalopathy, rhabdomyolysis, acute respiratory syndrome, acid-base disorders and electrolyte disturbances, intestinal infarction, and hemorrhagic complication (DIC) may occur.

The mortality rate for heat stroke ranges from 10 to 70% and depends on the age of the patient and the severity of the problem. The prognosis is poor when treatment is delayed more than 2 hours. Mortality rate and organ damage are directly proportional to the time that elapses between high body temperature and

---

COOLING METHODS

- Immersion of the body in cold or ice water.
- Use of ice packs on scalp, neck, axillae, and groin.
- Use of ice slush over the body.
- Cooling blanket.
- Undressing the patient, using fan after spraying the body with tepid water or covering it with a wet sheet.
- Heat-stroke commercial units.
- Iced gastric or peritoneal lavage (rarely used).
- Antipyretics are not effective.

---

s. talia alenabi and farzin halabchi

initiation of cooling therapy. There are some reports of heat-stroke occurrence in a cool-to-moderate environment, although most cases are seen in extreme heat. A long-distance endurance runner's body temperature may reach 40.6°C after a race.

Treatment

Advanced cardiac life support should be followed; rapid cooling is the first priority after CAB stabilization. Prompt fluid replacement with isotonic sodium chloride solution should be initiated. Ringer's solution is not used, as the liver cannot metabolize lactate effectively. As mentioned before, quick cooling therapy is the mainstay of better prognosis. There are different cooling methods, as shown in the box. Core body temperature should be monitored in the field continuously via a rectal thermometer or tympanic probe. The goal is to decrease body temperature to below 38.8°C within 30 minutes, ideally with a 0.2°C/minute reduction. The patient's clothing should be removed for better air flow over the skin. Some studies have shown that the most effective method of reducing core body temperature appears to be immersion in iced water, although the practicalities of this treatment may limit its use. Peripheral vasoconstriction may occur when the skin temperature reaches temperatures lower than 30°C, which may lead to shivering and increased internal heat production. Evaporative cooling is another effective method. The patient can be sprayed with lukewarm or cool water, and then a fan causes evaporative cooling. There are also some commercial units. An alcohol bath should be avoided, especially in children, as the alcohol can be absorbed by dilated cutaneous vessels. Using ice packs on the scalp, neck, axillae, and groin, ice slush over body, and a cold blanket are all effective. Sometimes, a combination of different techniques may be used to facilitate rapid cooling. More studies are needed to compare the effectiveness of different cooling methods.

Antipyretics are not effective. Salycilates can worsen existing coagulopathies, and acetaminophen can precipitate hepatic damage. To control shivering and seizure, benzodiazepines may be used.

Unfortunately, in about 25% of cases, tissue damage can continue to occur, even after the patient is cooled. Hospitalization is necessary.

Exertional hyponatremia

Exertional hyponatremia is a relatively rare condition. It occurs in prolonged events that take more than 4 hours. The serum sodium is below 130 mmol/l and results from either drinking water beyond sweat losses (water intoxication) or insufficient replacement of sweat sodium losses. In this situation, the extracellular water flows into the cells, producing intracellular swelling that causes potentially fatal neurologic and physiologic dysfunction.

The athlete's mental status will change, with disorientation, headache, nausea and vomiting, lethargy, hand and foot swelling, and, finally, pulmonary and cerebral edema and seizures. The patient may be dehydrated, normally hydrated, or overhydrated. A team physician should differentiate hyponatremia from heat stroke. In the former, the core body temperature is less than 40°C. Sometimes, the serum sodium can be measured in the field with a sodium analyzer. Considering the fluid intake and sweat and urine loss and using fluids containing enough sodium are all necessary for preventing exertional hyponatremia. If hyponatremia is suspected, the patient should be transferred to a hospital immediately with an intravenous line.

Prevention

Some prevention strategies for reducing the risk of heat-related injuries have been listed in Box 13.1. Also see the preventive recommendations in Chapter 23.

BOX 13.1 PREVENTIVE STRATEGIES FOR REDUCING HEAT INJURIES

- Identify the athletes who are prone to heat-induced injuries.
- The acclimatization procedure should be settled gradually for the athletes over 10–14 days.
- Check the environmental conditions before and during the activity and modify activity under high-risk conditions.
- Minimize the amount of clothing and equipment in hot and humid conditions.
- Provide an adequate supply of fluids, ice, and medical equipment needed in the field for management of heat illnesses.
- The athlete should drink adequate fluids during the 24-hour period before an event.
- Fluids should be readily available and served in containers that allow adequate volumes to be ingested with ease and with minimal interruption of exercise. The fluids should be cooler than ambient temperature, 15–22°C.
- It is recommended that individuals drink about 500 ml of fluid, about 2 hours before exercise.
- During exercise, athletes should start drinking early and continue at regular intervals.
- Inclusion of sodium and carbohydrates in the rehydration fluid is recommended for exercise events lasting more than 1 hour.
- Weight loss should not be more than 2–3% of body weight during exercise, and it is recommended that the athlete consume 1–1.5 l of fluid for each kilogram of weight loss.

---

s. talia alenabi and farzin halabchi

COLD-RELATED PROBLEMS

Humans normally maintain a steady core temperature by balancing heat production and heat loss. Radiation heat loss is maximal when the body is unclothed and erect and minimal when it is curled up and insulated. Conduction is the major route for heat loss during immersion in very cold water; even on land, wet clothing increases conductive loss. Evaporative heat loss occurs from the skin through insensible moisture loss and active sweating, through evaporation from wet clothing, and from the respiratory tract through warming and humidifying the inspired air. Convective heat loss is increased by limb movement and shivering. Both convective and evaporative heat losses are increased in windy conditions. The "wind chill index" was developed to describe the relative discomfort/danger resulting from the combination of wind and temperature (Figure 13.2).

Humans adapt less readily to cold than to heat. Even inhabitants of cold regions show only limited evidence of adaptation, such as a higher metabolic rate. Most cold-related injuries result from insufficient protection against the environment.

Cold-related injuries

The four commonest cold injuries are hypothermia, frostbite, immersion foot, and chilblains. The first two are medical emergencies that may eventually result in death.

Hypothermia

Hypothermia is defined as a subnormal body temperature ($< 35°C$). It occurs when the body is unable to preserve a steady core temperature.

Temperature (°F)

Calm	40	35	30	25	20	15	10	5	0	−5	−10	−15	−20	−25	−30	−35	−40	−45
5	36	31	25	19	13	7	1	−5	−11	−16	−22	−28	−34	−40	−46	−52	−57	−63
10	34	27	21	15	9	3	−4	−10	−16	−22	−28	−35	−41	−47	−53	−59	−66	−72
15	32	25	19	13	6	0	−7	−13	−19	−26	−32	−39	−45	−51	−58	−64	−71	−77
20	30	24	17	11	4	−2	−9	−15	−22	−29	−35	−42	−48	−55	−61	−68	−74	−81
25	29	23	16	9	3	−4	−11	−17	−24	−31	−37	−44	−51	−58	−64	−71	−78	−84
30	28	22	15	8	1	−5	−12	−19	−26	−33	−39	−46	−53	−60	−67	−73	−80	−87
35	28	21	14	7	0	−7	−14	−21	−27	−34	−41	−48	−55	−62	−69	−76	−82	−89
40	27	20	13	6	−1	−8	−15	−22	−29	−36	−43	−50	−57	−64	−71	−78	−84	−91
45	26	19	12	5	−2	−9	−16	−23	−30	−37	−44	−51	−58	−65	−72	−79	−86	−93
50	26	19	12	4	−3	−10	−17	−24	−31	−38	−45	−52	−60	−67	−74	−81	−88	−95
55	25	18	11	4	−3	−11	−18	−25	−32	−39	−46	−54	−61	−68	−75	−82	−89	−97
60	25	17	10	3	−4	−11	−19	−26	−33	−40	−48	−55	−62	−69	−76	−84	−91	−98

(left axis: Wind (mph))

Frostbite Times ☐ 30 minutes ▨ 10 minutes ■ 5 minutes

Wind Chill (°F) = $35.74 + 0.6215T − 35.75(V^{0.16}) + 0.4275T(V^{0.16})$
Where, T = Air Temperature (°F) V = Wind speed (mph)

Figure 13.2 Wind chill temperature index in Celsius

environmental problems

Risk factors

Children are more prone to heat loss during cold exposure than adults, because of their larger ratio of surface area to body mass and smaller amount of subcutaneous fat. Regarding gender, there are no distinct differences in cold tolerance when genders are matched for fitness at the same relative workload. Alcohol blunts mental awareness of cold and prevents shivering, possibly by causing hypoglycemia. Hypothermia may occur particularly rapidly when wet conditions are added to cold weather, but a severely cold environment is not always necessary for hypothermia to ensue, and it may occur during any season. Hypothermia is most likely to involve infants (whose large body surface area predisposes them to rapid heat loss) and the elderly (who may have impaired ability either to sense decreasing temperature, to limit heat loss by peripheral vasoconstriction, or to shiver). Infants and the elderly also have lower metabolic rates and so produce less heat. Drugs acting on the central nervous system (e.g., barbiturates, phenothiazines) may dull the body's response to cold and therefore increase susceptibility to cold. Other predisposing factors include malnutrition, hypoglycemia, hypothyroidism, neuropathies, hypopituitarism, peripheral vascular disease, smoking, adrenal insufficiency, diabetes, sepsis, and head injury.

RISK FACTORS OF HYPOTHERMIA

- Age (infants, children, elderly).
- Sex (female).
- Alcohol consumption.
- Medications: barbiturates, phenothiazines.
- Hypoglycemia.
- Malnutrition.
- Smoking.
- Chronic diseases (e.g., diabetes, hypothyroidism, neuropathies, peripheral vascular disease, hypopituitarism).
- Head injury.

Clinical presentation

There are several systems for describing the level of hypothermia. A common approach to classification includes core temperature (Tco) and functional characteristics. In the mild hypothermia range (35–32°C), thermoregulatory mechanisms (e.g., shivering) still operate fully. Patients are pale, cool, and have maximally vasoconstricted blood flow to the skin. Patients may shiver uncontrollably, have varying degrees of confusion, disorientation, ataxic gait, and dysarthria, and be unable to perform fine movements of the hand. These patients have tachycardia, tachypnea, and cold diuresis due to increased cardiac output and resultantly raised renal perfusion.

s. talia alenabi and farzin halabchi

HYPOTHERMIA

Mild

- Core body temperature = 35–32°C.
- Presentation: Patient is pale and cool, may shiver, may have confusion, disorientation, ataxic gait, and dysarthria. The sign of tachycardia, tachypenea, and cold diuresis are present.

Moderate

- Core body temperature = 32–28°C.
- Presentation: Severely impaired judgment, muscle rigidity, areflexia, dilated pupils, decrease of blood pressure, heart rate, and respiration, and arrhythmia may occur; J wave in EKG.

Severe

- Core body temperature = < 28°C.
- Presentation: Loss of consciousness, shivering absence, indiscernible blood pressure, areflexia, dilated pupils, deep coma, VF, or asystole.

In moderate hypothermia (32–28°C), the effectiveness of the regulatory system is reduced until it fails, and the primary effect of body cooling becomes evident. Shivering is reduced. Symptoms are more severe and may include severely impaired judgment, apathy, drowsiness, slurred speech, amnesia, ataxia, slowed reflexes, dilated pupils, and decreases in blood pressure, heart rate, and respirations. There is a progressive decrease in the level of consciousness, and atrial fibrillation and other dysrhythmias may occur. Electrocardiography may show the pathognomonic J point elevation or Osborne wave.

In severe hypothermia (< 28°C), consciousness is completely lost, shivering is absent, and acid-base disturbances develop. Blood pressure is undiscernible, respiration is extremely slow, the patient is in deep coma, pupils are dilated and fixed, and areflexia may be seen in muscles. The heart is prone to ventricular fibrillation (even if the patient is moved slightly) or asystole as well. Ventricular fibrillation resists pharmacologic or electrical cardioversion without core rewarming. Often, the recommended treatment depends on the severity of the hypothermia.

In the field, the degree of hypothermia can be predicted by noting the level of consciousness and whether the patient is shivering. A shivering patient probably has a core temperature of > 32°C and less-severe hypothermia; patients who are not shivering or who have impaired consciousness generally have a core temperature < 32°C and more-severe hypothermia.

Prevention

There are several measures that can be taken to prevent heat loss (see Box 13.2). Some prevention strategies have also been explained in Chapter 23.

Treatment

The goal of initial treatment for hypothermia is prevention of further heat loss. Basic life-support protocols (e.g., ensuring adequate airway and circulation) should be used as needed. Severe peripheral vasoconstriction in hypothermic patients typically makes pulses difficult to palpate. Furthermore, CPR may cause a fatal cardiac rhythm in hypothermic patients whose pulse is discernible. Therefore, pulse should be examined for a full minute to avoid inappropriate chest compression. Standard advanced cardiac life support (ACLS) protocols are often ineffective when core body temperature is < 30°C. If the first attempt at defibrillation does not reverse ventricular fibrillation, circulatory support should be given until core temperature is > 30°C; defibrillation may then be reattempted. Oxygen and intravenous fluids should be warmed before being given to hypothermic patients. Patients suffering from more chronic hypothermia are susceptible to hypotension (rewarming shock) during rewarming. Normal saline should be warmed and given as soon as possible. Dopamine may successfully reverse hypotension not corrected by intravenous fluid infusion. Rewarming may be passive or active. Passive rewarming (e.g., moving patients into a warm, sheltered environment and covering with dry blankets) should be attempted primarily in all hypothermic patients and may be sufficient for mildly hypothermic patients who are otherwise healthy. Dry blankets may create the warming rate of 0.5–2°C per hour, depending on shivering thermogenesis. Active rewarming can be external or internal. Active external rewarming techniques can supplement passive rewarming and include application of exogenous heat sources (e.g., heating blankets, heat lamps, hot packs), or even warm-water immersion. Although non-invasive, these techniques have potential complications. "Afterdrop" in core temperature can occur, as peripheral vasoconstriction is reversed, and blood is circulated through cold extremities, returning cold blood to the core; this peripheral vasodilation and venous pooling can lead to relative hypovolemia and hypotension (rewarming shock). Active core-rewarming techniques deliver direct heat internally and avoid the problems that may occur when external rewarming is used. These techniques may be simple or invasive. The simple core-rewarming techniques may be initiated immediately and include intravenously administering fluid warmed to a maximum of 40–43°C (which will modestly increase core temperature) or administering heated humidified air or oxygen through a mask or endotracheal tube. These two techniques together warm at a rate of 1–2°C per hour.

Hypothermic patients have a decreased basal metabolic rate (BMR), which decreases oxygen requirements. For this reason, the usual criteria for establishing death or irreversibility of disease are not valid for hypothermic patients; indeed,

---

REWARMING METHODS

Passive rewarming
- Move patient into a warm, sheltered environment and cover with dry blankets.

Active rewarming

External:
- Exogenous heat sources (e.g., heating blankets, heat lamps, hot packs).
- Warm-water immersion.

Internal:
- Simple:
  - intravenous administration of fluid warmed to a maximum of 40–43°C;
  - administration of heated humidified air or oxygen through a mask or endotracheal tube.
- Invasive:
  - peritoneal dialysis, hemodialysis, thoracostomy lavage, and use of esophageal warming tubes;
  - extracorporeal blood rewarming: arterial and venous femoral catheters connected to a countercurrent fluid warmer; venovenus rewarming.

many hypothermia patients survive prolonged periods despite a non-perfusing cardiac rhythm. Efforts at resuscitation, therefore, must be continued until rewarming is complete.

Frostbite

Frostbite may be defined as the acute freezing of tissues when exposed to ambient temperatures of below 0°C. In this situation, a local anatomic area loses so much heat that ice crystals form in the extracellular spaces. Frostbite most often affects the exposed skin (nose, ears, cheeks, exposed wrists), but also occurs in the hands and feet, because peripheral vasoconstriction significantly lowers tissue temperatures.

FROSTBITE

First degree

- White plaque with surrounding erythema.
- Edema, waxy appearance, and sensory deficit may be present.

Second degree

- Blister formation filled with clear or milky fluid surrounded by erythema and edema.

Third degree

- Blood-filled blisters progress to hard black eschar.

Fourth degree

- Muscle, tendon, or bone are affected, with resultant necrosis and tissue loss.

Frostbite is a disease of morbidity, not mortality. However, when combined with hypothermia or wound-related sepsis, death is possible. The severity of injury is related to the temperature gradient at the skin surface and the duration of exposure. Although tissue freezes more quickly at lower temperatures, the degree of irreversible damage is related to the length of time that the tissue remains frozen; therefore, either a delay in presentation or extended exposure to cold will greatly worsen the prognosis.

Environmental risk factors for frostbite include low ambient temperatures, high humidity, wind chill, high altitude, and prolonged exposure. Persons exposed to these conditions may also have pre-existing medical problems that compound the problem. Morbidity of frostbite can be increased by any process that impairs local circulation, thermoregulation, or mental status, e.g., atherosclerosis, diabetes mellitus, Raynaud's disease, peripheral vascular disease, thyroid disease, use of some drugs, whether therapeutic (e.g., anticholinergics, antihistamines, beta blockers, diuretics, and laxatives) or illicit (e.g., nicotine, amphetamines, cocaine, LSD, marijuana, opiates), and constrictive clothing. Alcohol consumption has been identified as a particular risk factor, because of its vasodilatory effects as well as suppression of an individual's judgment. Previous cold injury may be a predisposing factor for the next occurrence.

Clinical presentation

Patients with frostbite usually feel cold and numb during the early stages. Extreme throbbing pain usually begins 48–72 hours after the frostbite has occurred. Residual tingling from ischemic neuritis can last from a week to a month or, in rare cases, as long as 6 months. The skin may have a waxy-yellow or a mottled-blue appearance and becomes flushed and red with rewarming. Vesicles or bullae may form within 6–24 hours. A black, dry scar may be seen after 9–15 days, and mummification and auto-amputation can occur in about 22–45 days. In the long term, cold sensitivity, sensory loss, and hypopigmentation may persist in the affected part for years.

At the time of initial evaluation, most true frostbite injuries appear similar. For this reason, classification of frostbite is applied after rewarming. Historically, frostbite has been categorized into four degrees. In first-degree frostbite, there is a numb, central, white plaque with surrounding erythema. Edema, waxy appearance, and sensory deficit also may be present. Second-degree injury causes blister formation surrounded by erythema and edema. These blisters fill with clear or milky fluid in the first 24 hours. Third-degree injury is characterized by blood-filled blisters that may progress to a hard black eschar over a matter of weeks. Fourth-degree injury produces full-thickness damage, affecting muscles, tendons, and bone with resultant necrosis and tissue loss.

Some authors prefer to describe just two classes of injury, superficial (first and second degree) and deep (third and fourth degree), which appear to predict outcome more accurately. Superficial frostbite affects the skin and subcutaneous tissues; deep frostbite also affects bones, joints, and tendons. Deep frostbite is more serious, less common, and rarely occurs in well-managed sporting events.

Physical examination of the injured part can reveal favorable prognostic criteria, such as sensation to pinprick, healthy-appearing skin color, and blisters that fill with clear, rather than milky, fluid. In addition, the ability of the skin to deform under direct pressure is taken as a sign of dermal viability and, hence, a good prognosis. On the other hand, dark fluid-filled blisters, cyanotic skin color, more proximal vesicles on the extremities, and hard, non-deforming skin herald a poor prognosis.

Prevention and treatment

Proper clothing has a key role for prevention. A ski cap, facemask, and neck warmer can protect the face and ears from frostbite. Ski goggles can protect the

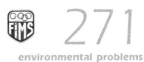

eyes. They must be well ventilated to prevent fogging, and can also be treated with antifog preparations. Polypropylene gloves or, in extreme temperatures, woolen mittens can be worn with windproof outer mittens of Gore-Tex or nylon. Sports shoes should be large enough to accommodate an outer pair of heavy wool socks. It is important to avoid getting wet, because heat loss can be increased by evaporation. The insulating ability of clothing can be decreased by as much as 90% when saturated either with external moisture or condensation from perspiration. If weather conditions are bad enough, it is better to cancel the practice or event for the day.

Treatment can be divided into three phases: (1) pre-thaw field-care phase; (2) immediate emergency department (rewarming) phase; and (3) post-thaw care phase, which may last for several weeks or months.

1. *Pre-thaw field care*: Before evaluation in a hospital, care of the patient with a potential frostbite injury is focused on protection of the involved part from mechanical trauma and avoidance of thawing until definitive rewarming can be performed. Before and during frostbite treatment, hypothermia should be assessed and corrected until core temperature reaches > 34°C. Rubbing of the affected tissue with a warm hand or snow does not increase local blood flow and may cause adverse mechanical trauma. Repeated bouts of thawing and refreezing result in a worsening injury. It is better for patients to walk with frozen feet to shelter than to attempt rewarming at the scene; however, walking on frostbitten feet may cause tissue chipping or fracture. The extremity should be protected against slow, partial rewarming by the avoidance of patient contact with fires or heaters. The extremity should be padded and splinted for protection, but no other treatment should be initiated.

2. *Rewarming*: According to the current guidelines for hospital frostbite care, rewarming should be carried out in a whirlpool bath or tub, with a mild anti-bacterial agent, at the generally accepted temperature of 40–42°C. If a tub is not available, warm wet packs at the same temperature may be used as alternative. Adherence to this restricted temperature range is essential: Rewarming at lower temperatures is less valuable to tissue survival, and rewarming at higher temperatures may compound the injury by producing a burn wound. Rewarming should be continued for 15–30 minutes, until thawing is complete. A red/purple appearance and pliable texture of the involved part indicate the end of vasoconstriction and are signs that warming should cease. Active motion during rewarming is beneficial, but massage should be avoided. Intravenous-fluid resuscitation is not generally mandatory for frostbite injury itself, although there are case reports of rhabdomyolysis and subsequent renal failure. In addition, the hypothermic patient may exhibit a cold diuresis that warrants compensation with intravenous fluid. Some patients may need analgesics for pain.

3. *Post-thaw care*: Rapid rewarming does reverse the direct effects of ice-crystal formation within the tissue, but it can do nothing to prevent the progressive dermal

s. talia alenabi and farzin halabchi

TREATMENT OF FROSTBITE

1. **Pre-thaw field care**
   - protection of the involved part and avoidance of thawing until definitive rewarming;
   - padding and splinting of the extremity.

2. **Rewarming**
   - hospital care, rewarming in whirlpool bath or tub or warm wet packs for 15–30 min;
   - active motion during rewarming;
   - avoidance of massage.

3. **Post-thaw care**
   - wrapping the body part in sterile sheets, elevation, and splinting;
   - debridement of white or clear blisters;
   - leaving hemorrhagic blisters intact;
   - medications.

ischemia seen in the post-thaw phase. Wrapping the body part in sterile sheets, elevation, and splinting are recommended, immediately after thawing. White or clear blisters represent superficial injury and require debriding to prevent further contact with the high levels of prostaglandin F2α and thromboxane A2 in the exudate. Hemorrhagic blisters, however, represent structural damage to the superficial dermal plexus, and, although it may be beneficial to aspirate the exudates from these blisters, the risk of desiccation has led most authors to advocate that they be left intact. In the past, aspirin has been given as a systemic antithromboxane agent. Aspirin inhibits the synthesis of prostaglandins, including some prostaglandins that are beneficial to wound healing. For these reasons, aspirin has been superseded by ibuprofen for this application.

Aloe vera is used as a topical inhibitor of thromboxane and, when used in conjunction with ibuprofen and prophylactic penicillin, has been shown to result in less tissue loss.

Adults should be given tetanus and diphtheria toxoids, depending on their immunization records. If severe or deep tissue damage has occurred, intravenous penicillin G should be administered every 6 hours for 48–72 hours.

A number of adjunctive therapeutic modalities have been examined in attempts to prevent or reduce the progressive dermal ischemia. These include low molecular weight Dextran, anticoagulation, vasodilators (Reserpine), thrombolytics, sympathectomy, hyperbaric oxygen, and surgical treatmen (e.g., escharotomy, fasciotomy, and amputation).

Non-freezing, cold-induced injuries

Frostnip

Frostnip is a non-freezing injury of the skin tissues, usually of the fingers, toes, ears, cheeks, and chin. Numbness, swelling, and erythema are present, but no tissue injury occurs. Usually, the skin tissues affected with frostnip do not feel painful. Tissues affected with frostnip are soft and resilient. Symptoms develop when blood vessels supplying the affected tissues narrow because of the cold temperature. Frostnip occurs at temperatures of about 15°C.

The only treatment needed is rewarming of the area for a few minutes. The affected extremity can often be rewarmed by being placed against another person's underarm or abdomen. During warming, the area may hurt or itch intensely. No permanent damage results, and full recovery is expected, although sometimes the area is particularly sensitive to cold for months or years afterward.

Trench foot (immersion foot)

Trench foot is a cold injury that occurs gradually over prolonged exposure to cold and humid, but not freezing, temperatures (usually at ambient temperatures of 0–10°C). In the natural history of a typical case of immersion foot, there are four stages: the period of exposure, and the pre-hyperemic, hyperemic, and post-hyperemic stages. During exposure and immediately after rescue, the feet are cold, numb, swollen, and pulseless. It seems that intense vasoconstriction sufficient to arrest blood flow is the leading factor during this phase. This is followed by a period of intense hyperemia, increased swelling, and severe pain. Severe cases may develop blisters (after 2–7 days), cellulites, and gangrene. The latter is usually superficial, and massive loss of tissue is rare. Within 7–10 days, the intense hyperemia and swelling subside, and pain diminishes in intensity. The extent of anesthesia at this time has been found a useful guide for classification of severity. A lesser degree of hyperemia may persist for several weeks. Objective disturbances of sensation and sweating, muscular atrophy, and paralysis now become apparent. These findings are correlated with damage to the peripheral nerves. After several weeks, the feet become cold sensitive; when exposed to low temperature, they cool abnormally and may remain cold for several hours. Hyperhidrosis frequently accompanies this cold sensitivity. The hands may be affected, but seldom as severely as the feet.

Immersion foot can often be prevented by changing socks and drying the feet at least daily. The main aims of first aid are rewarming the affected areas, relieving pain, and preventing complications such as infection or tissue death. Treatment consists primarily of gently warming, drying, and cleaning the foot, elevating it, and keeping it dry and warm. Rewarming needs to be done carefully, as over-heating of tissue may result in tissue infarction and gangrene. Some physicians give antibiotics to prevent infection. Sympathectomy and other measures designed to increase the peripheral circulation should not be employed immediately after rescue, but may have a place in the treatment of the later cold-sensitive state.

s. talia alenabi and farzin halabchi

Chilblains (pernio or cold sores)

Prolonged exposure to ambient temperatures of 0–16°C, in the presence of high humidity, can cause local itchy erythematous or cyanotic skin lesions and, in rare cases, discolored areas or blisters, usually on the dorsum of the foot. This represents a mild form of cold injury and should be considered separately from true frostbite. These lesions can also appear as plaques, nodules, vesicles, bullae, or ulcerations. The condition is uncomfortable and recurrent but self-limiting. Treatment is supportive, with gentle rewarming of the affected skin, elevation, and application of a dry bandage. The drug nifedipine may be used orally and sometimes relieves symptoms.

Other cold-related disorders

Cold also may cause or exacerbate specific syndromes in persons with underlying disorders. These include Raynaud's syndrome, lupus erythematosus, urticaria/anaphylaxis, and cold-induced asthma. The detailed description of these syndromes is beyond the scope of this chapter.

HIGH-ALTITUDE ILLNESS

Travel to a high altitude requires that the human body acclimatize to hypobaric hypoxia. Failure in acclimatization results in three common but preventable maladies, known as high-altitude illness.

High-altitude illness is the collective term to describe the cerebral and pulmonary syndromes that can affect unacclimatized persons shortly after ascent to high altitude. The term encompasses the mainly cerebral syndromes of acute mountain sickness (AMS) and high-altitude cerebral edema (HACE), and the pulmonary syndrome of high-altitude pulmonary edema (HAPE).

As there is an increasing number of people who choose to sojourn or retire to the mountains, altitude-related illnesses are a frequent cause of morbidity and occasional mortality, about which health-care providers, especially team physicians, should have greater awareness. In this part of the chapter, we will discuss the definitions, clinical aspects, and treatment of the primary high-altitude illnesses.

Acute mountain sickness

AMS is the most common form of the acute altitude illnesses.

Clinical presentation

AMS is a syndrome of non-specific symptoms and is therefore subjective. The Lake Louise Consensus Group defined AMS as the presence of headache in an unacclimatized person who has recently arrived at an altitude above 2,500 m,

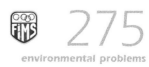

plus the presence of one or more of the following: gastrointestinal symptoms (anorexia, nausea, or vomiting), sleep disturbance, dizziness, and lassitude or fatigue (Table 13.2). Rarely, AMS occurs at altitudes as low as 2,000 m. Headache is deemed the cardinal symptom, but the characteristics are not sufficiently distinctive to differentiate it from other causes of headache. The symptoms typically develop within 6–12 hours after ascent, but sometimes as early as 1 hour. The symptoms are usually maximal on day 2 or 3, often disappearing by day 5. Peripheral edema may be seen, but there are no diagnostic physical findings, except in the few cases that progress to cerebral edema. The presence of abnormal neurological or respiratory signs can show progression to, or development of, HACE or HAPE.

Risk factors

The most important risk factors for the development of high-altitude illness are the rate of ascent, the altitude reached, the altitude at which an affected person sleeps (referred to as the sleeping altitude), and individual susceptibility.

Other possible risk factors for high-altitude illness include previous history of high-altitude illness, permanent residence below 900 m, exertion, and certain pre-existing cardiopulmonary conditions. Although exertion is a risk factor, lack of physical fitness is not. Obesity seems to be associated with the development of AMS, which may be partly related to greater nocturnal desaturation with altitude exposure. Children and adults seem to be equally affected, but people older than 50 years may be somewhat less susceptible to AMS than younger people. There is generally thought to be no significant difference in susceptibility to AMS between the sexes. Common conditions, such as hypertension, coronary artery disease, mild chronic obstructive pulmonary disease, diabetes, and pregnancy, do not appear to affect susceptibility to high-altitude illness. Neck irradiation or surgery and respiratory tract infection are potential risk factors that warrant further study. Although an association between AMS and dehydration has been noted, it is unclear whether dehydration is an independent risk factor for AMS. Diverse inter-actions between genetic factors and the environment most likely explain individual susceptibility or relative resistance to these hypoxia-induced illnesses.

Prevention

Gradual ascent is the cornerstone of prevention. The best strategy for avoiding AMS is to adopt a slow, flexible ascent profile with regular rest days, allowing time for acclimatization. However, determining an ideal ascent rate is difficult, and it differs among individuals. One rule of thumb is that, at altitudes higher than 3,000 m, never sleep more than 500 m above the previous night's altitude and have a full rest day each 3–4 days. For many people, this ascent rate is too slow, and guidelines now state that the height difference between consecutive sleeping sites should not be more than 600 m per day on average. The altitude at which a person sleeps (i.e. sleeping altitude) is of key importance. Therefore, it is per-missible to ascend more than the recommended daily rate, as long as descent is

Table 13.2 Lake Louise score (LLS) for the diagnosis of AMS

A diagnosis of AMS is based on:

1. A rise in altitude within the last 4 days

2. Presence of a headache

PLUS:

3. Presence of at least one other symptom

4. A total score of 3 or more from the questions below.

Note: A self-assessment score of up to 3 is often seen on arrival at a new altitude and will improve with acclimatization.

Self-report questionnaire

Add together the individual scores for each symptom to get the total score

Headache:	0	None at all
	1	Mild headache
	2	Moderate headache
	3	Severe, incapacitating headache
Gastrointestinal symptoms:	0	Good appetite
	1	Poor appetite or nausea
	2	Moderate nausea or vomiting
	3	Severe, incapacitating nausea and vomiting
Fatigue and/or weakness:	0	Not tired or weak
	1	Mild fatigue/weakness
	2	Moderate fatigue/weakness
	3	Severe fatigue/weakness
Dizziness/light-headedness:	0	None
	1	Mild
	2	Moderate
	3	Severe, incapacitating
Difficulty sleeping:	0	Slept as well as usual (the previous night)
	1	Did not sleep as well as usual
	2	Woke many times, poor night's sleep
	3	Could not sleep at all

Clinical assessment

All responses obtained by interview to the self-assessment questions, plus the following:

Sign score: _____

| Change in mental status: | 0 | No change |
| | 1 | Lethargy/lassitude |

continued

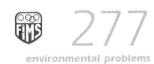

Table 13.2 continued

	2	Disorientated/confused
	3	Stupor/semiconscious
	4	Coma
Ataxia (heel–toe walking):	0	None
	1	Balancing maneuvers
	2	Steps off the line
	3	Falls down
	4	Unable to stand
Peripheral edema:	0	None
	1	One location
	2	Two or more locations

Functional assessment (assigned by investigator, not self-assessment)

Grade	Swelling	Tenderness	Function	Stability
I. Mild stretch	Minimal	Minimal	Normal/near normal	Normal
II. Partial tear	Moderate	Moderate	Difficulty toe walking	+ Anterior drawer −Talar tilt
III. Complete tear	Marked	Marked	Significant loss +Talar tilt	+ Anterior drawer

made before sleeping (climb high, sleep low). A night spent at an intermediate altitude (1,500–2,500 m) before ascent to high altitude will also aid acclimatization. Moderate activity, with day hikes to higher altitudes, and a high-carbohydrate diet seem to accelerate acclimatization, whereas physical exhaustion, consumption of alcohol, or use of sedative hypnotics will predispose a person to altitude illness.

In some situations, pharmacological prophylaxis may be warranted. These situations include rapid ascent (1 day or less) to altitudes greater than 3,000 m, rapid gain in sleeping altitude (higher than 900 m), or a past history of AMS or HAPE.

Acetazolamide is the preferred drug. The standard recommendation is 125 mg twice daily. It should be taken from 1 day before ascent and continued for 1–3 days, depending on clinical symptoms.

Dexamethasone may be used as an alternative in individuals with a prior history of intolerance of or allergic reaction to acetazolamide. The recommended adult doses are 2 mg every 6 hours, or 4 mg every 12 hours. Dexamethasone should not be used for prophylaxis in the pediatric population, owing to the potential for serious side effects.

POTENTIAL RISK FACTORS OF HIGH-ALTITUDE ILLNESS

- Rapid rate of ascent.
- Improper sleeping altitude.
- Previous history of high-altitude illness.
- Heavy labor in high altitude.
- Obesity.
- Younger age.
- Respiratory tract infections.
- Dehydration.
- Individual susceptibility.

With respect to headache, prophylactic aspirin (325 mg every 4 hours, for a total of three doses) reduced the incidence from 50 to 7%. Reports suggest various Chinese herbal preparations might prevent high-altitude illness, but there is a paucity of controlled studies in this regard. The notion that overhydration prevents acute mountain sickness has no scientific basis. However, maintenance of adequate hydration is important, because symptoms of dehydration can mimic those of AMS.

Treatment

The principles of treatment for AMS are to avoid further ascent until symptoms have resolved; to descend if there is no improvement or if symptoms worsen; and to descend immediately at the first signs of cerebral or pulmonary edema. In most cases of mild AMS, it is sufficient to rest and remain at the same altitude for another day, and symptoms will improve. Exertion should be minimized during this period, but occasional light exercise can be encouraged, as it increases SaO_2. Descent and supplementary oxygen (1–2 l per minute by nasal cannula) are the treatments of choice for moderate to severe AMS. Even a descent of only 300–1,000 m usually leads to relief of the symptoms. Additional pharmacotherapy may be used, especially if descent is impossible, and oxygen and hyperbaric chamber are unavailable. Acetazolamide (250 mg twice or three times daily) and dexamethasone (8 mg initially, followed by 4 mg four times daily) help lessen the severity of symptoms of AMS. Simulated descent in a portable hyperbaric chamber is also effective, and may be particularly useful when descent is impossible. With the use of these chambers at a pressure of 2 psi (13.8 kPa), the equivalent altitude is roughly 2,000 m lower than the ambient altitude.

Analgesics and antiemetics may afford symptomatic relief. Sedative hypnotic agents should be avoided, because of the risk of respiratory depression and associated drop in SaO_2.

High-altitude pulmonary edema (HAPE)

HAPE is a medical emergency and accounts for most deaths from high-altitude illness.

Clinical presentation

HAPE typically occurs at night, 1–3 days after arrival at altitudes higher than 2,500 m, and is not necessarily preceded by AMS. This syndrome rarely occurs after more than 4 days at a given altitude, owing to adaptive cellular and biochemical changes in pulmonary vessels.

Risk factors for HAPE are the same as for AMS and HACE. Additional sympathetic nervous system stimulation from exertion and cold will also contribute to increased pulmonary-artery pressure and an increased risk for developing HAPE. Abnormalities of the cardiopulmonary circulation that are associated with increased pulmonary blood-flow pressure, such as unilateral absence of a pulmonary artery or primary pulmonary hypertension, or both, increase the risk of HAPE, even at moderate altitudes. Upper respiratory tract infection or bronchitis may be precipitating factors, especially in children.

Early diagnosis is critical. Decreased performance and a dry cough should raise suspicion of HAPE. The first symptoms are generally dyspnea on exertion and reduced exercise tolerance that is greater than expected for the given altitude. Cough, dry and annoying at first, becomes productive later, with pink or blood-stained sputum and respiratory distress. Tachypnea and tachycardia are present at rest as the illness progresses. Orthopnea and frank hemoptysis are uncommon. Approximately 50% of HAPE cases may have AMS, and 14% have HACE. Fever is common, although rarely exceeds 38.3°C. Crackles typically originate in the right axilla and become bilateral as the illness progresses.

Prevention

A gradual ascent is the primary method for preventing HAPE. Drug prophylaxis should only be considered for individuals with a prior history of HAPE, and nifedipine is the preferred option in such situations. Although data are lacking, acetazolamide may be a sensible alternative, and clinical experience supports this. Salmeterol should only be considered as an adjunct treatment to nifedipine in high-risk individuals with known history of recurrent HAPE.

Treatment

Early recognition is the first, key step in the treatment of HAPE. Descent and supplementary oxygen are the most effective therapies. Descent is the mainstay of treatment. Descent of even a few hundred meters may be beneficial.

Breathing supplemental oxygen (4–6 l per minute) reduces pulmonary-artery pressure by 30–50%, which is sufficient to reverse the effects of the illness rapidly. Mild-to-moderate HAPE can be treated with rest and supplemental oxygen for

s. talia alenabi and farzin halabchi

48–72 hours. Patients with severe HAPE, indicated by the failure of arterial oxygen saturation to improve to more than 90% within 5 minutes of the initiation of high-flow oxygen, and those with concomitant HACE must be moved to a lower altitude and possibly hospitalized.

If oxygen is unavailable and descent is impossible, treatment in a portable hyperbaric chamber may be life saving.

Nifedipine, which can reduce pulmonary-artery pressure, is necessary only when supplemental oxygen is unavailable or descent is impossible. Sixty milligrams of the sustained-release version are administered daily in divided doses, without a loading dose. There is no recognized role for acetazolamide, beta-agonists, or diuretics in the treatment of HAPE.

Minimizing exertion and keeping the victim warm may help slow the progression of symptoms. A repeat ascent should not be attempted soon after the episode, because up to 2 weeks may be required for the person to regain full strength. After an episode of HAPE, a person should be advised subsequently to ascend to high altitudes more slowly, recognize symptoms of high-altitude illness early, and consider nifedipine prophylaxis, especially after multiple episodes.

High-altitude cerebral edema (HACE)

HACE is widely regarded as the end stage of AMS and is normally preceded by symptoms of AMS. HACE may occur in 2–3% of climbers at altitudes of 5,500 m, but the symptoms may occur at any altitude higher than 2,500 m.

Clinical presentation

HACE is a clinical diagnosis, characterized by the onset of ataxia, altered consciousness, or both, in someone with AMS or HAPE.

Initially, subjects will have symptoms that are indistinguishable from severe AMS. Prodromal symptoms of early mental impairment or a change in behavior may be ignored by patients and their companions. Severe headache, ataxic gait, lassitude, confusion, drowsiness, stupor, and coma characterize the clinical manifestations of HACE. Other signs and symptoms that may occur include nausea, vomiting, disorientation, hallucinations, cranial nerve palsy, hemiparesis, hemiplegia, and seizures (rarely). Ataxia is a common early feature and is almost pathognomonic. The skin may have a gray pallor or cyanotic appearance, as some degree of pulmonary edema is almost always present in HACE. Other associated findings of HACE may include papilledema and retinal hemorrhage (a common incidental finding). Focal neurologic signs are rare. Global encephalopathy rather than focal findings characterizes HACE.

Severe illness due to HACE may develop over a few hours, especially if the prodromal signs are ignored or misinterpreted. However, HACE usually requires 1–3 days to develop. The symptoms of HACE, like HAPE, are worse at night.

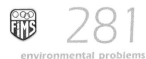

Treatment

As with AMS, slow ascent will reduce, although not remove completely, the risk of HACE. Careful management of AMS will prevent its progression to HACE. Early recognition of HACE is essential for successful treatment. Any evidence of HACE, including ataxia or change in consciousness, necessitates rapid descent (by at least about 600 m) and close supervision, because the victim's symptoms may progress during descent. Oxygen should be given if available, along with dexamethasone (initially 8 mg IV, IM, or PO, followed by 4 mg every 6 hours). Portable hyperbaric chambers should be considered if the patient is incapable of descending or if weather conditions prohibit descent, but descent as soon as possible must remain the first priority.

If descent is not feasible owing to logistical issues, supplemental oxygen or a portable hyperbaric chamber should be considered. Persons with HACE should also be started on dexamethasone, and consideration can be given to adding acetazolamide. No further ascent should be attempted until the victim is asymptomatic and no longer taking dexamethasone.

Sequelae from HACE can last weeks, but eventually patients usually recover completely. Overall mortality in untreated patients is 13%, which rises to 60% if coma occurs.

Other altitude-related problems

There are many conditions where high altitude may bear extra risks for patients involved. Some of the most important ones include ischemic and congestive heart disease, pregnancy, sickle-cell anemia or other hemoglobinopathies, bronchial asthma, and pulmonary diseases. In these cases, patients should be referred to an expert specialist for further assessment and recommendations.

AIR POLLUTION AND EXERCISE

Many chemicals are added to the air by industry, motor-vehicle traffic, and the use of energy for domestic or recreational purposes. Various air pollutants may affect physical performance.

Airborne pollutants are categorized as primary and secondary. Primary pollutants are those that affect directly from the source of pollution, whereas secondary pollutants are formed through chemical reactions between primary pollutants and other compounds, ultraviolet light, or with each other. Sulphur dioxide (SO_2), carbon monoxide (CO), nitrogen oxides (NO and NO_2), benzene, lead, and particulates such as dust and smoke are among the primary pollutants. Secondary pollutants include aerosols, ozone (O_3) and peroxyacetyl nitrate (PAN). CO is the most significant primary pollutant, as it changes the ability of erythrocytes to carry oxygen. Maximal exercise performance appears to be inversely affected by CO

HIGH-ALTITUDE ILLNESSES

AMS

Clinical presentation:

■ Headache at an altitude above 2,500 m, plus the presence of one or more of the gastrointestinal symptoms (anorexia, nausea, or vomiting), sleep disturbance, dizziness, and lassitude or fatigue.

Treatment:

■ Mild AMS: Avoid further ascent, rest one day more at the same altitude. Exertion should be minimized.
■ Moderate-to-severe AMS: Descent and supplemental oxygen.

Medication:

■ 250 mg acetazolamide twice daily.
■ 4–8 mg dexamethasone at first, then 4 mg four times/day.
■ Hyperbaric chamber is effective.

HAPE

Clinical presentation:

■ Dyspnea on exertion, reduced exercise tolerance, cough (dry at first and productive later), tachypnea, orthopnea, low-grade fever, crackles or wheezing (unilateral or bilateral).

Treatment:

■ Mild to moderate: descent, supplemental oxygen for 48–72 hours.
■ Severe: Descent to a lower altitude and hospitalization, 60 mg of sustained release nifedipine daily in divided doses, without a loading dose, if oxygen is not available or descent is impossible.

HACE

Clinical presentation:

■ Presence of ataxia or altered consciousness or both in someone with AMS or HAPE.

Treatment:

■ Immediate descent (at least about 600 m) and supplemental oxygen, dexamethasone (initially 8 mg IV, IM, or PO, followed by 4 mg every 6 hours).

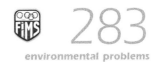

concentration in blood. Significant decrements in maximal exercise time, leg tiredness, and perceived exertion have been reported.

The CO level is high near motorways with heavy traffic, which cyclists or runners may use for training purpose. Low-level NO_2 inhalation can irritate the upper respiratory tract and impair mucociliary activity. Indoor ice-skating arenas are the most important source of NO_2 in sports environments. Poisoning with NO_2 and CO has been reported in ice-hockey players and referees. The source was an ice-resurfacing machine that was powered by gasoline. Switching to battery-powered ice-maintenance machines is recommended.

SO_2 is an airway irritant, with potentially harmful effects on epithelial cells. The level affecting pulmonary function should be high and, with current ambient levels, it cannot affect endurance exercise.

Environmental levels of lead have decreased since the introduction of unleaded petrol in motor vehicles. It has been suggested that high blood-lead levels influence homeostasis and nervous system function. Serious lead poisoning has been reported in instructors at an indoor pistol range. Lead oxide fumes can be produced by fragmentation of bullets when fired.

Ozone is a major airway irritant that causes irritation to the airways in resting and moderately exercising individuals. Ozone is one of the main constituents of smog. The O_3 level peaks near midday and is four or five times higher in summer. Adaptation to O_3 may occur after 2–5 days exposure to it.

PAN has been recognized as an eye irritant with a distinctive odor that results in blurred vision and eye fatigue. Younger men are more affected than older men. PAN exposure does not have any significant effect on exercise performance.

An aerosol is a suspension of ultramicroscopic solid or liquid particles in air or another gas, such as smoke, fog, or mist.

The precise effects of many air pollutants on human performance have not been explored yet. As air is a mixture of gases, and the pollutants are produced continuously, it is difficult to distinguish the effects of individual pollutants outside laboratories. On the other hand, the interaction of pollutants may have additive or synergistic effects on humans, with a greater threat to health and exercise performance than each single pollutant. Nevertheless, it is clear that the quality of air breathed in can have impact on exercise performance. In addition, air pollution can exacerbate respiratory conditions such as asthma and nasal allergies.

Athletes are at risk from inhaling air pollutants

The reasons are:

- as ventilation increases with exercise, the amount of pollutants inhaled will increase accordingly;

- the increase in airflow velocity transports pollutants further into the respiratory system; and
- during exercise, more air is inhaled through oral breathing rather than nasal breathing, and so the nasal filtering mechanisms will be bypassed.

Some prevention strategies for air pollution are listed in Box 13.3.

BOX 13.3 PREVENTION STRATEGIES FOR AIR POLLUTION

- Be informed of the air quality by following the meteorological news.
- Training should be scheduled at times associated with the least air pollution.
- When ambient O_3 level is high, exercise in the morning or at night. The peak O_3 level is around 3 p.m.
- Do exercise preferably in parks or alongside the ocean.
- On the way to an event, minimize exposure to pollutants by closing the windows of the vehicle.
- Minimize the warm-up period to limit the exposure time.
- During training on highways, keep 10–15 m distance from the exhaust pipes of cars.
- Consider wind direction and run or ride on the up-wind side of the road.
- Modify exercise intensity when the air-pollutant level is high.
- Do not exercise on days reported as hazardous or unhealthy.
- If the symptoms of chest pain or tightness, coughing, or wheezing occur, exercise should be stopped.
- Avoid cigarette smoke before and after exercise.
- Activated carbon facemasks can be used in urban environments.
- Ingesting antioxidants such as vitamins C and E is recommended, as they may have some protective effects against ozone-induced physiological changes.
- Inhaled beta-agonists can reverse ozone-induced bronchospasm in asthmatics.

JET LAG

See Chapter 8.

ACKNOWLEDGMENT

The editors acknowledge the assistance of Wendy Holdan, MSPT, of Boston Children's Hospital, for contributing to, and reviewing, this chapter.

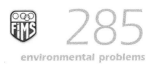

SUGGESTED READING

Armstrong L.E., Casa D.J., et al. American College of Sports Medicine position stand. Exertional heat illness during training and competition. *Med. Sci. Sports Exerc.* 2007; 39(3):556–72.

Bartsch P., Bailey D.M., et al. Acute mountain sickness: Controversies and advances. *High Alt. Med. Biol.* 2004; 5(2):110–24.

Basnyat B., Murdoch D.R. High-altitude illness. *Lancet* 2003; 361(9373):1967–74.

Biem J., Koehncke N., et al. Out of the cold: Management of hypothermia and frostbite. *CMAJ.* Feb. 4, 2003; 168(3):305–11.

Binkley H.M., Beckett J., et al. National Athletic Trainer's Association Position Statement: Exertional heat illnesses. *J. Athl. Train* 2002; 37(3):329–43.

Carlisle A.J., Sharp N.C.C. Exercise and outdoor ambient air pollution. *Br. J. Sports Med.* 2001; 35(4):214–22.

Castellani J.W., Young A.J., et al. American College of Sports Medicine position stand: Prevention of cold injuries during exercise. *Med. Sci. Sports Exerc.* 2006; 38(11):2012–29.

Coris E.E., Ramirez A.M., Van Durme D.J. Heat illness in athletes, the dangerous combination of heat humidity and exercise. *Sports Med.* 2004; 34(1):9–16.

Council on Sports Medicine and Fitness and Council on School Health. Policy Statement – Climatic Heat Stress and Exercising Children and Adolescents. *Pediatrics.* Aug. 8, 2011.

DeFranco M.J., Baker C.L. 3rd, et al. Environmental issues for team physicians. *Am. J. Sports Med.*, 2008; 36(11):2226–37.

Gallagher S.A., Hackett P.H. High altitude illness. *Emerg. Med. Clin. North Am.* 2004; 22(2):329–55.

Gavin T.P. Clothing and thermoregulation during exercise. *Sports Med.* 2003; 33(13):941–7.

Giesbrecht G.G. Prehospital treatment of hypothermia. *Wilderness Environ. Med.* 2001; 12(1):24–31.

Hamilton R., Paton B.C. The diagnosis and treatment of hypothermia by mountain rescue teams: A survey. *Wilderness Environ. Med.* 1996; 7(1):28–37.

Luks A.M., McIntosh S.E., et al. Wilderness medical society consensus guidelines for the prevention and treatment of acute altitude illness. *Wilderness Environ. Med.* 2010; 21(2):146–55.

Marshall S.W. Heat injury in youth sport. *Br. J. Sports Med.* Jan. 2010; 44(1):8–12.

Mason N. The pathology of high altitude: An introduction to the disease states of high altitude, current anesthesia and critical care. *Current Anaesthesia & Critical Care* 2000; 11(2):104–12.

Maughan R.J., Shirreffs S.M. Dehydration and rehydration in competitive sport. *Scand. J. Med. Sci. Sports* 2010; 20(Suppl. 3):40–7.

Maughan R.J., Shirreffs S.M., et al. Living, training and playing in the heat: Challenges to the football player and strategies for coping with environmental extremes. *Scand. J. Med. Sci. Sports* 2010; 20(Suppl. 3):117–24.

Murphy J.V., Banwell P.E., et al. Frostbite: Pathogenesis and treatment. *J. Trauma* 2000; 48(1):171–8.

Noakes T.D. Exercise in the heat: Old ideas, new dogmas. *Int. SportMed. J.* 2006; 7(1):58–74.

Roche-Nagle G., Murphy D., et al. Frostbite: Management options. *Eur. J. Emerg. Med.* 2008; 15(3):173–5.

Rodway G.W., Hoffman L.A., Sanders M.H. High-altitude-related disorders – Part I: Pathophysiology, differential diagnosis, and treatment. *Heart Lung* 2003; 32(6):353–9.

Rodway G.W., Hoffman L.A., Sanders M.H. High-altitude-related disorders – Part II: Prevention, special populations, and chronic medical conditions. *Heart Lung* 2004; 33(1):3–12.

Sallis R., Chassay C.M. Recognizing and treating common cold-induced injury in outdoor sports. *Medicine & Science in Sports & Exercise* 1999; 31(10):1367–73.

Santee W. Windchill index and military applications. *Aviat. Space Environ. Med.* 2002; 73(7):699–702.

Sawka M.N., Montain S.J. Fluid and electrolyte supplementation for exercise heat stress. *Am. J. Clin. Nutr.* 2000; 72(Suppl. 2):564S–72S.

Schoene R.B. Illnesses at high altitude. *Chest* 2008; 134(2):402–16.

Seto C.K., Way D., O'Connor N. Environmental illness in athletes. *Clin. Sports Med.* 2005; 24(3):695–718.

Smith J.E. Cooling methods used in the treatment of exertional heat illness. *Br. J. Sports Med.* 2005; 39(8):503–7.

Sunderland C., Morris J.G., Nevill M.E. A heat acclimation protocol for team sports. *Br. J. Sports Med.* 2008; 42(5):327–33.

Taylor N.A.S., Cotter J.D. Heat adaptation: Guidelines for the optimisation of human performance. *Int. Sport Med. J.* 2006; 7(1):33–57.

Ungley C.C., Channell G.D., Richards R.L. The immersion foot syndrome. *Wilderness Environ. Med.* 2003; 14(2):135–41.

Ziaee V., Yunesian M., et al. Acute mountain sickness in Iranian trekkers around Mount Damavand (5671 m) in Iran. *Wilderness Environ. Med.* 2003; 14(4):214–9.

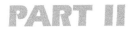

PART II

MUSCULOSKELETAL INJURIES

Diagnosis, treatment, and rehabilitation

INTRODUCTION

Angela D. Smith

The following chapters summarize international consensus for managing common musculoskeletal injuries in sport. The guidelines herein are not only intended for use by sports physicians or sports physiotherapists on the sports field or in sports injury clinics, but also serve well as a handbook for GPs, registrars, and students involved in sports and sports medicine education.

Appropriate *management* depends on a proper *diagnosis*, which in most cases starts with a thorough history and clinical examination. As a team medic, your specialty and competence may vary. If you are not an orthopedic specialist but feel confident to handle these injuries by yourself, your main task is to handle the acute situation, distinguish "emergencies" from "benign" conditions, and determine when and to whom the athlete should be referred for further investigations and treatment. You will always be asked, by the athlete, when and how training can be resumed. These chapters therefore address such issues, keeping in mind that competence and regimen may vary among different countries and levels of sport.

The approach to managing most sports injuries includes several components in addition to the treatment of the injury. If possible, immobilization should be minimized, to decrease the severity of disuse atrophy and general deconditioning. The athlete should perform cross-training activities, if possible, to maintain cardio-pulmonary fitness, strength, and flexibility. Strength and functional stability of the core (trunk) muscles are important parts of rehabilitation of almost all sports injuries. The athlete should strengthen, not only the core muscles, but also the entire kinetic chain for the injured region. For example, a pitcher with an injured elbow should obtain full strength, flexibility, and endurance of the entire upper extremity, as well as scapula–thoracic control, core stability, and support of lower-extremity function.

Athletes are often able to resume some aspects of training before their injuries have healed completely. One set of guidelines for playing while injured is known by the acronym PLAY, which is slightly modified below. It is applicable to most situations, with the aim of returning the athlete to play as rapidly and safely as possible.

- Pain may be present at the end of activity, but should be gone by the next morning, indicating that healing is progressing well.
- Limping, or favoring the injured limb, indicates it is too risky to return to full training or play.
- Ability to perform at expected level. If you have a lot of discomfort during or after sport activities, it indicates that the injury has not healed, or rehabilitation is not complete.
- You should not use pain-masking drugs to enable training or playing, so that you can monitor your body's signals of pain. Also, the doping aspect must be considered.

GENERAL OBJECTIVES

The following chapters aim to describe:

1. how to evaluate the athlete's history and injury mechanism;
2. how to conduct an initial clinical examination;
3. how to provide first aid from a musculoskeletal point of view;
4. when and to whom to refer the athlete for further investigations and treatment;
5. what advice to give regarding continuation of training and return to play.

The material will provide a theoretical basis for proper management and hands-on training of clinical examination techniques for diagnosing common sport injuries.

SPECIFIC OBJECTIVES

With respect to common sports injuries, these chapters will aim to:

1. exemplify typical history you may expect and common clinical symptoms and signs you may recognize from common sports injuries;
2. introduce hands-on techniques for proper clinical examination of common sports injuries;
3. provide hands-on tips for on-field first-aid treatment of acute sports injuries;
4. guide further investigations and referrals;
5. exemplify how to advise the injured athlete until full recovery.

GENERAL CLINICAL APPROACH TO ATHLETES PRESENTING WITH INJURY/PAIN

History

Consider age, gender, physical appearance, training status, and previous injury. How did the current symptoms occur? Let the athlete demonstrate! How does the athlete describe the symptoms, with regard to duration, intensity, and location?

Principles of clinical examination

- Always compare the injured with the non-injured side.
- Inspection and palpation: look for ecchymosis/laceration, swelling, muscle symmetry, local tenderness on palpation, neurovascular status.
- Range of motion: are there any restrictions? Does the limiting factor have an intra-articular pathology?
- Muscle function: is there muscle pathology or muscle guarding?
- Special tests: use tests for joint stability, tests for intra-articular disorders, and provocative tests.

Imaging

- Plain X-ray.
- Ultrasound.
- Magnetic resonance imaging (MRI).
- Computed tomography (CT) scan.
- Special imaging indications to be discussed in coverage of specific injuries.

When and to whom to refer

Refer whenever you are not comfortable with confirming a specific diagnosis/ treatment plan, including rehabilitation and return to play.

Treatment

- Acute or on-field treatment.
- Non-operative/functional treatment.
- Surgical treatment.

Return to play

- Formulation of a rehabilitation plan or program.
- Return to play criteria, objective, and subjective tests of function.

CHAPTER 14

SHOULDER INJURIES

Peter G. Gerbino

ACUTE SHOULDER INJURIES

Acute injuries about the shoulder include fractures of the clavicle, humerus, or scapula; acromioclavicular (AC) and sternoclavicular (SC) separation; and shoulder subluxation and dislocation. Occasionally, an athlete will sustain an acute rotator cuff tear, tendon rupture, or muscle tear (Figures 14.1 and 14.2).

Fractures

Fieldside assessment

The athlete has severe pain following a fall on to the lateral shoulder or an axial load to the humerus. Local, severe tenderness likely indicates a fracture. The injured limb should be supported with a sling, with ice applied to the injured region, until X-rays are completed, and the specific diagnosis is confirmed.

Diagnosis

Some fractures, such as clavicle or humeral-shaft fracture (Figure 14.3), can be palpated readily, and the diagnosis is made. Others, such as scapula fractures, may not be apparent to palpation in a muscular athlete. Once the diagnosis of fracture is suspected, the athlete is removed from the field and sent for radiographs. Splinting, strapping, or bracing can be used for comfort and to minimize motion. Plain radiographs consist of an anteroposterior view of the glenohumeral joint, a trans-scapular or scapular-Y lateral, and an axillary view.

Protected axillary views are done when the arm cannot be abducted. Special views can be used to assess the supraspinatus outlet, the anterior–inferior glenoid rim, and the clavicle. If doubt exists about bony anatomy, computed tomography (CT) is best for detailed evaluation.

Treatment

As the shoulder has a large range of motion, reduction of proximal humerus fractures does not have to be perfect. In adolescents or adults, the angulation

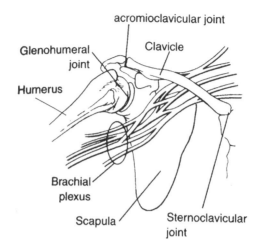

acromioclavicular joint

Glenohumeral joint

Clavicle

Humerus

Brachial plexus

Scapula

Sternoclavicular joint

Figure 14.1 Shoulder anatomy

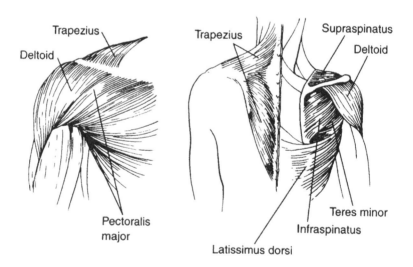

Trapezius

Deltoid

Pectoralis major

Trapezius

Supraspinatus

Deltoid

Teres minor

Infraspinatus

Latissimus dorsi

Figure 14.2 Shoulder anatomy

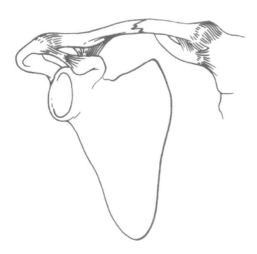

Figure 14.3 Clavicle fracture

should be less than 30°, and the reduction should be stable. Consideration should be given to ensuring anatomic reduction in the dominant shoulder of a throwing athlete, gymnast, or swimmer, who is prone to develop overuse shoulder injury even with a normal shoulder. Surgical reduction and internal fixation may be required to achieve this. Clavicle fractures nearly always heal acceptably when a sling or figure-of-eight brace is used for comfort (Figure 14.4). The figure-of-eight brace does not reduce the fracture. Exceptions include open fractures, those in which there is interposed muscle, and fractures with the skin at risk for perforation.

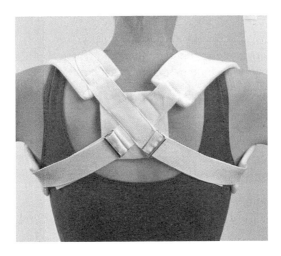

Figure 14.4 Figure-of-eight brace

These are reduced and internally fixed. The 2-mm-type clavicle fracture frequently needs to be repaired operatively, as well. Scapula fractures are usually high-energy injuries. Unless the glenoid is fractured and displaced more than 2 mm, scapula fractures can be treated by immobilization in a soft dressing, such as a sling and swathe. Check for associated injuries to the ribs, lung, and heart.

Rehabilitation

Once the fracture has healed, strength, range-of-motion, and proprioception must be restored before play is resumed. A typical progression includes early passive motion, followed by active motion and rotator-cuff strengthening. Periscapular stabilization and major shoulder muscle strengthening follow, in conjunction with shoulder proprioceptive training.

Return to play

When the bone is healed and the shoulder rehabilitated, as above, the athlete may return to competition. The time frame is variable, depending on the sport. A soccer player (except the goalkeeper) can return as soon as the bone is strong, whereas a wrestler needs complete rehabilitation before putting the shoulder at risk in competition.

SHOULDER FRACTURES

History

- Direct blow or axial load.

Examination

- Local tenderness and swelling, possible deformity.

Treatment

- Reduction/internal fixation/immobilization where appropriate.
- Rehabilitation to include periscapular stabilization.

Return to play

- When athlete can meet demands of sport.

Glenohumeral dislocation

Fieldside assessment

Shoulder dislocation generally occurs when the upper extremity is forced into extreme external rotation and abduction (Figure 14.5). The athlete with an anteriorly dislocated shoulder will hold the extremity in external rotation, adducted if possible. The athlete should be removed from play. On rare occasions

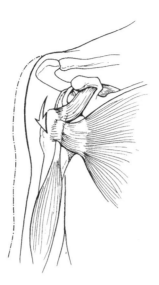

Figure 14.5 Glenohumeral dislocation

(particularly with recurrent dislocations), the shoulder can be reduced by the athlete, and some athletes can return to the contest after such dislocations. Muscle relaxation (often requiring medication) is usually needed for reduction, which should be performed by a trained clinician, but sometimes a reduction can be done with no medication. Fracture must also be ruled out by complete evaluation at an appropriate facility.

Diagnosis
The physical examination will localize the site of dislocation. More than 90% of traumatic shoulder dislocations occur in the anterior direction. In addition to the abnormal arm position, a posterior hollow space in the shoulder may be apparent. The axillary nerve may be injured, causing decreased sensation and deltoid muscle weakness. Posterior dislocations occur less frequently, and this diagnosis is sometimes missed initially. Consider performing X-rays before any reduction maneuver, particularly in the skeletally immature athlete. What appears to be a shoulder dislocation may actually be a proximal humerus physeal fracture. X-rays also show glenoid and humeral head fractures that may influence treatment. At a minimum, X-rays should be obtained following reduction.

Treatment
A physician who witnesses a shoulder dislocation and is experienced at reduction may, on occasion, attempt to reduce the shoulder in the locker room, before pain and muscle spasm are prohibitive. Later, using muscle relaxants and analgesics, the shoulder can be reduced. Radiographs should be taken of all shoulder

dislocations to confirm reduction and to identify fractures of the humeral head (Hill–Sachs lesion) and glenoid rim that can accompany these injuries. Prereduction films are not always necessary. Treatment of dislocations is controversial. Following first-time anterior glenohumeral dislocation, up to 90% of competitive athletes will redislocate if not repaired surgically. Despite this, the usual recommendation for first-time dislocation remains conservative, with 4–6 weeks of rest in a sling, followed by therapy to restore motion and strength. Immobilization in external rotation has not been found to be helpful. Depending on the athlete's situation, however, primary repair, usually arthroscopic, should be considered. Recurrent dislocations are stabilized surgically, by open or arthroscopic means.

Rehabilitation

Whether treated non-surgically or surgically, 3–4 months of rehabilitation are required to achieve pre-injury status. In all cases, attention is paid to restoring the rotator cuff and periscapular muscle strength, before working the larger shoulder girdle muscles.

Return to play

Following operative repairs, 4 months is usually necessary to achieve adequate healing, strength, and proprioception to return to sports safely. Shoulder dislocations treated non-operatively may return to sport after pain subsides and full motion and strength are restored.

GLENOHUMERAL SHOULDER DISLOCATIONS

History

- Fall, or fall combined with separate impact (such as from another player).
- Athlete often feels shoulder pop out of joint.

Examination

- Usually athlete holds shoulder adducted and externally rotated.
- Obvious deformity.

Treatment

- Consider immediate reduction.
- Consider surgical stabilization.

Return to play

- When athlete can meet demands of sport (non-operative).
- After 4 months of rehabilitation (operative).

---

peter g. gerbino

Shoulder separations

Fieldside assessment

The mechanism of injury for AC and anterior SC separation is usually a fall directly on the lateral shoulder (Figures 14.6 and 14.7). The mechanism of posterior SC separation may be the same, or result from a direct blow. The severity of pain is related to the severity of injury, but typically athletes are unable to continue to play. Local tenderness and deformity (in more severe degrees of injury) provide the likely diagnosis. If fieldside examination shows a posterior SC separation, emergency cardiopulmonary evaluation and treatment are required.

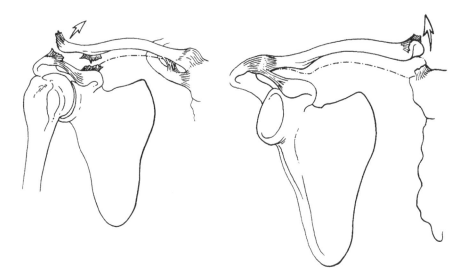

Figure 14.6
Acromioclavicular separation

Figure 14.7
Sternoclavicular separation

If the injury is AC or anterior SC separation, a sling will provide comfort until full assessment is completed.

Diagnosis

The physical examination will localize the site of dislocation. Inspection, palpation, and the cross-arm test (Figure 14.8) are usually adequate to assess AC or SC injuries. To visualize the severity of AC joint injury, with the athlete seated and relaxed, the examiner can passively pull downward on both arms and observe the space created between the acromion and the distal clavicle on the injured side. X-rays may be obtained to help assess the degree and direction of AC and SC separations.

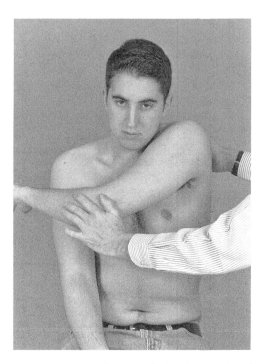

Figure 14.8 The "cross-arm" test that axially loads the clavicle, causing pain if either the AC or SC joint is injured

SC injuries are particularly difficult to image and may require CT for the pathology to be seen well. In the skeletally immature athlete, physeal fracture is more likely than actual AC or SC joint dislocation.

These physes may not fuse until after 20 years of age. Depending on the athlete's age, the epiphysis, which typically maintains its ligamentous attachments to the acromion or the sternum, respectively, may be difficult to visualize on X-ray if it is still primarily cartilage rather than bone.

Treatment

AC separations are usually treated non-operatively. Some grade III separations are repaired with reconstructions of the coracoclavicular ligaments, especially in weightlifters or athletes who must wear shoulder pads. These are relative indications for surgery, however. Chronic, symptomatic, mild AC separations are treated with distal clavicle resection and stabilization. Grade III or higher AC dislocations are treated by reconstructing the coracoclavicular ligaments. SC separations are usually anterior and are treated non-operatively. Posterior SC dislocations may compromise pulmonary and neurovascular structures and are reduced and stabilized operatively. Growth-plate fractures heal rapidly, and these deformities may remodel completely with time.

Rehabilitation

An AC separation or an anterior SC separation can be rehabilitated with general shoulder strengthening as soon as pain permits. Operative AC and SC repairs require 4–6 weeks of healing before motion and strengthening can be started. Whether treated non-surgically or surgically, 3–4 months of rehabilitation are required to achieve pre-injury status. Rotator cuff and periscapular muscle strength should be restored before the larger shoulder girdle muscles are worked.

ACROMIOCLAVICULAR SHOULDER SEPARATION

History
- Impact to lateral shoulder (from fall or blow).

Examination
- Local tenderness, elevated clavicle.

Treatment
- Sling: surgery rarely indicated.

Return to play
- When pain permits and athlete can meet demands of sport.

STERNOCLAVICULAR SHOULDER SEPARATION

History
- Direct blow to the lateral shoulder.

Examination
- Tenderness and palpable deformity.

Treatment
- Anterior SC separation: consider closed reduction; rarely stays reduced, but surgical stabilization rarely indicated.
- Posterior SC separation: requires emergent evaluation and generally needs reduction.

Return to play
- When athlete can meet demands of sport.

Return to play

Athletes with AC and SC separations that are treated non-operatively can return to play as pain permits. Depending on the sport, the injury can be strapped or padded, and the athlete can return within days or weeks. Following operative repairs, 4 months is usually necessary to achieve adequate healing, strength, and proprioception for the athlete to return to sports safely.

Glenohumeral subluxation

Partial dislocation (subluxation) of the glenohumeral joint can occur after single or repetitive trauma to the anterior, inferior, or posterior capsule. The glenoid labrum can be torn during dislocation or subluxation. Glenohumeral subluxations and multidirectional laxity are treated non-operatively, with rotator cuff and periscapular strengthening. Only if conservative therapy fails is surgical stabilization considered. This can be performed open or arthroscopically, and the labrum should be repaired at the same time.

Acute muscle or tendon rupture

Fieldside assessment

Sudden, severe pain in the region of a muscle following a forceful contraction – usually as the muscle is actually lengthening – suggests muscle or tendon rupture. Strength is immediately markedly decreased, and local pain and swelling, with muscle spasm, occur rapidly. The athlete is removed from play. Ice and an elastic compressive wrap decrease symptoms at fieldside.

Diagnosis

Muscle or tendon rupture to pectoralis major, biceps long head, subscapularis, and other rotator cuff muscles can occur (Figure 14.9). Palpation for defects along the muscle tendon course or a prominent biceps or pectoralis major muscle bulge inconsistent with the contralateral side should raise suspicions of complete tear. Weakness in internal rotation should raise suspicions for a subscapularis tear. Physical examination will identify most of these ruptures. Magnetic resonance imaging (MRI) or ultrasound can confirm the diagnosis.

Treatment

For all of these except the biceps long head tendon, operative repair is necessary. Biceps long head rupture is frequently degenerative, and it is difficult to achieve satisfactory repair. The resulting weakness has not been found to be significant. Tenodesis to the humeral shaft, rather than repair, can be considered for the biceps.

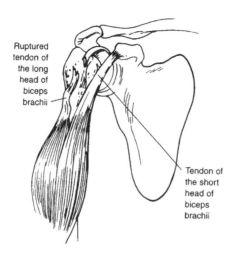

Ruptured
tendon of
the long
head of
biceps
brachii

Tendon of
the short
head of
biceps
brachii

Figure 14.9 Rupture of the long head tendon of the biceps

Rehabilitation

After rotator cuff or pectoralis tendon repair, passive motion is begun immediately, followed by active motion at 6 weeks postoperatively. Strengthening can also be started at 6 weeks.

Return to play

Following biceps long head rupture, the athlete may return to play as soon as pain and swelling resolve. Most athletes wait 4–6 months following rotator cuff or pectoralis repair to allow adequate healing and strengthening.

ACUTE MUSCLE OR TENDON RUPTURE

History
- Sudden forcible contraction followed by severe pain.
- May hear or feel a "pop."

Examination
- Weakness, palpable defect.

Treatment
- Surgical repair generally indicated, depends on severity and location.
- Strengthen when sufficiently healed.

Return to play
- When athlete can meet demands of sport.

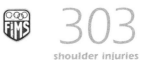

303

NON-ACUTE SHOULDER INJURIES

Non-acute or overuse injuries of the shoulder include impingement, glenohumeral pain associated with mild ("micro-") instability, and neurologic pain such as thoracic outlet syndrome. Chronic impingement can lead to a "traumatic" rotator cuff tear from relatively minor trauma. Labral tears can be acute or chronic.

Rotator cuff impingement

Diagnosis

When the rotator cuff muscles are disproportionately weak compared with the large shoulder muscles, the humeral head translates too far anteriorly or superiorly, and the greater tuberosity can impinge upon the acromion or coracoacromial ligament through the rotator cuff. The resulting friction can lead to bursitis, tendinitis, tendinosis, and tears. In throwing athletes, impingement and subclinical instability with or without labral tear are common. The impingement is frequently a secondary manifestation from glenohumeral laxity and labral pathology.

Reproducing the impingement (Figure 14.10) confirms the diagnosis, but it is more important to discover why the muscle imbalance exists. Causes include training error (developing only the large muscles), rotator cuff tear (such as from a violent throw or fall), or repetitive motion (such as occurs in swimmers, as they pull the humeral head against the coracoacromial ligament with every stroke).

The history and visual inspection of the shoulder will focus the examiner on those areas requiring detailed testing. Shoulder range of motion can be simply

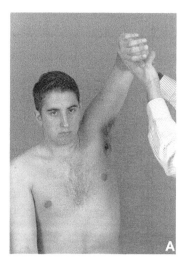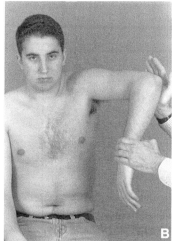

Figure 14.10 Shoulder subacromial impingement as described by (A) Neer and (B) Hawkins

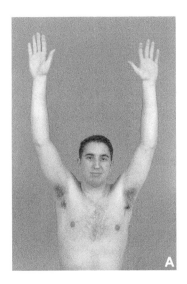
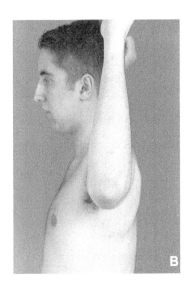
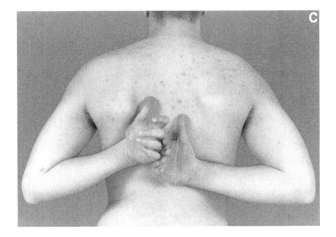

Figure 14.11 Measuring shoulder range of motion. (A) Overhead elevation measures shoulder extension, abduction, and scapulothoracic motion. (B) External rotation in 90° of abduction. (C) Noting the spinous process that can be reached with the thumb and comparing with the opposite side assesses internal rotation and adduction

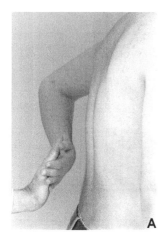

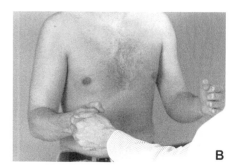

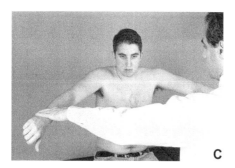

Figure 14.12 Measuring rotator cuff strength. (A) Internal rotation minimizing
pectoralis major effects best isolates subscapularis. (B) External
rotation assesses infraspinatus and teres minor. (C) Resisted
abduction with thumbs down (increased impingement) and arms
30° anterior to coronal plane best assesses supraspinatus pain and
strength

evaluated by measuring elevation, forward flexion, adduction, external rotation
in 90° of abduction, and the height along the spine that can be reached by the
thumb (adduction, internal rotation) (Figure 14.11). Testing internal rotation in
90° of abduction allows detection of tight posterior capsule and external rotator
muscles. The tests for subacromial injury are depicted in Figures 14.10A and
14.10B.

Evaluating internal rotation, external rotation, and adduction, as shown in Figure
14.12, assesses rotator cuff strength. Glenohumeral joint problems are assessed
with three special tests. The apprehension test leads to pain and apprehension
with forced abduction and external rotation (Figure 14.13). A positive test indicates

peter g. gerbino

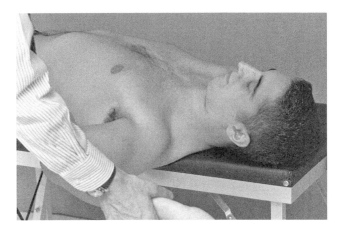

Figure 14.13 The "apprehension" test for anterior dislocation. Painful sensation that the shoulder is about to dislocate is considered positive

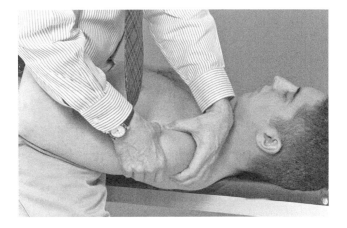

Figure 14.14 Glenohumeral translation is assessed in the anterior, posterior, and inferior directions. The test can be performed sitting or supine

anterior glenohumeral instability or pain. Glenohumeral translation (Figure 14.14) is checked in the anterior, posterior, and inferior directions. This is always compared with the contralateral side. Finally, loading the anterior, posterior, or superior capsule and rotating the humeral head, trying to elicit a painful "pop" (Figure 14.15), can assess the labrum. Many named tests have been described to assess the labrum. None is perfect for all athletes. Scapular dyskinesis frequently results from shoulder injury. Assessing dyskinesis requires evaluation of scapular motion.

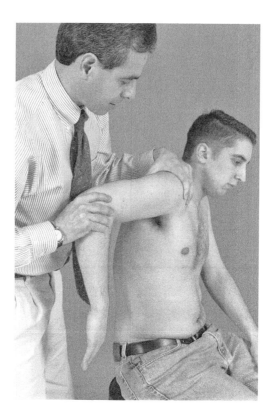

Figure 14.15 The "crank" test axially loads the joint, and rotation stresses the labrum, to bring out painful pops or clicks indicating a labral tear

Imaging

The best study for evaluation of rotator cuff tears and other soft-tissue injury is MRI. Even MRI, however, is poor at evaluating labral tears. Use of gadolinium with the MRI or use of a CT arthrogram is better at finding labral irregularities. In many countries, ultrasound is used routinely for soft-tissue evaluation of shoulder problems. Its use is growing rapidly in the United States. The technique used should be based more on local availability and the skill of the ultrasonographer, rather than on a specific set of rules.

Treatment

Treatment of impingement first requires rotator cuff and periscapular strengthening. Treating scapular dyskinesis requires a skilled physiotherapist who understands the subtle changes that occur with this problem. A subacromial injection of corticosteroid may be necessary to decrease inflammation and gain sufficient pain relief to permit stretching and strengthening. If resolution does not occur or is transient, glenohumeral pathology must be considered, and arthroscopic evaluation may be indicated. Further treatment may include labral repair or debridement and capsular tightening by arthroscopic or open means. Thermal capsular shrinkage has been used in the past, but results have been unacceptable.

Rehabilitation

As impingement is classically caused by relatively weak rotator cuff muscles, strengthening the subscapularis, supraspinatus, infraspinatus, and teres minor is mandatory. The scapular stabilizers, including rhomboids, trapezius, levator scapulae, and serratus anterior, must be strengthened as well. Especially important are the lower trapezius muscles. These periscapular muscles must be strengthened in non-operative treatment of shoulder instability, as well as following operative glenohumeral repairs. The strengthening program should include the entire kinetic chain, particularly the trunk muscles. Shoulder proprioception refers to control of the shoulder at all points of motion. Following capsular injury or surgery, proprioception must be restored prior to return to play. In general, this is accomplished by practicing the activities necessary to the particular sport, especially if throwing is involved (Figure 14.16). Resumption of throwing is accomplished by slow relearning of the muscle firing sequences as strength is restored. Restoration of muscle balance and endurance are fundamental principles of rehabilitation. In the shoulder, this refers to balance between cuff and major muscles and between internal and external rotators. Any imbalance can lead to excessive translation in one direction and instability or impingement.

Likewise, muscle endurance needs to be improved, so that asymmetries do not develop as the athlete becomes fatigued. This concept is especially important in

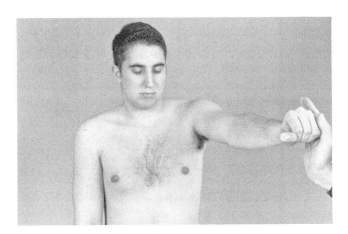

Figure 14.16 One type of proprioception training for the injured shoulder requires the patient to resist unexpected (eyes closed) attempts to move the upper extremity in different directions

throwers and racquet-sport athletes, who will alter their mechanics as one muscle group fatigues prematurely. Alteration of technique can lead to impingement, tendinitis, and instability for swimmers. If the internal rotators are much stronger than the external rotators, an impingement on the coracoacromial ligament can develop that is very difficult to correct.

Return to play

Return to play following overuse shoulder injury is governed by two factors. The first is pain within the range of motion required for the sport. The second is adequate strength and proprioception to perform the movements of the sport without risk of re-injury. Ideally, the shoulder (including trunk/scapulothoracic region) has a full, pain-free range of motion, with balanced strength and endurance and normal proprioception. In reality, if the shoulder is relatively well balanced and pain-free, and if extreme or painful motions (e.g., external rotation) can be restricted, the athlete can return to play.

Swimmer's shoulder

Diagnosis

Swimmer's shoulder is anterior impingement at the coracoacromial ligament from overdevelopment of the pectoralis major and anterior deltoid. Frequently, there is decreased internal rotation and a tight posterior capsule. The prolonged imbalances and abnormal motions of swimmer's shoulder can lead to subclinical instability and anterior labral degeneration. Associated biceps tendinitis occurs frequently.

Treatment

Initial treatment is stretching of the posterior capsule and external rotators and strengthening of the rotator cuff. Restoration of normal scapulothoracic strength and smooth motion is required. This requires trunk (core) strengthening as well. Surgical subacromial decompression alone, without balancing of the cuff and major muscles of the shoulder, will have a low success rate.

Rehabilitation

Swimmer's shoulder is rehabilitated much the same as impingement, with special emphasis on maintaining normal rotation and preventing an imbalance from developing between the strong pectoralis major and deltoid and the small stabilizer muscles. Recent studies have shown that the serratus anterior and lower trapezius are key to stabilizing the scapula.

Return to play

As in the other shoulder overuse injuries, anterior impingement that has resolved should not recur if technique and muscle balance have been optimized. If the athlete is not compulsive about maintaining range of motion and periscapular strength, the condition will recur. Swimming is allowed when symptoms are gone.

Microinstability

Microinstability is a term used to describe the situation where minor excess (usually anterior) motion has developed. This increased translation can be seen as a labral tear, labral "peel-back," stretching of the rotator interval part of the capsule, or a combination of these. All of these occur from repeated strain of the humeral head against the anterior capsule and labrum. Peel-back refers to gradual attenuation of the labral attachment to the glenoid, resulting in a larger than normal sublabral cleft.

Microinstability should be suspected in throwers and racquet-sport athletes with anterior shoulder pain during use. A click indicates a labral tear or peel-back lesion. Imaging studies are usually unrewarding.

Treatment is as for labral tear or instability: repairing the labrum, restoring normal labral peel-back, and closing the rotator interval as needed. Rehabilitation and return to play are the same as for dislocation repair.

SHOULDER PAIN, NON-ACUTE

History
- Gradual onset of pain.
- Single specific location, multiple locations, or diffuse.
- Consider pre-existing strength/flexibility deficits.

Examination
- Determine specific locations of tenderness.
- Shoulder hyper-mobility.
- Pain with special tests.
- Flexibility; strength of shoulder and shoulder stabilizers; check scapulo-thoracic motion, scapular dyskinesis.

Treatment
- Make specific diagnoses where possible.
- Strengthen entire kinetic chain.
- NSAIDs, RICE.

Return to action
- Normal strength and flexibility, preferably pain-free.

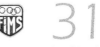

Neurologic problems

Overuse nerve injuries about the shoulder include thoracic outlet syndrome and suprascapular nerve entrapment. Suprascapular entrapment occurs at the scapular notch and can result in severe infraspinatus atrophy. Surgical decompression at the notch is usually curative.

In the absence of abnormal anatomy, thoracic outlet syndrome is caused by poor posture, weak trapezius, and weak levator scapulae. This syndrome presents as pain, paresthesias, and/or weakness in the brachial plexus distribution. Strengthening of the supporting muscles will improve the neurological component of the syndrome.

Vascular problems

Vascular injuries about the shoulder include thoracic outlet syndrome, traumatic intimal tears to the axillary or subclavian vessels, or deep vein thrombosis. Deep vein thrombosis typically presents as massive swelling of the arm, often following exercise. It is treated with anticoagulation for up to 6 months, or by pharmacologic thrombolysis. The vascular component of thoracic outlet syndrome will respond to trapezius and levator scapulae strengthening. In cases of additional cervical rib or other anatomic cause, surgical decompression may be required. The vascular surgeon treats intimal tears to shoulder girdle arteries or veins. Minor tears can be followed closely with Doppler, MRI, or contrast angiography. Large tears must be repaired or excised.

ACKNOWLEDGMENT

The editors acknowledge the assistance of Grover Price, PT, of Boston Children's Hospital, for contributing to, and reviewing, the rehabilitation sections in this chapter.

SUGGESTED READING

Andrews J.R., Wilk K.E., Reinold, M. (Eds.) *The athlete's shoulder.* New York: Churchill Livingstone; 2008.
Hawkins R.J., Misamore G.W. (Eds.) Shoulder injuries in the athlete. *Surgical Repair and Rehabilitation.* New York: Churchill Livingstone; 1996.
Kibler W.B., McMullen J. Scapular dyskinesis and its relation to shoulder pain. *J. Am. Acad. Orthop. Surg.* 2003; 11(2):142–51.
Krishnan S.G., Hawkins R.J., Warren R.F.(Eds.) *The shoulder and the overhead athlete.* Lippincott Williams & Wilkins; 2004.

peter g. gerbino

CHAPTER 15

ELBOW, FOREARM, WRIST, AND HAND INJURIES

James A. Whiteside and James R. Andrews

ACUTE ELBOW INJURIES

Acute traumatic elbow injuries are not uncommon among athletes. Fall, direct contusion, or collision injuries can cause dislocations or fractures around the elbow. Fractures may involve the radial head, olecranon, distal humerus, medial epicondyle, capitellum, or trochlea around elbow joints. Emergent orthopaedic referral is necessary for any athlete with a fracture or dislocation, evidence of brachial artery injury, or nerve injury. Management of elbow fractures in children differs from those in adults.

Elbow dislocation

Fieldside assessment
Usually, the athlete sustains a fall injury on an outstretched hand, with the elbow extended (75% result from a fall injury). There is severe pain. The athlete supports his/her forearm with the other hand. Look for gross swelling and deformity, which are usually very obvious (Figure 15.1A). Although anterior and divergent elbow dislocations do occur, the vast majority of dislocations are posterior (Figure 15.1B). Feel for the posteriorly displaced olecranon process. A thorough neurovascular examination is mandatory, especially of the ulnar nerve. Because of the high incidence of associated fractures (20–50%), pre-reduction radiographs must be taken. The elbow is splinted in a comfortable position, and the athlete is transported to hospital for proper assessment and management.

Diagnosis
With typical history and obvious elbow deformity, clinical diagnosis of posterior elbow dislocation is not difficult. Differential diagnoses include fractures of the distal humerus. Associated injuries are not uncommon; these include radial head fractures, olecranon fractures, coronoid process fractures, and medial epicondyle avulsion fractures (common in adolescents).

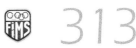

Treatment

A team physician with proper training and experience can attempt closed reduction of a simple posterior elbow dislocation in the field, provided that there is no significant swelling, spasm, or any obvious associated injury. By an hour or so after the injury has occurred, closed reduction under proper sedation is necessary. For simple elbow dislocation, the best results are obtained with conservative treatment. However, surgery is considered for the following conditions: (a) an unstable

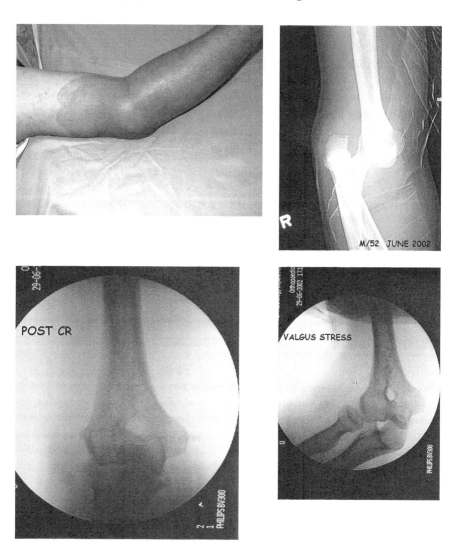

Figure 15.1 (A) Posterior elbow dislocation: gross. (B) Posterior elbow dislocation. (C) Posterior elbow dislocation: gross instability upon valgus stress

314

james a. whiteside and james r. andrews

elbow after reduction (Figure 15.1C); (b) a competitive throwing athlete; or (c) associated fractures. Surgery for unstable elbows includes repair or reconstruction of the damaged collateral ligaments, with or without use of a hinged external fixator.

Rehabilitation

Shoulder and finger exercises are begun at once. Simple posterior elbow dislocation should be treated conservatively, aiming for early range-of-motion (ROM) training within a stable arc of motion. Immobilization should be kept minimal. Full flexion and extension in a hinged brace, with the forearm immobilized in pronation, are advisable. An extension block can be added to ensure the elbow range is confined within the stable arc of motion. Once stability is improved, attention should be turned to regaining full ROM.

Return to play

Normal daily activities are permitted when the ROM is functional and the arm strength reaches 80% of normal. Sport activities are allowed when the athlete's confidence in elbow strength and the required technical skills have returned.

Distal humerus fracture

Distal humerus fractures include intra-articular or extra-articular fractures. Intra-articular fractures can be classified as single column (medial or lateral condyle fractures) or two column (T-shaped or Y-shaped intercondylar fractures) (Figure 15.2A). Extra-articular fractures can be classified into extra-capsular (supracondylar (Fig. 15.3), medial epicondylar, or lateral epicondylar fractures) or intra-capsular

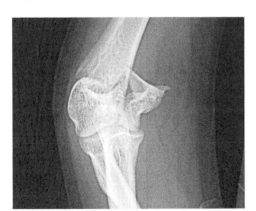
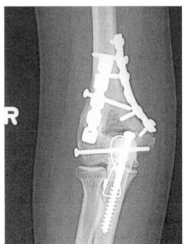

Figure 15.2 (A) T-shaped intercondylar fractures. (B) T-shaped intercondylar fractures treated with open reduction and rigid internal fixation

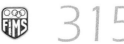

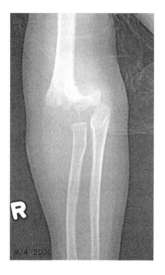

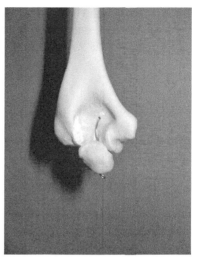

Figure 15.3
Supracondylar fracture
X-ray

Figure 15.4
Bony landmarks of the medial
epicondyle and tip of olecranon process
normally form an equilateral triangle

(transcondylar fractures). Young athletes may sustain a supracondylar fracture, with posterior displacement of the distal fragment.

Fieldside assessment

Following a fall, collision, or direct contusion to the elbow, the athlete has severe elbow pain, sometimes with obvious deformity. Look for swelling, which develops rapidly and diffusely. Feel for bony landmarks of the medial epicondyle, lateral epicondyle, and tip of the olecranon process, which normally should form an equilateral triangle (Figure 15.4). Check for neurovascular function of the upper limb. The elbow is splinted in its resting position, and the athlete is transported to hospital for proper assessment and management. Frequent monitoring of the vascular status during transfer is important.

Diagnosis

Clinical diagnosis of distal humerus fracture is not difficult, given the typical presentation and physical findings. Radiographic examination with plain anteroposterior (AP) and lateral X-rays of the elbow are mandatory for proper assessment.

Treatment

Operative treatment, open reduction, and internal fixation are usually indicated. Open reduction allows anatomical reduction of fragments, to ensure accurate alignment of the distal humerus (Figure 15.2B). Rigid internal fixation provides immediate stability to allow early rehabilitation and minimize residual stiffness.

Rehabilitation

If the fracture is stable after rigid internal fixation, ROM exercises can be started. The elbow joint can be protected with a removable splint. Strengthening exercises are added when bone healing is sufficient, to include triceps, forearm supination, pronation, biceps, and periscapular musculature in both closed and open chain positions, to promote weightbearing within a pain-free range. Then, the patient should be advanced to sport-specific functional training for return to sport.

Return to play

The expected time for bone to heal depends on the fracture pattern and fixation methods, but is usually not fewer than 8 weeks. The expected duration of rehabilitation usually takes not fewer than 12 weeks.

Radial head or neck fracture

Fieldside assessment

The athlete sustains a fall injury on the outstretched hand, with the forearm in pronation, which occurs frequently during contact sports. Look for elbow effusion, which is usually present. There is usually no obvious deformity. Feel for sharp, localized bone tenderness over the radial head, as this is a reliable clinical finding. There is pain with elbow flexion or extension and forearm rotation. Check for any bone block to motion. It is important to look out for Essex–Lopresti fracture by checking any associated wrist and/or central forearm pain.

Diagnosis

There is usually no obvious deformity, except for the presence of an elbow effusion. Definite local tenderness at the radial head makes the diagnosis obvious. Radiographic examination with plain AP and lateral X-rays of the elbow are employed to determine the type of radial head or neck fracture (Figure 15.5), any comminution, degree of displacement, and any associated injury. Classification by Mason for radial head fractures is commonly used: (I) undisplaced, (II) displaced, (III) comminuted, and (IV) radial head fracture with associated dislocation (Figure 15.6).

Treatment

Athletes with non-displaced fractures can be treated conservatively, with early ROM. Aspiration of the hemarthrosis and instillation of local anesthetic for pain relief under strict sterile condition are often useful. This brings dramatic pain relief and allows assessment for any mechanical block. A long arm posterior splint with the elbow at 90° is applied for 5–7 days. Displaced fractures should be treated with open reduction and internal fixation with screws or mini-plates.

317

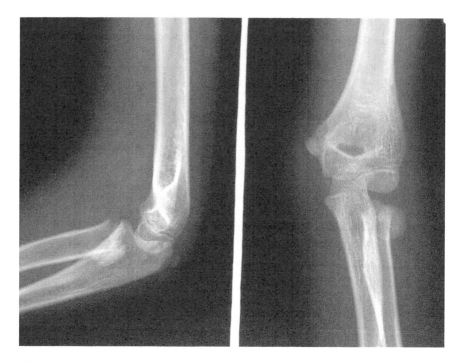

Figure 15.5 Displaced radial neck fracture

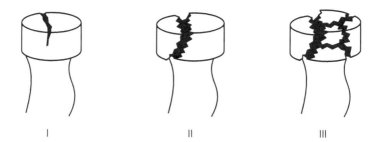

Figure 15.6 Classification of radial head fractures by Mason: (I) undisplaced; (II) displaced; (III) comminuted

Rehabilitation

Repeat radiographs should be obtained to look for any displacement during follow-ups. Active ROM exercises, including forearm supination and pronation, flexion, and extension, should be performed, as pain is tolerated. Ice application is helpful. Strengthening exercises can be added, as tolerated, when full ROM is attained, and clearance is given by the supervising physician. Strengthening exercises should

318

emphasize elbow extension in both open and closed chain positions, as well as supination. Throughout the strengthening period, the physiotherapist (PT) should continue to monitor the patient's ROM, so that it does not regress. In addition, closed chain exercises are helpful to promote weightbearing through the joint, to decrease osteopenic conditions post injury and to promote bone healing. Most athletes can expect good-to-excellent function after 2–3 months of rehabilitation.

Return to play
As radial head fracture is an intra-articular fracture, bathed in synovial joint fluid, complete bone healing is expected to take about 6–8 weeks. In some sports, which require little use of the arms, the athlete is allowed to return limited training as soon as a few days following the injury, with an appropriate brace for protection.

Separation of medial epicondylar epiphysis

In adults, isolated medial epicondylar fractures are uncommon. In children, the medial epicondyle usually begins to ossify at the age of 5 and is fully ossified by the age of 16. Normal throwing imparts large medial distraction, and a repetitive throwing action can result in chronic apophysitis. Medial epicondyle avulsion is usually preceded by chronic apophysitis. A hard throw may result in medial epicondyle avulsion fractures in these young throwing athletes.

Fieldside assessment
If the elbow is dislocated, deformity is, of course, obvious. But, even without dislocation, the diagnosis should be suspected if a young athlete presents with severe medial elbow pain after a hard throw. ROM of the elbow joint is decreased. There is localized swelling and tenderness over the medial epicondyle region. Pain may be accentuated with elbow and wrist flexion or forearm pronation. Check for ulnar nerve function, because of its proximity to the medial epicondyle. The arm is supported with a sling, and the athlete is transported to hospital for proper assessment and management.

Diagnosis
Typical history and presence of localized tenderness at the medial epicondyle region mean clinical diagnosis is not difficult. An AP X-ray of the elbow is necessary to determine the amount of displacement of the medial epicondylar epiphysis, ranging from minimal to marked displacement (Figure 15.7A). X-ray of the opposite elbow may be required also. Beware that the fragment may be trapped within the elbow joint.

Treatment
Fractures with minor displacement can be treated conservatively, with a long arm cast and the elbow in flexion for 3–4 weeks. If the medial epicondylar epiphysis

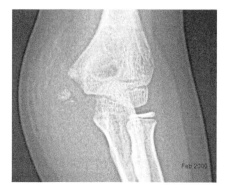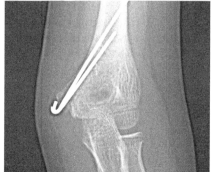

Figure 15.7 (A) Medial epicondyle avulsion fracture. (B) Medial epicondyle avulsion fracture: open reduction and internal fixation with two Kirschner wires

is displaced, open reduction and internal fixation, with a screw or two Kirschner wires, is indicated (Figure 15.7B). A trapped fragment in the elbow joint must be freed. After fixation, the integrity of the medial collateral ligaments should be evaluated.

Rehabilitation

Assisted ROM is initiated early if rigid internal fixation allows. After wound healing, controlled biceps, triceps, periscapular and shoulder, and hand strengthening is begun, while the elbow is protected against valgus stress by a hinged elbow brace for about 4 weeks. Continue to monitor and stretch wrist and finger flexors, avoiding excessive forces on the medial aspect of the elbow. At 6–8 weeks following injury, forearm and wrist strengthening exercises could be started. Look out for late ulnar nerve palsy.

Return to play

Most athletes regain full ROM and good strength after 12 weeks of rehabilitation. Forceful throwing activities are discouraged for a full year.

Olecranon fracture

The triceps muscle inserts by a broad tendinous expansion on to the posterior aspect of the olecranon. The olecranon process is susceptible to direct trauma, because it is essentially a subcutaneous bone. Fractures may be extra-articular (an avulsion fracture among the elderly) or intra-articular (involving the trochlea notch), displaced (greater than 2 mm separation between fragments) or non-displaced. These fractures can be classified as transverse (due to traction), oblique, or comminuted (due to direct trauma), stable or unstable (with elbow joint subluxation or dislocation). Displaced-stable fractures account for 85% of olecranon

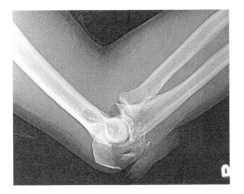

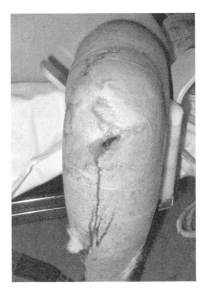

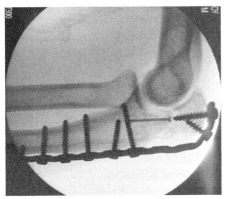

Figure 15.8 (A) Unstable olecranon fracture with comminution X-ray. (B) Unstable olecranon fracture with comminution soft-tissue injury. (C) Open reduction to achieve anatomical reconstruction, and internal fixation to allow early mobilization

fractures. Unstable fractures account for 5% of olecranon fractures, usually associated with radial head fractures and comminution (Figure 15.8A).

Fieldside assessment

Direct trauma to the elbow joint is a common mechanism causing olecranon fractures. These fractures are usually comminuted, with associated soft-tissue injury (Figure 15.8B). On the other hand, a fall on an outstretched hand, with the elbow in flexion, can cause a displaced transverse fracture owing to traction, resulting in failure of the extension mechanism. The athlete has severe pain and local swelling. The displaced olecranon appears prominent, and a defect may be palpable. ROM of the elbow joint is limited by pain and effusion. Check for any associated ulnar nerve injury. The athlete is removed from the field, and the elbow joint is properly splinted with a well-padded long arm splint, usually with the elbow joint flexed at 60° of flexion. Orthopaedic referral for proper assessment and management is indicated.

Diagnosis

Radiographic examination with a true lateral view of the elbow is employed to determine the type of olecranon fracture, any comminution, degree of displacement, and any associated injury. Fractures should be considered non-displaced when displacement of any fragment is less than 2 mm, and active extension against gravitational force is possible; non-displaced fractures account for 5% of olecranon fractures.

Treatment

Displaced olecranon fractures are indicated for open reduction and internal fixation, usually employing the principles of the tension band effect. Severely comminuted olecranon fractures often require open reduction and internal fixation with plating (Figure 15.8C).

Non-displaced and stable olecranon fractures can be managed conservatively by short-term immobilization (2–3 weeks), with early active, assisted motion. Follow-up radiographs should be taken to make certain there is no displacement of fragments. The athlete is transported to hospital for proper assessment and management.

Rehabilitation

Gradual elbow joint motion is allowed once healing and/or rigid internal fixation has been achieved. Strengthening exercises are permitted when union is achieved in 6–10 weeks. With range and strength, attention should be paid to avoiding end-range elbow extension, to promote proper healing of the olecranon fracture. Usage of tape or splinting to block end-ROM of elbow extension can be useful for patient feedback and prevention of complications.

Return to play

Progressive, pain-free activities are permitted once healing is complete. Full ROM is established by 8 weeks following injury. In most cases, return to sports may be expected at 3–5 months.

Rupture of the distal biceps brachii

Athletes involved in strength sports, rugby, and weight lifting are prone to this injury. The tendons usually fail at the insertion sites to the radial tuberosity.

Fieldside assessment

The athlete gives a history of sudden onset of severe elbow pain in the antecubital region after lifting or pulling a heavy object. Sometimes, a "pop" is also felt. Look for proximal migration of the biceps muscle belly, especially when compared with the non-injured side. Feel for local tenderness over the distal biceps. Pain and weakness with elbow flexion and supination are noted. In athletes with complete

james a. whiteside and james r. andrews

rupture, normal distal migration of the biceps muscle belly upon pronation is not present. Beware of partial rupture, which should be suspected with the presence of crepitus with forearm rotation. Immediate treatment consists of local ice application and supporting the forearm with a sling.

Diagnosis

Rupture of the distal biceps brachii is a clinical diagnosis. Bruising is usually seen after a few days. Plain radiographs are universally negative. MRI can demonstrate the lesion but is usually not indicated in a typical case with complete rupture.

Treatment

In an athlete with complete rupture, early primary repair, with reattachment of the tendon to the radial tuberosity, is desirable. Non-operative treatment may result in loss of strength at both elbow flexion (about 20%) and supination (about 40%). Occasionally, delayed primary repair is feasible when the lacertus fibrosis is intact, which can minimize the extent of proximal migration.

Rehabilitation

Postoperatively, the elbow is splinted at 90° flexion and neutral rotation. Active pronation and supination are allowed 1 week after the repair. Active ROM exercises are employed to reestablish normal ROM over the next 6 weeks, in a controlled fashion. Strengthening exercises are added when nearly full ROM is achieved. Strengthening should be initiated with isometric exercises, with progression to active ROM, and later with progressive resistive training. Physical therapy routines for the shoulder, wrist, and hand are maintained throughout this time.

Return to play

Unlimited activity is permitted when the elbow is pain free, with normal ROM and full strength. Usually, it takes more than 3 months to return to strength sports.

NON-ACUTE ELBOW INJURIES

Lateral epicondylitis

Runge first described lateral epicondylitis in 1873 as "writer's cramp." The condition is characterized by localized tenderness and chronic pain near the lateral epicondyle and is now commonly referred to as "tennis elbow." Causative factors include repetitive overuse, poor mechanics, and insufficient muscle conditioning, causing damage to the common wrist extensors at the lateral epicondyle. There is micro-tearing of the musculotendinous portion of the extensor carpi radialis brevis (ECRB). The condition is common among athletes taking part in golf, fencing, and throwing sports, but is still most commonly seen in racquet sports.

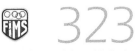

Diagnosis

Diagnosis of lateral epicondylitis is basically clinical. The athlete shows no visible atrophy, swelling, or bruising. There is localized tenderness over the extensor mass, 1–2 cm distal to the lateral epicondyle. Pain is aggravated by resisted wrist extension or passive wrist flexion. Weakness of handgrip should be pain related. Radiological examination is not necessary; occasionally, it is ordered to exclude other pathology.

Treatment

Conservative treatment gives a cure rate of 75–90% and should always be tried first. Initial treatment goals are to decrease pain and to encourage healing of the injured tendon by reduction of overload and activity modification. Together with other treatment measures, including use of counterforce bracing, local physical therapy, ice application, topical NSAID, and occasional oral medications with NSAID, symptoms should be controlled well in most cases. Steroid injections are reserved for patients whose status does not improve after 6–8 weeks of therapy. The effectiveness of other treatment modalities, such as acupuncture, extra-corporeal shock wave therapy, and botulinum toxin injection, needs to be confirmed. Surgery is rarely required.

Return to play

In the acute phase, the focus should be on stretching the usually short wrist and finger flexors. Afterwards, attention can be shifted to restoring biceps and supinator muscle strength over overused wrist extensors. Additionally, correction of faulty scapular alignment may be indicated to improve the chance of a full return to sport. Use of modalities, i.e. phonophoresis, iontophoresis, and cryotherapy, may be helpful to progress the patient. Also, manual treatment, to include cross-friction massage and use of a Chopat strap, can also help promote healing and a return to sport. Overall, exercises to increase muscular strength and endurance are important. An interval return to full activity is allowed. Emphasis on maintenance is important to avoid recurrence of pain.

Osteochondrosis/Osteochondritis dissecans

During the late cocking and early acceleration phases of throwing, there is increased valgus stress of the elbow and load stress at the radiocapitellar joint. A repetitive throwing action, common among young throwing athletes and gymnasts, may result in osteochondrosis (Panner's disease/Haas disease), osteo-chondritis dissecans (OCD) of the capitellum, or, rarely, OCD of the radial head. Current opinion favors the theory that these lesions are different. Panner's disease typically resolves with growth. OCD may, and all too often does, lead to loose body formation, residual deformity of the capitellum, and degenerative elbow arthritis.

james a. whiteside and james r. andrews

Diagnosis

Age, onset, loose body formation, radiographic findings, and deformity of the capitellum all aid in differentiating these two conditions. Panner's disease is a disease of the ossification centers in young children that begins as necrosis of the capitellum and is followed by regeneration and recalcification. It affects a younger population, and onset is usually acute, with fragmentation of the entire ossific nucleus. The athlete presents with activity-related lateral elbow pain. Swelling may be negligible, or slight effusion may be present. Flexion and extension are generally limited. OCD of the capitellum often affects the preadolescent and adolescent group of athletes, after ossification of the capitellum has been completed. It typically involves the lateral or central portion of the capitellum. The child, in the 13–16-year-old age group, usually presents with lateral elbow pain and has a flexion contracture of 15° or more. Plain radiographs show radiolucency of the capitellum. Loose body formation and secondary changes of hypertrophy of the radial head may also be observed.

Treatment

In the athlete with osteochondrosis, initial treatment should consist of rest, avoidance of throwing, and, occasionally, bracing until pain and local tenderness have subsided. In the athlete with OCD of the capitellum, the status of the lesion directs treatment methods. A non-displaced, in situ OCD lesion may heal with rest and protection. Throwing (or whatever the offending activity) should be eliminated until pain, tenderness, and stiffness have completely resolved. A partially detached OCD lesion may be salvaged by operative reattachment and internal fixation. A loose or displaced OCD lesion is managed by surgical excision of the loose fragment and curettage of the base.

Return to play

An interval return to full activity is permitted under supervision when the elbow motion is pain-free, arm strength is normal, and the osseous lesion has healed. The program should be guided by symptoms.

Chronic medial (valgus) instability

Chronic medial instability is usually associated with overuse activity, including throwing and pitching. Repetitive valgus stress to the elbow results in medial collateral ligament attenuation, radiocapitellar joint compression, and postero-medial ulno-humeral compression (Figure 15.9A). Associated ulnar nerve traction neuritis, resulting from repetitive stretching, is noticed in up to 40% of throwing athletes with chronic medial instability. Posteromedial olecranon impingement causes inflammation, chondromalacia, osteophytes, and loose bodies formation, leading to development of flexion contracture and pain upon extension (Figure 15.9B).

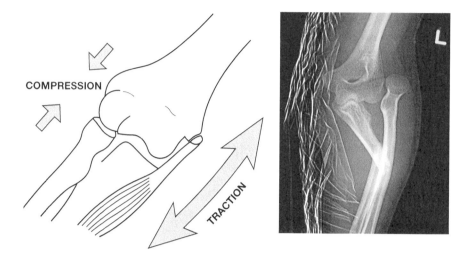

Figure 15.9 (A) Repetitive valgus stress results in medial collateral ligament attenuation and radiocapitellar joint compression. (B) Posteromedial olecranon impingement

Diagnosis

The athlete presents with medial elbow pain during or after throwing, along with decreased throwing efficiency. Rest may improve symptoms, which tend to recur after repetitive throwing. There is local tenderness 1 cm distal to the medial epicondyle. Valgus stress, with the elbow in a flexed position, causes significant medial elbow pain. In some cases, there is medial joint line opening. Check for Tinel's sign of the ulnar nerve at the cubital tunnel, which may be positive. Posteromedial impingement is demonstrated by eliciting posterior elbow pain at full extension and is accentuated with valgus stress. Plain X-rays of the elbow are usually negative. Look for small avulsion fractures, ossification within the medial collateral ligaments, loose bodies in the posterior or lateral compartments, marginal osteophytes, or olecranon hypertrophy. Gravity stress radiographs may be helpful. MRI can help confirm the clinical diagnosis.

Treatment

Rest and rehabilitation constitute initial treatment. The recreational, low-demand athlete does not necessarily require reconstruction. The high-performance throwing athlete cannot tolerate decreased performance and may benefit from surgical reconstruction of the anterior band of the medial collateral ligaments, with an ipsilateral palmaris longus tendon graft, combined with anterior ulnar nerve transposition if indicated.

Return to play

Full athletic activity is generally not permitted for a full year. Pitchers usually require 2 years before peak performance is regained.

Medial epicondyle apophysitis

Normal throwing imparts a large medial distraction force at the elbow; repetitive throwing actions may result in physeal microfractures and widening, known as chronic apophysitis. The condition is a result of "too much throwing" with excessive valgus stress across a skeletally immature elbow.

Diagnosis

A young pitcher presents with progressive medial elbow pain over the dominant arm, diminished throwing effectiveness, and decreased throwing distance. There is no visible atrophy or bruising. Feel for localized tenderness over the medial epicondyle. Resultant elbow flexion contracture of more than 15° is not uncommon. Resisted wrist flexion and pronation should be painful. A plain AP X-ray of the elbow shows apophyseal widening and fragmentation, best confirmed by comparison with the opposite elbow.

Rehabilitation

Medial epicondyle apophysitis is treated conservatively with relative rest, along with local ice application and NSAID medications, until the physis becomes nontender. ROM for elbow flexion and extension should be initiated, followed by strengthening of wrist and finger flexors. Corrective postural exercises for throwing should be simulated to improve the biomechanics of throwing when appropriate. Examination of lower-extremity flexibility may be indicated – owing to the tendency to have short lower extremity muscles, primarily hip internal rotators – in order to prevent future excessive strain on the medial aspect of the elbow when the patient returns to sport. Also, factors including pitching-related factors, throwing-related factors, practice-related factors, and frequency of throwing are carefully evaluated. The number of outings per season and number of pitches per outing (or per week) should be restricted.

Return to play

A progressive throwing program is initiated at 8 weeks. Interval return to full activity is permitted under supervision when the motion is pain-free and arm strength is normal, and is guided by symptoms. Recurrence of pain indicates too rapid a return to full activity.

FOREARM INJURIES

Forearm fracture

Forearm fractures include fractures of the shaft of the radius, ulna, or both bones. Forearm fractures are further classified according to fracture location (metaphyseal, diaphyseal), fracture patterns (transverse, short oblique, spiral, comminuted), displacement, and angulations. A Monteggia fracture-dislocation is a proximal or middle ulna fracture associated with radial head dislocation (Figure 15.10A). A Galeazzi fracture-dislocation is a distal-third radius fracture associated with distal radioulnar joint dislocation. An Essex–Lopresti fracture-dislocation is a fracture of the proximal radius with complete disruption of the interosseous membrane.

Fieldside assessment

The athlete presents with forearm fractures, usually sustained in a fall injury on an outstretched hand, or a direct contusion injury. Clinical diagnosis is not difficult, because there is immediate severe pain, with obvious forearm deformity and rapid development of swelling. Neurovascular assessment is necessary. The elbow is splinted in a comfortable position, and the athlete is transported to hospital for proper assessment and management.

Diagnosis

A thorough neurovascular examination is essential. Plain AP and lateral X-rays of the forearm, including both the elbow and wrist, are mandatory for proper assessment. Monitor clinical signs related to compartmental syndrome.

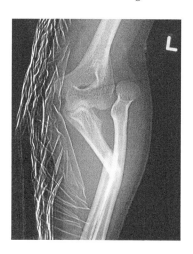
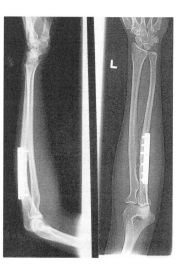

Figure 15.10 (A) Monteggia fracture-dislocation. (B) Monteggia fracture-dislocation treated with open reduction and internal fixation with plating

Treatment

Adult athletes usually require open reduction and rigid internal fixation with plating to maintain good position (length, angulations, and rotation of each bone) (Figure 15.10B). Malunion often leads to loss of forearm rotation. In children, a minor degree of overlap and angulation is acceptable and can be treated conservatively with a long arm cast after closed reduction. Repeat X-rays are essential to look for any displacement during healing.

Rehabilitation

Rigid internal fixation allows early mobilization exercises. In adults, the expected time of bone healing is about 8–12 weeks, and the expected duration of rehabilitation is about 12–24 weeks.

Return to play

The athlete must have near normal ROM and strength and is able to perform the necessary sport-specific activities.

ACUTE WRIST INJURIES

Distal radius fractures

A Colles' fracture (first described by Abraham Colles in 1814) is a distal metaphyseal fracture of the radius, usually 3–4 cm from the articular surface, with typical deformity (dorsal tilt, dorsal displacement of distal fragment, and radial shortening). An intra-articular variant involves the radiocarpal joint and/or the distal radioulnar joint. In adult athletes, these fractures can be comminuted and intra-articular, requiring open eduction to restore the normal anatomy and internal fixation and/or external fixation. In young athletes, the fractures are usually physeal fractures that do not involve the articular surface. The epiphysis is shifted and tilted dorsally, and usually carries with it a triangular metaphyseal fragment, a Salter type II physeal fracture.

Fieldside assessment

The athlete presents with severe wrist pain, with or without obvious deformity, following a fall injury on the outstretched hand. Classical silver-fork deformity (Figure 15.11) (with prominence on the back of the wrist and a depression in front) may be obvious, with definite local bone tenderness. Check for median nerve function. The wrist is splinted in a comfortable position, and the athlete is transported to hospital for proper assessment and management.

Diagnosis

Plain AP and lateral X-rays of the wrist are mandatory for proper assessment of the fracture. Assessment should include degree of deformity (radial shortening, amount of dorsal tilting), any intra-articular involvement (any gap or step), and any associated fracture (ulnar styloid or carpal bones).

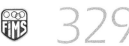

329

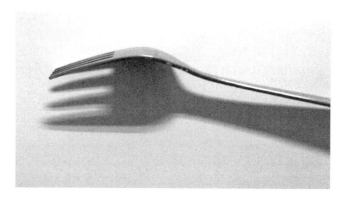

Figure 15.11 Classical silver-fork deformity

Treatment

In young athletes, the distal radius metaphyseal or epiphyseal fractures can be treated conservatively by closed reduction and immobilization (a long arm cast). In adult athletes, open reduction and fixation (internal and/or external fixation) are indicated when the distal radius fractures are considered unstable, or if closed reduction is unsatisfactory. Unacceptable deformity means a persistent articular step-off greater than 2 mm, a dorsal tilt greater than 10°, and/or uncorrectable radial shortening of greater than 3–5 mm.

Rehabilitation

Exercises aimed at restoring normal strength and ROM of the wrist joint are offered. The fracture unites in 6 weeks.

Return to play

Return to play is individualized, depending on the outcomes of the treatment and the functional demands of the sport.

Traumatic carpal dislocations

Traumatic carpal dislocations are manifestations of significant wrist-trauma injuries. Carpal dislocations can be classified into perilunar, radiocarpal, midcarpal, axial, and isolated carpal dislocations, based on common pathomechanics and anatomical patterns. By far the most frequent dislocations are perilunar dislocations. The magnitude of force required is considerable.

Fieldside assessment

The athlete presents with severe wrist pain after a high-energy accident, with the wrist having sustained a hyperextension injury, and the lunate having been pushed volarly. Pain and swelling are often severe. There are fullness on the volar aspect

james a. whiteside and james r. andrews

(Figure 15.12A), severe local tenderness, and limitation of wrist motion in all directions; all these make clinical diagnosis of a severe wrist injury obvious. Checking for median nerve function is mandatory. The wrist is splinted in a comfortable position, and the athlete is transported to hospital for proper assessment and management.

Diagnosis

Palmar lunate dislocation can be diagnosed on an AP X-ray of the wrist, with the lunate appearing triangular (instead of its usual trapezoid shape) (Figure 15.12B); on a lateral neutral-rotation view of the wrist, there is volar dislocation of the lunate (Figure 15.12C). Dorsal perilunate dislocation can be diagnosed on an AP X-ray of the wrist with a foreshortened carpus, overlap of the lunate and capitate, and disruption of the Gilula's lines; on a lateral neutral-rotation X-ray of the wrist,

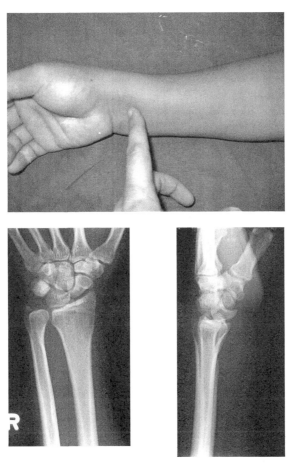

Figure 15.12 Palmar lunate dislocation: (A) fullness; (B) AP X-ray; (C) lateral X-ray

the capitate is displaced dorsally from the lunate. Always look for concomitant injuries from this high-energy trauma, especially a scaphoid fracture. However, depending on pre-reduction plain radiographs alone to assess the extent of osseous pathology is unreliable and sometimes difficult.

Treatment

The dislocation must be reduced early, which is best in the operating room under general anesthesia or adequate regional anesthesia. Use of intra-operative fluoroscopic control is essential. Be prepared for open reduction if closed reduction cannot be achieved. Appropriate ligament repairs and internal stabilization, usually with multiple K-wires, is required.

Rehabilitation

The arm is immobilized in a long arm–thumb spica for 6 weeks. This is followed by 4 weeks in a short arm–thumb spica. K-wires are removed after 10–12 weeks. Wrist mobilization and strengthening are then progressed as tolerated.

Return to play

Residual stiffness is not uncommon. Scaphoid (navicular) fractures are not uncommon, constituting about 70% of all carpal-bone fractures. The fracture line may be at the distal pole, waist, proximal pole, or the tubercle region. With a precarious blood supply being retrograde from the distal to proximal regions, fracture at the waist may lead to nonunion, and has a higher chance of developing osteonecrosis in the proximal fragment (Figure 15.13).

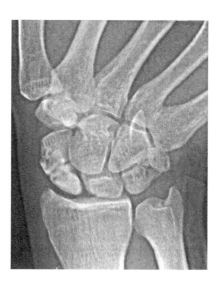

Figure 15.13 Scaphoid fracture: nonunion and osteonecrosis of the proximal fragment

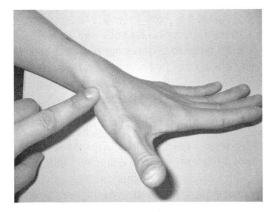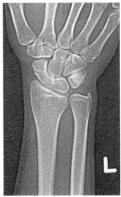

Figure 15.14 (A) Scaphoid fracture: local tenderness at anatomical snuffbox.
(B) Scaphoid fracture

Fieldside assessment

The athlete presents with pain at the radial side of the wrist, after a fall injury on the outstretched hand with the wrist in hyperextension. There should be no obvious deformity. Look for swelling, and feel for local tenderness at the anatomic snuffbox (Figure 15.14A). The athlete may feel little discomfort, and ROM is only slightly limited. Diagnosis is difficult and should always be suspected in a patient with typical presentation.

Diagnosis

Four radiographic views of the wrist should be obtained when evaluating a presumed scaphoid injury, including posteroanterior, scaphoid (posteroanterior view with 30° of ulnar deviation), true lateral, and oblique projection views. A radiolucent line is diagnostic of an acute scaphoid fracture (Figure 15.14B). Resorption at the fracture site and subchondral sclerosis are radiological evidence of delayed union or nonunion. Plain radiographs may not show the fracture line initially; CT, MRI, or repeat plain radiographs a few weeks later can be helpful in arriving at the diagnosis.

Treatment

Treatment can be controversial, depending on the location and stability of the fracture and the type of sports activity. Conservative treatment for a non-displaced fracture with a thumb spica cast is acceptable. Open reduction and internal fixation are indicated for a displaced fracture. Technological advances have improved union rates and accelerated healing time to union. For minimally displaced or non-displaced fractures, percutaneous screw fixation with a cannulated screw can provide better compression strength and rigid internal fixation, thus allowing an earlier recovery and return to sport.

Rehabilitation

Scaphoid fractures treated with cast immobilization typically require 8–12 weeks for bone healing. Nonunion is not uncommon for scaphoid fractures. Once healed or surgically stabilized, ROM exercises begin, followed by strengthening exercises.

Return to play

Return to play for an athlete with a scaphoid fracture should be individualized, depending on the type of sport (degree of physical contact, any wrist involvement) and treatment method (any internal fixation, which fixation method, any cast, which type of cast). For athletes with non-displaced scaphoid fractures, return to play in a non-contact sport with a well-applied thumb spica, before bone union, can be allowed. For athletes participating in contact sports, immediate fixation and return to play in a cast can be considered. These athletes should understand the associated potential risks concerning return to play before bone union. In sports that involve wrist action, return to play is not allowed until bone union is complete.

Scapholunate dissociation

Carpal stability is maintained by complex osseous and ligamentous architecture, including the ligaments between carpal bones (intrinsic ligaments) and between radius and carpus (extrinsic ligaments). Carpal instability is the resultant mal-alignment of the carpal bones under physiologic loads from ligamentous and bony injury that disrupts normal carpal equilibrium. Static carpal instability describes a condition with positive clinical examination and matching abnormal imaging. Dynamic carpal instability means a condition of load intolerance, where clinical examination makes the diagnosis, but corroboration by X-ray studies is negative. Scapholunate dissociation is the commonest form of carpal instability, with disruption of the scapholunate interosseous ligament (SLIL). Complete dissociation results in a palmar flexion position of the scaphoid and concomitant extension position of the lunate.

Fieldside assessment

The athlete presents with acute wrist pain after a fall on an outstretched hand, with the wrist in hyperextension and ulnar deviation. Grip strength is decreased. Wrist extension causes pain. Feel for local tenderness directly over the scapholunate region. The scaphoid shift test is positive in cases with a complete tear of the SLIL. Wrist instability is sometimes difficult to be certain of clinically.

Diagnosis

Plain X-rays, including stress roentgenograms, are helpful in diagnosis. An AP X-ray of the wrist shows height loss of the scaphoid (Figure15.15A). A lateral X-ray shows the vertical position of the scaphoid bone and subluxation of the proximal scaphoid on to the dorsal rim of the radius. An AP supinated view of the wrist

Figure 15.15
(A) Scapholunate dissociation.
(B) Open reduction and internal fixation are the preferred method of treatment

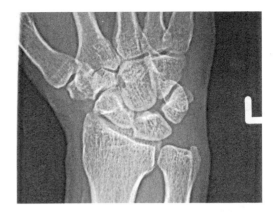

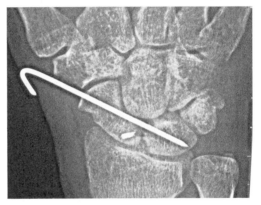

with maximum ulnar deviation while gripping should show a scapholunate gap greater than 5 mm. Further, additional investigations with cinearthrography, MRI, and, if necessary, wrist arthroscopy, can help confirm the diagnosis.

Treatment

Because scapholunate dissociation leads to progressive degenerative arthritis of the wrist, reduction and internal fixation form the preferred method of treatment, especially for athletes with acute injury. Treatment of the acute scapholunate ligament tear includes (a) open reduction and stabilization of the scapholunate relationship with K-wires, (b) direct ligamentous repair, and (c) augmentation with a dorsal capsulodesis (Figure 15.15B).

Rehabilitation

Wrist ROM is often slow to return after operative treatment. The K-wires are typically removed at 8–10 weeks; an individualized exercise program is then initiated.

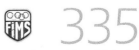

Return to play

Return to contact sports usually takes 4–6 months. Near-normal ROM and strength adequate for the demands of the sport are required before full participation is resumed.

NON-ACUTE WRIST SYNDROMES

Carpal tunnel syndrome

Carpal tunnel syndrome (CTS) is the commonest compressive neuropathy and involves compression of the median nerve by the transverse carpal ligament. Dysfunction is usually manifested by sensory changes such as pain, paresthesia, numbness, or a pins-and-needles sensation, with tingling in the three and a half radial digits. The most commonly involved finger is usually the middle finger. The condition is usually associated with repeated forced hand movements, or continuous flexion or extension of the wrist. The condition is noted in athletes participating in different kinds of sport, such as lacrosse, gymnastics, cycling, and racquet sports.

Diagnosis

Nocturnal paresthesia and pain are almost universal. Pain, tingling, and/or decreased sensation over the three and a half radial digits may be reproduced by maintaining the wrist in full flexion for a minute or two, because pressure inside the carpal tunnels can be significantly increased with the wrist in extreme extension

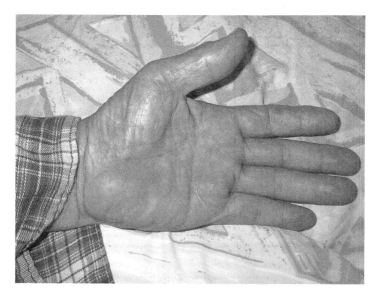

Figure 15.16 Carpal tunnel syndrome: thenar muscle atrophy

and flexion. Tinel's sign, over the transverse carpal ligament at the volar aspect of the palm, and the Phalen test are usually positive. Check the thenar muscles for any atrophy (Figure 15.16). Electrodiagnostic studies may be required for diagnosis, especially in mild cases, because these studies represent the only objective tests.

Treatment

Initial treatment of CTS consists of activity modification, rest, anti-inflammatory medications, splinting at night, and decreasing or eliminating the offending activity. Surgery is indicated if there is thenar muscle weakness and atrophy, progress of symptoms, or no improvement within 3 months. Release of the transverse ligament can be performed employing open carpal tunnel release (CTR) or endoscopically assisted surgery (ECTR).

Rehabilitation

Patients commonly present in acute, subacute, or chronic states of inflammation with carpal tunnel syndrome. Splinting, rest, and cryotherapy can be effective to reduce symptoms initially. Neural gliding exercises can be helpful in restoring range of motion at fingers and wrist in all stages of healing. In addition, stretching the adductor pollicis and extrinsic extensors may be indicated and should be addressed, as needed. After symptoms have resolved, any weakened muscles must be restrengthened before a return to unrestricted activity. Also, attention to work and sport ergonomics, aspects of daily living (ADLs), and leisure-activity bio-mechanics should be addressed, so that the patient returns to activity without reaggravating the problem.

Return to play

Once full strength and range of motion are established, return to play is permitted, usually by 3–4 weeks following surgery. Residual thenar muscle atrophy may persist.

De Quervain's disease

De Quervain's disease is a condition describing tenosynovitis of the abductor pollicis longus (APL) and extensor pollicis brevis (EPB) tendons in the first dorsal compartment of the wrist. The inflammation and irritation are caused by repetitive use or overuse, commonly seen in athletes participating in racquet sports, golf, javelin, and disc throwing.

Diagnosis

The athlete presents with pain and tenderness in the radial aspect of the wrist around the radial styloid region, aggravated by active and passive motion of the thumb. Local tenderness and swelling are noted. A positive Finkelstein's test (passive ulnar deviation of the hand at the wrist joint, with the thumb placed inside the palm) will reproduce radial wrist pain.

337

Treatment

As with any other tenosynovitis, treatment consists of RICE therapy in conjunction with physical therapy, occupational therapy evaluation, and elimination of the aggravating activity. Corticosteroid injection may be considered into the first dorsal compartment of the wrist.

Rehabilitation

Partial immobilization with a wrist/thumb splint can be offered. When out of the splint, the athlete performs active ROM and grip-strengthening exercises for the intrinsic muscles of the hand and fingers. NSAIDs, iontophoresis, and cryotherapy can be helpful to control inflammation prior to a return to sport. Work ergonomics and ADLs at home and in sport should be addressed.

Return to play

Daily activity in a splint is permitted early on. If possible, the splint should be worn even during full activity, in order to prevent exacerbation of symptoms. Use of NSAIDs prior to activity is effective.

HAND AND FINGER INJURIES

Laceration of the hand

Fieldside assessment

With elevation and direct pressure application, most bleeding stops quickly. Bleeding vessels should not be clamped at fieldside; other structures may be injured, making subsequent arterial microvascular repair difficult. After the athlete is removed from play and in a suitable environment, the wound may be cleansed and carefully evaluated. Check for function of the deep structures beneath the wound, in particular, finger movement for tendons, circulation for vessels, and sensation for digital nerves. X-ray for a foreign body (FB) if there is possibility of a retained FB. Always suspect an FB in a glass wound. Simple, non-contaminated lacerations can be cleaned and sutured. Dirty wounds should be thoroughly cleaned and left to heal by second intention, or delayed primary suture at about 3 days if the wound remains clean. Athletes with flexor tendon cut injuries, neurovascular trauma, or lacerations that cross the borders of zone II ("no man's land") should be referred to a hand specialist for proper repair and management.

Human bites to an athlete's hand may occur in contact or collision sports. These "benign"-looking injuries can lead to severe infection of skin, joint, and/or bone. Human bites should be thoroughly irrigated and debrided and should not be sutured primarily. Depending on the depth of the injury, antibiotics may be required.

Metacarpal fractures

The metacarpal bones are vulnerable to blows and falls upon the hand, or longitudinal force from a boxer's punch, resulting in fractures. Fracture can be at the base, shaft, neck, and head of the metacarpal bone. A blow may fracture the metacarpal neck, usually in the fifth finger (a boxer's fracture). Angular deformity is better compensated at the fourth and fifth metacarpal bones, as hyperextension at the metacarpophalangeal joints (MCPJs) is possible. A twisting force may cause spiral fractures of one or more shafts. Rotational deformity is serious and less acceptable.

Fieldside assessment

With a boxer's fracture, ask the athlete specifically if a punch on a tooth occurred. Look for local swelling or flattening of the fifth knuckle. The corresponding displaced metacarpal head can be palpated as a prominence in the athlete's palm. Feel for localized bony tenderness at the metacarpal neck region. Finger movement is minimally decreased.

With a shaft fracture, there is significant local pain and swelling. Look for a dorsal "hump" at the shaft region, if there is significant angular deformity. Checking for any rotational deformity is essential, by asking the athlete to close his/her hand with the distal phalanges extended. Malrotation causes "scissoring" of the finger: the finger may diverge and overlap with the other fingers. The athlete is removed from competition, and the hand is elevated. Ice and a splint or a bulky compressive bandage is applied. The athlete is transported to hospital for proper assessment and management.

Diagnosis

Clinical diagnosis is not difficult, given the classical presentation with typical physical findings. Radiographic assessment with plain X-rays should be made. Do not forget that there may be more than one fracture. Look for dislocation at the carpometacarpal joint (CMCJ), especially in cases with fractures at the base.

Treatment

Treatment of metacarpal fractures should be individualized, depending on the specific fracture patterns, site of the fracture, degrees of angulation and shortening, any associated rotational deformity, and the specific needs of the athlete. Rotational deformity should be fully corrected. Metacarpal head fractures are intra-articular and require anatomic reduction. Metacarpal neck fractures at the fifth metacarpal bone can accept angulations of up to 20°. However, in a throwing athlete's dominant hand, much lower angulations are acceptable. These fractures should then be reduced and internally fixed. Metacarpal neck fractures at the index finger should always be reduced, as deformity is less tolerated. Transverse shaft fractures with slight displacement can be treated conservatively with a cast or a removable splint. Oblique or spiral fractures with rotation, angulations, or significant displacement may need reduction and internal fixation.

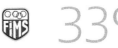

Rehabilitation

As soon as sufficient fracture stability is attained, usually by 3 weeks after the injury, the athlete begins ROM exercises, to include finger-gliding exercises. The athlete should then focus on strengthening intrinsic muscles of the hand, with attention to restoring functional grip, which takes place through the third, fourth, and fifth digits primarily. Therapeutic exercises for the elbow and shoulder should continue to include cardiovascular conditioning.

Return to play

The athlete may return to play when healing is complete. Depending on the demands of the sport, the athlete may resume training and even competition, using a plastic splint or soft cast for protection.

Bennett's fracture

A Bennett's fracture involves a fracture of the base of the thumb metacarpal, extends into the carpometacarpal joint, and is unstable.

Fieldside assessment

The athlete presents with pain and swelling of the base of the thumb after a punching injury. The thumb looks short, and the CMCJ region is swollen (Figure 15.17). The athlete is removed from competition, and the hand is elevated. Ice and a splint or bulky compressive bandage are applied. The athlete is transported to hospital for proper assessment and management.

Diagnosis

X-rays show that a small fragment of the metacarpal bone remains in place, and the remaining thumb is subluxed proximally (Figure 15.18A).

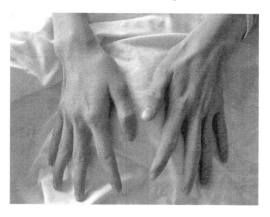

Figure 15.17 Bennett's fracture: the right thumb looks short, with local swelling at the base

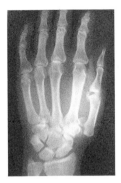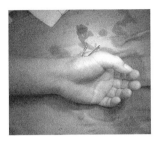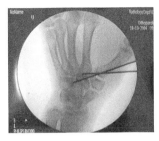

Figure 15.18 Bennett's fracture: (A) typical radiographic features; (B) Bennett's fracture treated with two Kirschner wires. (C) Intra-operative fluoroscopic control to confirm reduction

Treatment

Reduction is difficult to maintain in a plaster of Paris cast. Internal fixation is the recommended treatment choice, usually with two Kirschner-wires or a small screw, to stabilize these unstable fractures (Figures 15.18B and 15.18C). A POP cast is applied.

Rehabilitation

During immobilization in a cast, shoulder, elbow, and finger ROM exercises, with strengthening, are encouraged. As soon as early healing is sufficient, physical therapy begins. After any percutaneous wires have been removed, the athlete performs resistance hand therapy daily for 2–3 months.

Return to play

When the athlete's hand is pain free and has full ROM, with good hand/grip strength, full athletic activity is allowed. A padded splint may be necessary for more vigorous activity.

Ulnar collateral ligament sprain (Gamekeeper's thumb)

The ulnar collateral ligament (UCL) is essential for key pinching and opposition. A significant radially deviated force applied on an abducted thumb causes damage to the UCL and/or volar plate of the thumb MCPJ.

Fieldside assessment

The athlete presents with pain and swelling at the base of thumb after a fall on to an outstretched hand with the thumb abducted. It is common in skiing, with the thumb caught in the handle of the ski pole or in the gaps in the surface of a dry ski slope. Tenderness is localized to the ulnar aspect of the thumb MCPJ. Beware that one may not be able to elicit laxity in acute injuries because of pain.

 341

Diagnosis

X-ray is taken to rule out any avulsion fracture at the base of the proximal phalanx. If X-rays are negative for fracture, local anesthetic may be given to allow proper assessment by physical examination. The degree of any instability should always be compared with the contralateral uninjured thumb. With a sprain, there is an increased laxity of the MCPJ for a few degrees, but there is a definite "end point." Adduction stress applied with the MCPJ at 30° flexion causing more than 30° of radial deviation compared with the unaffected side, together with a lack of definitive end point, is indicative of a complete tear of the UCL. Radial instability with the MCPJ fully extended may indicate more extensive damage involving the volar plate. Complete tears can result in the abductor aponeurosis being trapped between the torn ends (termed Stener lesion) and prevent healing.

Treatment

Acute partial tears can be treated adequately with a thumb spica for 3–4 weeks, followed by exercises to increase ROM. The spica should be well molded and adjusted frequently, as swelling resolves with time. Complete tears are best treated with direct surgical repair or tendon graft reconstruction, followed by a thumb spica for about 6 weeks. Avulsion fracture should be fixed surgically.

Rehabilitation

Flexion and extension of fingers, elbow, and shoulder are begun early to prevent stiffness. Strengthening exercises for intrinsic hand muscles and thumb within the pain-free range are started at 6 weeks.

Return to play

The athlete may perform routine activities at 6–8 weeks following surgery, wearing a rigid or soft thumb splint. Full activity is allowed at 10–12 weeks following injury or surgery, when the thumb is pain free, with full ROM. For some activities causing stress at the MCPJ, the thumb spica should be worn for further protection.

Phalangeal fractures and dislocations

Fieldside assessment

The athlete presents after "jamming" a finger. There is moderate pain, considerable swelling, and local tenderness of the finger. If the deformity is consistent with dorsal dislocation of the proximal interphalangeal joint (PIPJ), immediate closed reduction may be carried out. The injured finger may then be protected with a dorsal splint and taped to an adjacent finger. If pain and joint stability allow, the athlete may return to competition. X-rays are indicated to rule out any associated fracture. If the tenderness is over the shaft of the phalanx, or varus/valgus/rotational deformity is apparent, the presumed diagnosis is a displaced shaft fracture, and the athlete is removed from play.

james a. whiteside and james r. andrews

Diagnosis

Differential diagnoses include fracture of the phalangeal shaft, sprain or dislocation of the interphalangeal joint (IPJ), and ligamentous injury combined with intra-articular fracture. Look for deformity, and especially rotational deformity. Dorsal dislocation of the PIPJ, which frequently occurs when a ball hits the athlete's fingertip and jams the finger into hyperextension, causes rupture of the volar plate and often concomitant collateral ligament injury. Isolated collateral ligament injuries are caused by abduction or adduction forces applied to an extended finger. Careful examination can localize the precise area of tenderness. Clinically, the amount of instability is measured by the extent to which there is opening with varus and valgus stress, carried out in both extension and slight flexion. Stress X-rays may be required to differentiate complete tears from incomplete disruption. X-rays determine the location of the fractures and any associated deformity (Figure 15.19).

Treatment

Fractures of the proximal and middle phalangeal shaft require accurate reduction and may require internal fixation. In skeletally immature athletes, slight angular deformity in the plane of flexion and extension resolves with growth through remodeling. Rotational deformity should not be accepted, as this deformity does not improve significantly with remodeling.

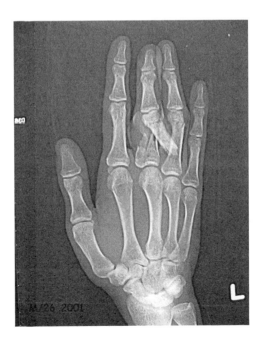

Figure 15.19 Comminuted fracture of proximal phalanx of middle finger

343

Fractures of the distal phalanx are often crush-type and are not angulated. Treatment usually is directed toward the associated soft-tissue injury. Subungual hematoma should be decompressed to relieve pain. Occasionally, the nail may be avulsed. Any significant nail-bed injury should be repaired, and the nail may be replaced into the nail fold as a stent.

Reduction of a dorsal dislocation of the PIPJ is accomplished by firm traction of the distal half of the finger. If the reduction is delayed, local anesthesia may be required to give sufficient pain control and relaxation to allow reduction. Use of a dorsal splint in a functionally flexed position allows the athlete to hold a ball without too much difficulty. The digit should be taped to an adjacent finger to provide further protection. The protection splint is maintained for about 3 weeks, and buddy taping is used for the next three weeks. Even with a small, volar plate avulsion fracture (less than one-third of the articular surface), treatment is usually the same. For more significant intra-articular fractures, open reduction and internal fixation are generally recommended.

Partial collateral ligament tears (sprains) are best treated by buddy taping for 3–6 weeks. For complete tears, there is controversy between simple, conservative buddy taping therapy and surgical intervention.

Rehabilitation

For stable injuries, the athlete should perform finger ROM exercises several times a day when out of the splint. Active finger flexion against increasing resistance is allowed. Finger abduction and adduction exercises are started at 1–2 weeks for stable injuries.

Return to play

Full activity is allowed when the finger is pain free with full ROM. Buddy taping is continued for at least 4–6 weeks, and occasionally for the entire season.

Mallet finger

Mallet finger typically occurs if there is sudden forceful flexion of an extended distal interphalangeal joint (DIPJ), resulting in disruption of the extensor tendon or an avulsion fracture of the distal phalanx. There is inability to extend the DIPJ. If the tendon is only stretched, the deformity lacks about 15–20° of full extension. If the tendon is torn off at the dorsal base, lack of full extension may exceed 30–40°. In the acute setting, full passive motion is typically preserved. X-rays should be obtained to look for any fracture at the base of the distal phalanx and joint subluxation.

Surgery is indicated if there is subluxation of the DIPJ, or if the avulsed fracture involves more than one-third of the joint surface. Conservative treatment involves continuous use of a mallet splint (to keep the DIPJ in slight hyperextension) for a minimum of 6 weeks, followed by night splinting for an additional 2 weeks.

Protection during athletic activities should continue for an additional 4 weeks. Splinting is still recommended, even if initiated up to 4 weeks following the injury.

Jersey finger

Jersey finger is a condition characterized by avulsion of the flexor digitorum profundus tendon from its insertion into the base of the distal phalanx, usually in the middle finger. This injury is caused by forced extension of a maximally flexed DIPJ, commonly as a result of getting a finger caught on the jersey of another player, who struggles to pull away quickly. The condition can be classified into three groups, according to Leddy: (1) when the tendon retracts into the palm, (2) when the tendon retracts to the level of the PIPJ, and (3) when there is an associated avulsion fracture that causes the torn tendon to be held up at the level of the DIPJ.

Diagnosis

The athlete presents with loss of the normal cascade of the fingers and inability actively to flex the DIPJ. Often the athlete does not recognize the severity of the injury and presents late.

Early surgical management to reattach the tendon is necessary to restore active flexion of the finger. Those injuries seen late can either be treated by "active neglect," DIPJ capsulodesis, DIPJ fusion, or, in a few, select cases, free tendon grafting.

Rehabilitation

After removal of sutures at 2 weeks, protected ROM exercises are started aggressively. Functional motion may not be attained until 3–4 weeks. Full strength may lag by 6–8 weeks.

Return to play

With padded-glove protection, the athlete may return to full competition 8 weeks after surgery. Residual limitation of full flexion and weaker flexion power are not uncommon. The deficit usually does not hinder athletic function.

ACKNOWLEDGMENT

The editors acknowledge the assistance of Wendy Holdan, MSPT, of Boston Children's Hospital, for contributing to, and reviewing, the rehabilitation sections in this chapter.

SUGGESTED READING

Bae D.S. Injuries to the wrist, hand, and finger. In: Michell L.J., Purcell L.K., Eds. *The Adolescent Athlete*. New York, NY: Springer; 2007:223–63.
Bell S. Elbow and arm pain. In: Brukner P., Khan K., Eds. *Clinical Sport Medicine*. 3rd ed. Sydney, Australia: McGraw-Hill Professional; 2007:289–307.

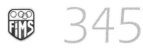

Burra G., Andrews J.R., Acute shoulder and elbow dislocations in the athlete. *Orthop. Clin. North Am.* 2002; 33(15):479–96.

Fleisig G.S., Weber A., Hassell N., Andrews J.R. Prevention of elbow injuries in youth baseball pitchers. *Curr. Sports Med. Rep.* 2009; 8(5):250–4.

Garcia-Moral, C.A., Green, N.E., Fox, J.A. Hand and wrist. In: Sullivan J.A., Anderson S.J., Eds. *Care of the Young Athlete*. American Academy of Orthopedic Surgeons and American Academy of Pediatrics; 2000:349.

Gerbino P.G. Elbow disorders in throwing athletes. *Orthop. Clin. North Am.* 2003; 34(3):417–26.

Hutchinson M.R., Andrews J.R. Preventing elbow injuries. In: Bahr R., Engebretsen L., Eds., *Sports Injury Prevention*. Wiley-Blackwell, Hoboken, NJ: 2009; 153–74.

Kocher M.S., Waters P.M., Micheli L.J. Upper extremity injuries in the pediatric athlete. *Sports Med.* 2000; 30(2):117–35.

Lee S.J., Montgomery K. Athletic hand injuries. *Orthop. Clin. North Am.* 2002; 33(15):547–54.

Letts M., Green N.E., Fox J.A. Elbow and forearm. In: Sullivan J.A., Anderson S.J., Eds. *Care of the Young Athlete*. Rosemont, IL: American Academy of Orthopedic Surgeons and American Academy of Pediatrics; 2000:309–22.

Luke A., Lee M., Safran M. Elbow and forearm injuries. In: Micheli L.J., Purcell L.K., Eds. *The Adolescent Athlete*. New York, NY: Springer; 2007:194–222.

Rettig A.C. Traumatic elbow injuries in the athlete. *Orthop. Clin. North Am.* 2002; 33(15):509–22.

Steinberg B. Acute wrist injuries in the athlete. *Orthop. Clin. North Am.* 2002; 33(15):535–46.

CHAPTER 16

HIP, SPINE, AND PELVIS INJURIES

Lyle J. Micheli, Dzovig S. Parsehian, and
Thomas C. Kim

ACUTE BACK INJURIES

Strains/sprains

Fieldside assessment
The athlete complains of pain in the back region, usually without radiculopathy.

Diagnosis
Muscle strain or ligamentous sprain is one of the common causes of back pain in adults, although it is less common in adolescents. Athletes at risk for back strain are constitutionally tight, especially those with tight lumbar fascia or tight hamstrings. Improper training or lifting technique may cause muscular strain. Sudden contraction or a direct blow may also lead to strain. Hyperflexion may result in ligamentous sprain to posterior structures, such as the posterior longitudinal or interspinous ligament. A combination of hyperextension, rotation, and side bending may lead to ligamentous sprain. In adolescents, an avulsion or sprain of the dorsal lumbar attachment to the apophysis of the iliac crest or spinous process may occur. Localized pain, tenderness, and muscular spasm may be seen.

Treatment
Generally, symptoms are treated with rest, NSAIDs, and eventually stretching (especially if tight thoracolumbar fascia or hamstrings are noted) and strengthening with a physical therapy program. Soft-tissue injuries to the back generally should resolve over 4–6 weeks. If symptoms do not resolve, further work-up may be warranted to look for other possible causes of back pain, especially in a pediatric or adolescent athlete.

Rehabilitation
Acute back strains respond best to cryotherapy for up to 72 hours after injury, along with avoidance of complete rest. Splinting may be useful initially to provide

compression and reduce forces on the involved back musculature. Restoring good movement patterns (i.e. cueing for lower-abdominal stabilization with emphasis on hip flexion vs. lumbar spine flexion when performing hands and knees rocking backward; cueing for lower-abdominal stabilization prior to leg movement with supine single knee to chest and with supine double knee to chest lumbar stretches), sleeping, and sitting modifications, and education on proper transitional movement patterns (i.e. moving in/out of bed via log-rolling) should be initiated to reduce stresses on the back. Gentle lower abdominal strengthening should be initiated, with gradual return of full body strengthening, stretching, and endurance training, as indicated.

Return to play

Return to play is individualized; the severity of pain and the range of motion help determine when the athlete may resume activities.

BACK STRAIN

Examination

- Back pain, with or without pre-existing back problem.
- No neurologic symptoms.
- Spine and/or paraspinal muscle tenderness, spasm.

Treatment

- Symptomatic, followed by stretching and strengthening.

Return to action

- When able to fulfill demands of specific sport.

NON-ACUTE BACK INJURIES

Lordotic back pain

Fieldside assessment

The athlete may complain of insidious back pain, which is present off the field as well as during play.

Diagnosis

Hyperlordotic back pain is frequently associated with a rapid growth spurt and is typically a diagnosis in adolescent rather than adult athletes. With growth, the patient develops a tight thoracolumbar fascia and relative tightness of the soft tissues, particularly the hamstrings.

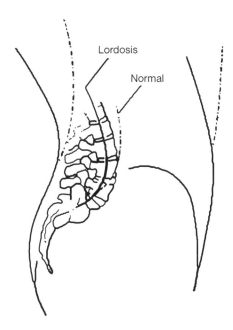

Figure 16.1 Athlete with lordosis

This lack of flexibility leads to hyperlordosis and also makes the individual more prone to injury. A flexion-type activity may cause apophyseal widening and traction apophysitis. Diagnosis is made by the finding of lumbar hyperlordosis accompanied by tight hamstrings and tight lumbar fascia (Figures 16.1 and 16.2). Often, the patient has a compensatory round back deformity of the thoracic spine.

Treatment

Treatment is conservative, with gentle stretching that may be facilitated by heat, contrast baths, and massage. Flexion exercises follow, including abdominal and spinal extensor strengthening, and eventually peripelvic strengthening. Associated

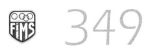

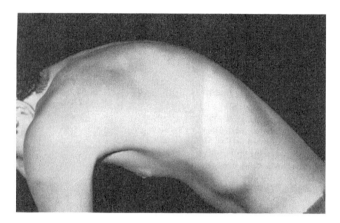

Figure 16.2 Adolescent athlete with tight thoracolumbar fascia

---

DIFFERENTIAL DIAGNOSIS OF HIP AND PELVIS PAIN

- Strains.
- Hip pointer.
- Avulsion fractures.
- Osteitis pubis.
- Sacroiliitis.
- Snapping hip.
- Stress fracture.

---

peripelvic contractures, such as tight hamstrings or hip flexion contractures, must be addressed with both stretching and strengthening exercises.

Rehabilitation

Formal physical therapy is helpful early, including therapeutic modalities such as massage, and cryotherapy in acute stages, rather then moist heat to promote healing. Attention should be placed on lower abdominal strengthening and stabilization. Correction of imbalances, particularly hip flexor inflexibility in relation to lower abdominal weakness, should also be addressed. Overall, rehabilitation should focus on achieving flexibility and return to full strength.

Return to play

Sports participation can usually continue while the athlete is undergoing therapy. Maintaining flexibility and strength is important to prevent reinjury.

Disk disease

Fieldside assessment

The athlete usually has chronic back pain, but sometimes the presenting symptom is an acute episode of back pain, with or without radiculopathy.

Diagnosis

Disk disease may take the form of a degenerative disk, disk bulge, or an actual disk herniation (Figure 16.3). A degenerative disk is more likely in adult athletes and is often a typical part of aging, but it can be seen in adolescent athletes, especially following repeated microtrauma. Risk factors include strenuous lifting and collision sports, as well as repeated flexion, axial loading, and extreme rotation (such as with golf). Gymnastics, in particular, is a sport where individuals have a high incidence of degenerative disks, as revealed by MRI (63% in Olympic-level female gymnasts in a study). Atypical Scheuermann's, which is discussed separately, can lead to early disk degeneration.

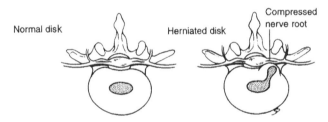

Figure 16.3 Normal/herniated disk

The athlete with degenerative disk disease generally presents with non-specific complaints of back pain. Range of motion may be limited, secondary to pain and muscle spasm. Plain films may demonstrate loss of disk height, but it is unclear whether this is itself a cause of back pain or is a pre-existing condition. If back pain is associated with radiculopathy, however, disk bulge or herniation should be considered. Radiculopathy generally warrants an MRI examination or computed tomography (CT) scan to rule out possible disk herniation.

Disk bulges may be found on MRI, but – like disk degeneration – their significance is often unclear. MRI examinations of a sample population between the ages of 20 and 39 years have shown 54% of the population having disk bulge (along with disk degeneration in 34% and disk herniation in 21%). Thus, disk bulges (and disk degeneration, or even disk herniation) can be found in many asymptomatic individuals. A discogram, with injection into a joint reproducing symptoms, may provide evidence that the involved disk is the source of pain, but generally is not performed unless surgical intervention is contemplated, and is not recommended as a stand-alone diagnostic measure, owing to somewhat conflicting results of its predictive value.

Tears of the disk's annulus fibrosus can lead to acute back pain. Actual disk herniation can lead to nerve root compression, with ensuing radicular pain, numbness, and weakness, but acute disk herniation is generally a rare source of back pain in the athlete. Disk herniation pain is typically worse with flexion and may be increased with coughing, sneezing, or sitting. A special case of annulus injury without disk herniation is a radial tear of the inner annulus, which may lead to inflammation of the outer annulus. Pain occurs with flexion. In this case, MRI will show a high signal on T2-weighted images in the posterior annulus, and a discogram will confirm the diagnosis. In adolescents, a posterior apophyseal avulsion fracture at the annular attachment may cause a unique type of disk herniation.

Treatment

Treatment of disk pathology is generally conservative, with a brief period of relative rest, NSAID medications, and physical therapy. If a herniated disk is present with radiculopathy, treatment generally consists of conservative treatment and, if necessary, a rigid orthosis in 10–15° of lordosis. If radiculopathy persists, epidural steroids may be warranted. Only if symptoms continue despite these interventions should surgery be contemplated.

Generally, 90% of athletes with disk disease improve over 12 weeks. Surgery is only performed for refractory pain (over 6–12 weeks) or progressive neurologic

---

HERNIATED DISK

History

- Acute or gradual onset of pain.
- Radicular symptoms.
- Presentation in adolescence often atypical.
- Pain worse with flexion, coughing, sitting.

Examination

- Pain with motion.
- Neurologic abnormality.

Treatment

- Non-operative, symptomatic, therapeutic exercises.
- Surgery when persistent or with progressive neurologic deficit.
- Bowel or bladder symptoms suggest caudaequina syndrome – a surgical emergency.

Return to action

- When pain free, with normal range of motion and strength.

---

deficit. If bowel or bladder symptoms are present, however, caudaequina syndrome must be considered, and emergent surgical evaluation is required. Bilateral lower extremity weakness or numbness should also alert the team physician to possible caudaequina syndrome.

Rehabilitation

Therapy focuses on establishing normal range of motion, flexibility, and strength. Special attention should be focused on improving sleeping, sitting, and transitional positions contributing to symptoms. Also, focus should be paid to stretching the likely short hamstrings, piriformis, ITB, rectus abdominus, and gluteus maximus musculature. Self, manual, and mechanical lumbar traction can be useful to decrease symptoms. Additionally, use of a lumbar support can be helpful.

Return to play

The athlete may return to play when pain has resolved and therapy has allowed for normal range of motion and strength.

Atypical (lumbar) Scheuermann's

Fieldside assessment

The athlete typically complains of back pain with gradual onset.

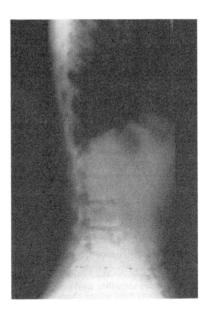

Figure 16.4 Relative thoracic hypokyphosis and lumbar hypolordosis, with resultant "flatback"

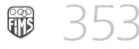

Diagnosis

Atypical Scheuermann's (or lumbar Scheuermann's disease) is a unique type of diskogenic back pain frequently seen in gymnasts, divers, and wrestlers, and in athletes whose activities involve hyperflexion and weight lifting. It is associated with a relative thoracic hypokyphosis and lumbar hypolordosis with resultant "flatback" (Figure 16.4). This contrasts with typical Scheuermann's kyphosis, the better-known entity of vertebral body repetitive injury, which occurs in the thoracic spine and results in a structural thoracic kyphosis. Flatback may be noted on physical examination or on standing lateral radiographs. Pain with hyperflexion suggests the diagnosis. MRI may show anterior disk herniation, Schmorl's node formation, end-plate avulsion, and/or apophyseal avulsions.

Treatment

Treatment is conservative, using a 10–15° lordosis brace to unload the injured vertebral bodies. The brace is worn for 4–6 months. Therapeutic exercise is incorporated during the recovery phase.

Rehabilitation

Along with bracing, physical therapy is initiated, involving stretching (especially hamstring stretching and piriformis muscles), strengthening of lower abdominals, serratus anterior, and periscapular musculature, and lumbar spine extension exercises can be helpful.

Return to play

The athlete may return to play with the brace when asymptomatic.

Spondylolysis/spondylolisthesis

Fieldside assessment

The athlete generally complains of back pain, usually with gradual onset. Increased pain with extension maneuvers, such as the back walkover in gymnastics, arabesque in dance, or the throw-in in soccer, is usually present.

Diagnosis

Spondylolysis is most frequently seen from hyperextension sports such as gymnastics, football, and figure skating. It is seen more frequently in adolescent than adult athletes and should be suspected if pain is elicited by provocative hyperextension, particularly hyperextension pain while the athlete stands on one foot (Figure 16.5). Unilateral pain suggests unilateral spondylolysis.

The rate of spondylolysis in adolescent athletes with back pain was found to be as high as 47% in one study. In athletes, spondylolysis is generally considered a stress fracture of the pars interarticularis, caused by repetitive hyperextension. Evidence suggests genetic risk factors for developing spondylolysis (e.g. a high

l.j. micheli, d.s. parsehian, and t.c. kim

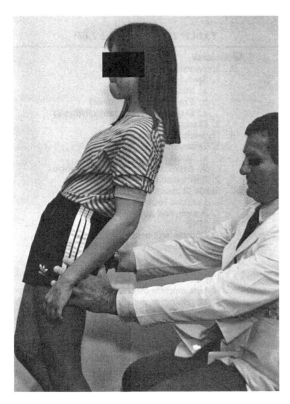

Figure 16.5 Provocative hyperextension test to help determine presence of posterior element injury

incidence found in Inuit populations), but this may represent another subset of this disease and is frequently asymptomatic. An association has been found between symptomatic spondylolysis and spina bifida occulta. Nevertheless, most evidence points to this condition being an acquired phenomenon from repetitive microtrauma, particularly extension. If physical examination suggests spondylolysis, AP and lateral radiographs may demonstrate a defect at the pars interarticularis. Oblique images may better demonstrate this defect, but a single-photon emission computerized tomography (SPECT) bone scan is the gold standard to confirm the diagnosis (Figures 16.6 and 16.7). Findings vary from unilateral stress reaction to bilateral pars fractures and spondylolisthesis. Bone scans may also be helpful to determine if the stress fracture is metabolically active. CT scans are best for assessing fracture healing during follow-up but MRI also may help both in the diagnosis and follow-up of this condition.

Spondylolisthesis is the forward slippage of the vertebra relative to the adjacent vertebral body (Figure 16.8). Spondylolisthesis has been categorized into several

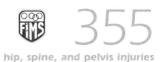

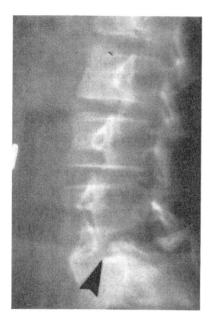

Figure 16.6
The initial imaging studies for a patient with extension back pain are the anteroposterior (AP), lateral, and collimated lateral view of the lumbosacral area. Plain radiographs have low sensitivity for identifying spondlolysis, although the standing lateral is the most useful film for identifying spondylolisthesis and can identify the grade of spondylolisthesis by percentage of slippage

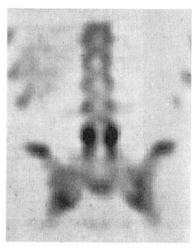

Figure 16.7
SPECT bone scan of L–S spine showing L4 spondylolysis. Plain radiographs, including obliques, were normal

types: congenital, isthmic, degenerative, traumatic, pathologic, and post-surgical. Bilateral pars interarticularis stress fractures can lead to the isthmic type of spondylolisthesis. The most frequently involved level is L5–S1. Grading is based on the percentage of the vertebral body that is displaced: grade I: 0–25%; grade II: 25–50%; grade III: 50–75%; grade IV: 75–100%; and grade V (spondyloptosis): 100%.

Treatment

We recommend the use of a 0° Boston overlapping brace for treatment of spondylolysis, although the use of bracing and its efficacy are a source of debate,

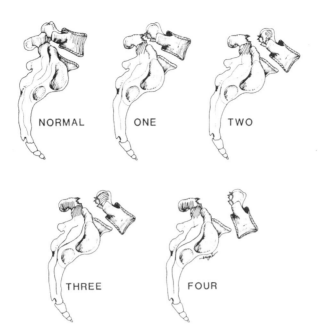

NORMAL   ONE   TWO

THREE   FOUR

Figure 16.8 Spondylolisthesis is graded into four degrees of severity, based on the extent of the forward slippage

and some recommend a period of activity modification without bracing. The athlete initially wears the brace for 23 hours a day. In addition, physical therapy is initiated. If a stress fracture is identified, bracing continues for a minimum of 4–6 months. Only short-term bracing is required if stress reaction, rather than a stress fracture, is found, as this generally resolves more rapidly than actual stress fractures. Healing may result from this treatment, especially if the diagnosis is made early in the course of the disease. Weaning from the brace begins when the CT scan shows healing, or the patient becomes asymptomatic. Resolution of symptoms may represent a fibrous nonunion if healing is not demonstrated on CT images. During the weaning phase, the athlete may use the brace for sports and at night, and ultimately curtail night-time usage. If the patient is still symptomatic following 6–9 months of treatment, and CT demonstrates the fracture not to be united, external electrical stimulation may be initiated. If severe pain persists beyond 9–12 months, posterolateral in situ fusion may be recommended.

Isthmic spondylolisthesis is generally stable and does not progress significantly. Grade I spondylolisthesis is treated like spondylolysis. Grade II treatment is individualized. For deformity of grade III or higher, neurologic symptoms, slip progression, or persistent pain may require posterolateral fusion. If surgical fusion is necessary, return to sports must be individualized, but single-level fusion is not a contraindication to sports participation.

Rehabilitation

Physical therapy is essential and focuses on peripelvic flexibility and antilordotic strengthening. Extension-type exercises for the back should be avoided. Also, care should be taken in avoiding strengthening in prone and four-point positions with patients with known spondylolisthesis to avoid excessive shear forces on the spine that could lead to worsening of spinal alignment. Core stabilization in standing, hook-lying, and supine positions are more appropriate for these patients.

Return to play

The athlete may return to sports when asymptomatic in the brace (generally at about 6 weeks) and pain-free with play.

Lumbar stenosis/facet arthropathy

Fieldside assessment

The athlete complains of back pain, which is usually of gradual onset.

Diagnosis

Lumbar spinal stenosis is narrowing of the spinal canal, which may cause compression of the spinal cord or nerve roots. Stenosis may be either congenital or degenerative. Compression of the cord or nerve roots may lead to symptoms such as claudication, paresthesias, and weakness, in addition to back pain.

Characteristically, the athlete describes intolerance to prolonged standing or walking, with a normal neurologic exam at rest. Facet arthropathy is more common in older athletes and has not been reported in children (although adolescents may develop a facet syndrome that is treated like a soft-tissue injury). The athlete may report stiffness, difficulty with bending or with rotation, and aching following activities. Findings may include specific focal tenderness or asymmetric range of motion. Facet joint pain often occurs with extension. Bone and CT scans may be normal. MRI has been found to be very useful in the diagnosis of lumbar stenosis.

Treatment

Treatment for both lumbar spinal stenosis and facet arthropathy is conservative, with NSAIDs, activity modification, rehabilitation, and, if necessary, steroid injections. If conservative measures fail to alleviate symptoms, a corticosteroid injection may be both diagnostic and therapeutic.

Rehabilitation

Initially, range of motion into lumbar spine flexion is promoted to relieve pressure on the spine. Later, functional training should be incorporated, with emphasis on keeping lower abdominals stabilized with walking. Stretches to hamstrings and gluteus maximus can be helpful.

Return to play

The athlete may continue to play with this condition. However, safe, unrestricted participation requires full range of motion and strength.

Transitional vertebrae

Fieldside assessment

The athlete generally complains of low-back pain in the low lumbar or upper sacral region of the spine, usually of gradual onset.

Diagnosis

Transitional vertebrae represent a congenitally incomplete segmentation of the low lumbar or upper sacral vertebrae, effectively a pseudoarthrosis. A rapid flexion or extension injury may cause inflammation at this pseudoarthrosis and lead to pain, stiffness, and limited range of motion.

Treatment

Initial treatment is rest and anti-inflammatory medication. An orthosis may help alleviate symptoms, as physical therapy is instituted. A corticosteroid injection may be both diagnostic and therapeutic for this condition. On rare occasions, fusion or resection of the impingement may be necessary.

Rehabilitation

Skilled physical therapy should focus on the individual impairments and on improving the lumbar spine active range of motion with correct biomechanics.

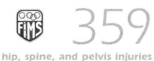

The athlete performs stretching, lower abdominal strengthening, and spinal stabilization exercises.

Return to play
The athlete may return to play when asymptomatic.

Other

In the workup of persistent back pain, further evaluation, such as bone scan, CT scan, and MRI, may also help delineate other possible sources of back pain. Conditions such as infection and neoplasm must be considered in the differential diagnosis. Scoliosis may also be noted, but rarely causes back pain unless severe.

An adolescent with idiopathic scoliosis may generally participate fully in athletics, even if brace treatment is required. Infectious etiologies include osteomyelitis and discitis. Infection should be suspected in cases with an appropriate history, and if symptoms such as fever and chills are found. Bone scan and MRI, as well as biopsy (surgical or CT-guided), may help confirm the diagnosis. Pain relieved by the use of NSAIDs should raise the suspicion of an osteoid osteoma. Other neoplasms, such as osteoblastoma, hemangioma, aneurismal bone cysts, giant-cell tumor, and malignancies, may be found in the spine. These findings should prompt a referral to a specialist.

ACUTE HIP/PELVIS INJURIES

Strains

Fieldside assessment
The athlete complains of sudden pain in the region involved. If a fracture is not suspected, the athlete may walk off the field for assessment, unless limited by pain (Figure 16.9).

Diagnosis
Adductor strains are usually caused by forced external rotation of an abducted leg, but also may occur when the adductors are repeatedly in use, as in hockey, skating, and tennis. The adductor longus is most frequently involved. The diagnosis is suspected if there is tenderness over the adductor tendons or musculature. Passive abduction causes pain, as does active, resisted adduction. Other conditions such as osteitis pubis, hernia, or even obturator nerve entrapment (diagnosed by electromyogram) should be suspected in longstanding cases. MRI may shows signs of a tear or hemorrhage, or may show chronic changes with longstanding cases, but radiographic studies may often not be helpful.

Hamstring strains result from a sudden stretch in the hamstring musculature, usually with the hip in flexion and knee in extension. Symptoms typically include spasm, swelling, and localized tenderness over the hamstrings.

l.j. micheli, d.s. parsehian, and t.c. kim

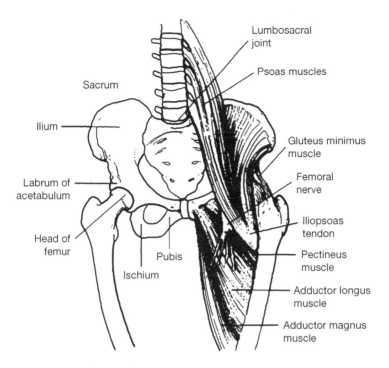

Lumbosacral joint

Psoas muscles

Sacrum

Ilium

Gluteus minimus muscle

Femoral nerve

Labrum of acetabulum

Iliopsoas tendon

Head of femur

Pectineus muscle

Pubis

Ischium

Adductor longus muscle

Adductor magnus muscle

Figure 16.9 Hip, pelvis, and groin anatomy

Treatment

Treatment of adductor and hamstring strains is generally conservative, with rest, ice, NSAIDs, and elastic wraps initially, followed by rehabilitation. Stretching exercises begin after acute symptoms resolve, followed by rehabilitative exercises. If symptoms continue following adductor strain, a steroid injection into the adductor insertion into the pelvis may be considered. If the condition still does not resolve, procedures such as adductor releases and rectus tightening have been described, but it has been reported that only about 60% of athletes undergoing an adductor tenotomy return to the same level of sports participation. With hamstring strains in athletes, recurrence is unfortunately relatively common. Often, reinjury is more severe, with a longer recovery time.

Rehabilitation

Rehabilitation in the acute phase that can prove helpful includes pulsed ultrasound, compression of soft tissue with hip spica wrapping, early gentle hip passive range of motion, and submaximal hip isometrics. In the subacute phase, ultrasound, whirlpool, and/or moist hot packs, active range of motion into hip abduction and adduction, single leg balance and prioprioceptive activities, gentle groin stretching, abdominal strengthening, and cardiovascular training on bike and/or elliptical

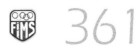

361

trainer can be started. Prior to return to sport, functional drills can be initiated, including lateral agility and cutting exercises, to include slideboard, Fitter, peripelvic stabilization with medicine ball, and protective wrapping, as needed, in preparation for return to sport. Additionally, dynamic eccentric strengthening can be particularly useful.

Return to play

The athlete may return to play when pain resolves. Running, jumping, and stairs should be avoided if they cause pain. Stretching before sport activity and limiting excursion of the muscle group with strapping or compression shorts may prevent injury recurrence.

ADDUCTOR AND HAMSTRING STRAINS

History

- Sudden eccentric contraction with sudden pain.

Examination

- Local tenderness, swelling, muscle spasm.

Treatment

- RICE; no stretching until acute symptoms have resolved.
- Emphasize dynamic eccentric strengthening.

Return to action

- When pain resolves.

Iliac crest contusion (hip pointer)

Fieldside assessment

The athlete complains of substantial pain in the iliac crest region from a direct blow or a fall. If a pelvic fracture is not suspected, the patient may walk or be assisted off the field for evaluation.

Diagnosis

"Hip pointers" is the athletic nickname for contusions of the iliac crest (Figure 16.10). These injuries are common in contact sports such as football, rugby, and soccer. Diagnosis is based on the mechanism of injury and the physical findings. Tenderness localizes to the iliac crest, and pain and muscle spasm may cause an antalgic gait. With the many muscle attachments to the iliac crest (abdominals from above, gluteals from below), muscle contractions may also elicit pain. Lateral

362

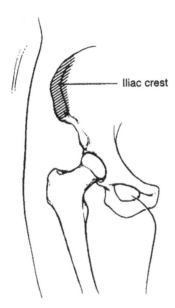

Figure 16.10 Iliac crest contusion/hip pointer

abdominal tenderness and pain with flexion of the trunk to the opposite side suggest strain of the external oblique aponeurosis. Radiographic evaluation may be warranted, if the diagnosis is in doubt or if a fracture is suspected. Apophyseal avulsion fractures in adolescents or fractures of the iliac wing may be identified. MRI may be useful to identify stress fractures and to demonstrate muscular edema.

Treatment

Treatment for hip pointers includes ice, rest, and compression in the acute phase following injury. Partial weight-bearing with crutches may be necessary for a few days, if pain is severe. Rehabilitation progresses once acute symptoms have resolved.

Iliac fractures are generally stable, but may need to be treated initially with bed-rest.

Rehabilitation

Acutely, heat, or aggressive physical therapy should be avoided, as these modalities may aggravate the hematoma and cause additional bleeding. Later, gentle therapy may be started with stretching and careful attention paid to abdominal streng-thening, starting with isometrics, with guidance by a supervising PT. The athlete then gradually resumes non-contact activities with initiation of sports conditioning and endurance training in the clinic, followed by a gradual return to sport-specific activities.

Return to play

The athlete may be cleared for sports when pain resolves, and the athlete is able to resume sport-specific activities. Additional padding may be necessary when the injured athlete resumes play. Iliac wing fractures typically require up to 12 weeks before a return to sports.

ILIAC CREST CONTUSION/"HIP POINTER"

History

- Direct blow.

Examination

- Point tender; often muscle spasm.

Treatment

- RICE; crutches as needed.
- Stretching particularly important.

Return to action

- When pain resolves and can meet demands of sport.
- May need special protective padding.

Avulsion

Fieldside assessment

The athlete complains of sudden pain in the region of an apophysis. The athlete is assisted or carried from the field, and further evaluation is performed.

Diagnosis

Apophyseal avulsion fractures are an injury of adolescent athletes, usually between the ages of 14 and 17. These injuries often occur following or during a growth spurt, when the soft tissues are typically tight. The mechanism of injury is generally a sudden forceful muscular contraction that pulls the muscle's bony attachment free from its bed. Musculoskeletally "tight" athletes are particularly prone to these injuries. In adults, this mechanism would instead cause an injury to the muscle–tendon junction. Avulsion fractures should be suspected if specific point tenderness is noted at an apophysis (Figure 16.11). Common sites of involvement are as follows:

- *Anterior superior iliac spine – sartorius attachment*: The athlete has anterior hip pain and point tenderness over the anterior superior iliac spine. Pain is

364

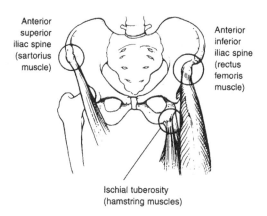

Anterior superior iliac spine (sartorius muscle)

Anterior inferior iliac spine (rectus femoris muscle)

Ischial tuberosity (hamstring muscles)

Figure 16.11 Avulsion fractures in the pelvic area

also elicited with resisted knee extension and hip flexion. Diagnosis can be confirmed by X-rays.

- *Anterior inferior iliac spine – attachment of the rectus femoris*: The athlete has anterior hip pain and point tenderness over the anterior inferior iliac spine, just inferior to the anterior superior iliac spine. Injury is usually caused by a powerful quadriceps contraction, as with a forceful soccer kick. This bony prominence may be difficult to palpate. X-rays confirm the diagnosis.
- *Ischial tuberosity – hamstring attachment*: The athlete has buttock pain and pain with sitting. Point tenderness is directly over the ischial tuberosity. Plain radiographs confirm the diagnosis.
- *Iliac apophysis – attachment of the abdominal musculature*: This injury may occur with violent contraction of the abdominal musculature while the trunk is forced to the contralateral direction. The athlete has pain and tenderness along the iliac crest. Pain occurs with bending to the opposite side.
- *Lesser trochanter – iliopsoas attachment*: The athlete has pain in the medial hip near the adductors, typically following forceful hip hyperextension. Plain X-rays show the avulsion fracture.

Treatment

Treatment of apophyseal avulsion fractures is generally conservative, with rest, ice, and compression. The athlete may need to use crutches for a few days. When flexibility improves, the athlete begins a regular exercise program of gentle stretching, followed by progressive resisted exercises.

Displaced ischial tuberosity avulsion fractures may require open reduction and internal fixation to avoid late pain and sciatic nerve irritation, but this is still a point of some controversy. If the athlete presents with symptoms weeks or months following a non-reduced displaced ischial tuberosity fracture, then surgical excision (rather than reduction and internal fixation) may help to relieve symptoms of the nonunion. Displaced anterior inferior iliac spine fractures may block hip motion

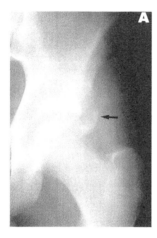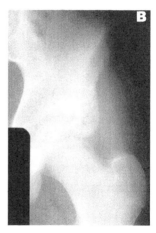

Figure 16.12 (A) Anterior inferior iliac spine avulsion fracture. (B) Anterior inferior iliac spine avulsion fracture after healing

AVULSION FRACTURES

History

- Usually adolescent.
- Sudden pain in apophyseal region following forceful muscle contraction.

Examination

- Local tenderness.
- Hip usually held in flexion.

Test for specific point of injury by having athlete contract attached muscle, i.e.:

- anterior superior iliac spine – sartorius attachment;
- anterior interior iliac spine – rectus femoris;
- iliac apophysis – abdominals;
- lesser trochanter – iliopsoas;
- ischial tuberosity – hamstrings.

Treatment

- Crutches as needed.
- RICE.
- Gentle stretching as pain decreases.

Return to action

- Normal range of motion and strength.
- Usually 4–8 weeks.

l.j. micheli, d.s. parsehian, and t.c. kim

if the fragment is displaced by more than 2 cm. CT scans may help to delineate the relationship of these fragments to the hip joint.

Rehabilitation

The athlete's physical therapy typically starts with gentle stretching, followed by initiation of isometric strengthening, followed by active range of motion, and finally progressive resistive strengthening. As muscle strength returns, conditioning and sport-specific activities may be gradually introduced.

Return to play

The athlete may return to play when full range of motion and strength are normal, usually after 4–8 weeks.

NON-ACUTE HIP/PELVIS INJURIES

Osteitis pubis

Fieldside assessment

Osteitis pubis is generally a chronic and progressive condition. The athlete typically presents with chronic pain in the region of the symphysis pubis, which is aggravated by activity (Figure 16.13).

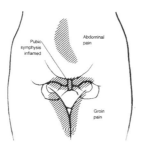

Figure 16.13
Osteitis pubis

Diagnosis

Osteitis pubis is thought to be caused by repetitive microtrauma in the region of the symphysis pubis and occurs most commonly in running sports, as well as soccer, football, and hockey. Forces across the symphysis are exerted by the rectus abdominis and adductors. It can be difficult to differentiate osteitis pubis from adductor strain, but athletes with osteitis pubis are tender directly over the symphysis. The athlete may have a painful lateral compression test, where applying force on the iliac wing, with the athlete in the lateral decubitus position, may elicit pain in the region. X-rays may show bone resorption near the symphysis, and a radionuclide bone scan may show increased uptake in the region. MRI may show signal changes in the region and is helpful in confirming the diagnosis.

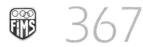

Treatment

Treatment is rest, NSAIDs, and heat. A brief period of bed rest followed by progressive crutch-ambulation may be necessary in severe cases. Steroid injections under fluoroscopy may be useful if symptoms fail to resolve. Operative arthrodesis and debridement procedures have also been described.

Rehabilitation

Rehabilitation with physical therapy often involves modalities to alleviate inflammation, followed by gentle stretching, possible need for muscle energy and other manual techniques to correct imbalances in pelvic alignment, and core strengthening. Physical therapy is generally successful, but often is prolonged for 3–9 months for resolution.

Return to play

The athlete may return to activities when symptoms allow. Symptoms may persist for a prolonged period.

OSTEITIS PUBIS

History
- Chronic, progressive pubic/groin pain.

Examination
- Tenderness directly over symphysis.

Treatment
- Rest, NSAIDs, heat.
- Prolonged rehabilitation (typically 3–9 months).

Return to action
- When symptoms allow.

Sacroiliitis

Fieldside assessment

Symptoms of sacroiliitis are usually insidious, and the athlete may complain of back, buttock, or leg pain, which is usually chronic in nature.

Diagnosis

The sacroiliac joint acts to dissipate forces between the spine and lower extremities. Motion at the sacroiliac joint is limited, with minimal amounts of rotation and translation occurring at this joint. Forces across this joint can thus be increased

l.j. micheli, d.s. parsehian, and t.c. kim

with particularly strong muscular contractions. The athlete with sacroiliitis may complain of back pain, buttock, and leg pain. The patient is tender over the sacroiliac joint and often will have a positive FABER test (the ipsilateral hip that is flexed, abducted, and externally rotated (FABER) causes pain in the sacroiliac region or the buttock). A bone scan may be helpful to rule out a possible sacroiliac stress fracture. Other conditions that may cause similar symptoms are stress fractures of the joint, infection, and inflammatory conditions such as ankylosing spondylitis.

Treatment
Treatment for sacroiliitis is rest, NSAIDs, and ice. This is usually accompanied by physical therapy. An injection into the sacroiliac joint under fluouroscopic guidance may be both diagnostic and therapeutic, but is used only in refractory cases. Stress fracture is treated with partial weight-bearing for 4–6 weeks.

Rehabilitation
Physical therapy may be incorporated for peripelvic strengthening, use of muscle energy techniques to improve sacroiliac joint (SIJ) alignment, muscle flexibility, and usage of SIJ belts and/or taping for symptom reduction. Strengthening with a focus on bilateral lower extremities, with progression to unilateral activities, works best, as most complaints arise from pain with unilateral stance activities that exacerbate and/or cause the injury in the first place.

Return to play
The athlete may return to play when full range of motion and strength return.

Snapping hip

Fieldside assessment
The symptoms are usually of gradual onset and rarely require on-field attention.

Diagnosis
Snapping hip most commonly consists of snapping of the iliotibial band or the iliopsoas tendon over a bony prominence – the iliotibial band snapping over the greater trochanter (external snapping hip) and the iliopsoas tendon snapping over the pectineal eminence and/or femoral neck (internal snapping hip). The athlete has localized tenderness of the tendon or the underlying bursa. The athlete can usually reproduce the snapping symptom voluntarily.

Lateral snapping hip and greater trochanteric bursitis often coexist. Tenderness localizes to the region of the greater trochanter, often to the posterior aspect. The Ober test is usually positive, indicating iliotibial band tightness. Adduction of the flexed hip also typically causes pain. Athletes with a prolonged history of painful snapping hip typically have significant contractures of the hip flexors and hamstrings.

The snapping iliopsoas tendon is frequently seen in dancers, gymnasts, and soccer players. This snapping may cause painful stenosing tenosynovitis near the iliopsoas insertion on the lesser trochanter. The athlete can usually reproduce the snapping, which can be localized by the examiner. Diagnosis is confirmed by pain on three provocative tests. First, progressive passive hyperflexion of the involved hip will elicit pain. Second, with the leg in a "frog" position, the athlete flexes and adducts the hip against resistance. Third, the examiner hyperextends and abducts the hip, flexes the knee, and internally rotates the hip. Internal snapping hip must be differentiated from intra-articular causes such as labral tears, loose bodies, and osteochondral injuries. Radiographic studies such as X-ray, CT scan, and MRI may help in differentiating an internal snapping hip from an intra-articular cause.

Treatment

Treatment for snapping hip includes stretching any tight lower-extremity muscles and improving spinal stability by appropriate strengthening exercises. Rest, ice, and NSAIDs help the athlete control pain sufficiently to follow the therapeutic exercise program.

Greater trochanteric bursitis can be treated by massage, ultrasound, and iliotibial band stretching. If symptoms do not resolve, a steroid injection should be considered, and, if symptoms still persist, surgical bursectomy may be considered. Surgical partial release of the iliotibial band for snapping hip and/or greater trochanteric bursitis is rarely required. Treatment for recalcitrant iliopsoas tendinitis may include injection of corticosteroid into the tendon sheath. If symptoms still persist, surgical release or lengthening may be considered.

SNAPPING HIP

History
- Usually gradual onset.
- Generally either iliotibial band or iliopsoas tendon.

Examination
- Iliotibial band: local tenderness; positive Ober test.
- Iliopsoas tendon: palpable snapping anteromedial hip region with flexion/extension.

Treatment
- Iliotibial band: RICE, stretch iliotibial band.
- Iliopsoas tendon: rest, NSAIDs, heat, core strengthening.

Return to action
- When able to meet demands of sport.

Rehabilitation

For snapping secondary to the iliotibial band, physical therapy consisting of ultrasound and iliotibial band stretching may be effective. Posterior gluteus medius and lower abdominal strengthening should be addressed, in order to improve neuromuscular (NM) control in the peripelvic region. Stretching of the hip flexors should also be addressed. Formal physical therapy for both snapping-hip conditions generally consists of improving postural alignment, spinal stabilizer muscle endurance, and peripelvic flexibility.

Return to play

The athlete may return to play when symptoms permit, and strength and range of motion are sufficient to meet the demands of the sport.

Femoroacetabular impingement

Fieldside assessment

The athlete will complain of anterior, or anterolateral, hip pain, usually insidious.

Diagnosis

Femoroacetabular impingement encompasses cam and pincer impingement, but usually is combined. Cam impingement refers to a prominence at the femoral head–neck junction, which causes microtrauma to the anterosuperior acetabular rim. This can lead to chondral injuries and labral pathology. Pincer impingement refers to acetabular overcoverage of the femoral head, which again can lead to damage to the labrum and the articular cartilage. Besides pain, locking and catching may occur, especially in cases with chondral or labral tears. Physical exam will usually elicit pain with adduction and internal rotation with the hip flexed to 90°. Radiologic evaluation consists of radiographs, but a CT scan or MRI/MRI arthrogram may be necessary.

Treatment

Unfortunately, non-surgical treatment often fails to alleviate symptoms. Arthroscopic treatment may be necessary in cases of impingement, as well as for chondral and labral lesions. Chondral lesions may be treated with abrasion chondroplasty and, if necessary, microfracture, while labral tears may be addressed with debridement or repair. Impingement may necessitate treatment of the overlying acetabular rim or the prominence at the femoral head–neck junction.

Rehabilitation

Despite low success rates with rehabilitation to prevent arthroscopic surgery, pre-habilitation can be helpful and should emphasize symptom reduction, to include joint mobilization (i.e. long axis joint distraction), restoration of muscle imbalances in preparation for surgery, to include gluteus maximus, posterior gluteus medius, deep hip external rotators (ERs), and lower abdominal strengthening, being careful to avoid excessive hip flexor activation, and stretching of the hamstrings, piriformis, and psoas.

After arthroscopic treatment, the athlete is usually one-sixth weight-bearing for 3 weeks (longer, if a microfracture is performed). Physical therapy is initiated on the first day post-operation for gait and stair training, restoration of active range of motion in internal rotation in supine and hook-lying positions, along with isometric strengthening of gluteus maximus and lower abdominals. At this time, extension and external rotation of the hip are limited to reduce stress on the femoral head. In later stages of the rehabilitation, the focus is placed on restoration of NM timing of gluteus maximus, posterior gluteus medius, and deep hip ER, strengthening of involved lower extremity with avoidance of excessive hip flexor strengthening to prevent a tendency for psoas tendinitis, and flexibility of LEs as needed. The bike can be added in the second week post-operation, and the elliptical trainer approximately six weeks post-operation. Physicians often differ in opinion when initiating running on a rubberized track only, vs. allowing treadmill usage, following surgery with this patient population. This controversy stems from variabilities in neuromuscular timing activation post-operatively. Patients resume gentle, supervised running and more sport-specific training approximately 3–4 months post-operation, based on the individual. Most patients return to sport at around 6 months plus post-operation, generally, on clearance by their physician.

Return to play

Athletes are often able to return to sports after recovery, although the presence of arthritis was found to be a limiting factor in some participants in one recent study. The time to return to sports depends on the nature of the procedure performed, but should be expected to be at least 6 weeks.

Hamstring syndrome

Fieldside assessment

Hamstring syndrome is usually a chronic condition. The athlete complains of buttock pain centered over the ischial tuberosity, especially with sitting and stretching of the hamstring, along with referred pain to the back of the thigh and knee.

Diagnosis

Hamstring syndrome is caused by the tight tendinous structures of the hamstring, particularly the biceps femoris tendon, compressing or irritating the sciatic nerve as it passes underneath the tendons and over the ischial tuberosity. Hamstring syndrome is most commonly seen in track athletes and can be precipitated by chronic or acute proximal hamstring strains. Athletes complain of pain during sprinting and hurdling, as the hamstring is stretched, and especially with sitting.

It is important to rule out back injury as a cause of sciatic pain before making the diagnosis of hamstring syndrome. On examination, the athlete is tender over the ischial tuberosity and complains of pain with hip flexion range of motion, and it is often possible to palpate the taut hamstring tendons on examination. The athlete can have a positive straight-leg raise test, but most often the neurological examination is normal.

Treatment

Initial treatment is conservative, using rest, physical therapy, and NSAIDs. Steroid injection under fluoroscopy may be useful if symptoms do not resolve using therapy and NSAIDs. Surgical hamstring release and sciatic decompression are indicated if conservative treatment is not successful. Neoprene shorts can be helpful for compression and support with conservative treatment or post-surgically.

Rehabilitation

Physical therapy emphasizes RICE, use of hamstring isometrics, followed by use of bike, modalities (i.e. ultrasound, electrical stimulation, and moist heat), proprioceptive training, and hamstring stretching and strengthening, particularly eccentric strengthening.

Return to play

The athlete may participate with conservative treatment, as tolerated, when symptoms decrease and he/she has full range of motion and strength. Post-surgically, the athlete requires rest, physical therapy, and a gradual progression back into sport activity.

HAMSTRING SYNDROME

History
- Most often gradual onset buttock pain in area of ischial tuberosity.
- Referred pain to back of thigh or knee.
- Pain with sitting.

Examination
- Tenderness over ischial tuberosity.
- Pain with hip-flexion range of motion.

Treatment
- Rest, therapy, NSAIDs.
- Corticosteriod injection.
- Hamstring release and sciatic decompression.

Return to action
- When symptoms decrease and full range of motion and strength return.

373

Stress fracture

Fieldside assessment

The athlete complains of activity-related hip pain. Occasionally, the athlete may have sudden pain on the field and be unable to bear weight. In this situation, fracture should be suspected, and the athlete should not be allowed to bear weight, but should be transported for further evaluation and treatment.

Diagnosis

Stress fractures of the proximal femur are relatively rare, but they occur most commonly in endurance sports such as running and result from repetitive micro-trauma. Stress fractures can also occur in the pelvis and the sacrum. The athlete feels pain in the hip, anterior thigh, or groin with running, or with any weight-bearing. Range of motion is usually painful and limited, especially internal rotation. Plain radiographs may be normal. If the diagnosis is suspected, a bone scan should be obtained. CT scan may further delineate the anatomy of the fracture. MRI has been found to be the most sensitive imaging technique to detect occult fractures of the proximal femur.

Treatment

Compression-type fractures involve the inferior portion of the femoral neck. They can usually be treated with non-weight-bearing until pain resolves, then partial weight-bearing, and finally full weight-bearing and rehabilitation. Frequent X-ray follow-up is necessary to ensure that displacement at the fracture site does not occur during the course of treatment. Prolonged symptoms or displacement are indications for surgical fixation. Transverse or tension-type fractures may also be treated conservatively, but, if symptoms become worse or the fracture extends or displaces, internal fixation is usually required. Pelvic stress fractures are usually treated conservatively, with rest followed by rehabilitation.

Rehabilitation

When healing is sufficient and the athlete is pain-free, gradually increasing rehabilitation is started, first with aquatic therapy, then walking, followed by jogging. The athlete must remain pain-free. When able to jog, the athlete may then gradually resume sport-specific activities.

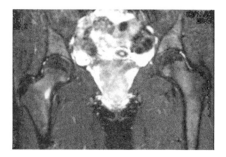

Figure 16.14
Stress fracture of the femoral neck

Sports hernia

Fieldside assessment

The athlete usually presents with insidious unilateral anterior hip or deep groin pain, which is exacerbated by activity or a Valsalva maneuver and resolves with rest.

Diagnosis

Sports hernias, also referred to as athletic pubalgia, must be considered in the differential diagnosis of groin pain in athletes, particularly with sports that involve quick, twisting maneuvers. They are caused by a tear or a weakness of the posterior inguinal wall, mostly occur in males, and can be associated with adductor tendinopathy. Physical examination fails to find a traditional hernia, but often presents with point pubic tenderness. Ultrasound and MRI may help rule out other sources of pathology, but radiologic studies cannot confirm the diagnosis and are often normal.

Treatment

Non-surgical treatment consisting of physical therapy is often the initial treatment utilized, but rarely resolves symptoms. Initial treatment would consist of NSAIDS, massage, contrast (heat and cold), and rest. Open or laparoscopic hernia repairs are often necessary after a course of non-operative management, and may be performed in conjunction with an adductor tenotomy.

Rehabilitation

Modalities of therapy would include deep massage, contrast, and rehabilitation focusing on core and pelvic strengthening, along with rest and a gradual return to activities.

Return to play

If therapy is successful, expect about 6 weeks of rehabilitation to return to sport-specific activities. Once the patient can resume these activities, he/she may be cleared to play. Results of surgical repair are generally excellent, with over 90% of athletes able to return to sports, with recovery times ranging from 2 weeks to 6 months.

OTHER CAUSES OF PAIN IN THE HIP AND PELVIS AREA

As with back injuries, it is important to consider other possible, non-traumatic causes of hip and pelvis pain in the athlete. In the young athlete, other causes of hip pain include Legg–Calve–Perthes, slipped capital femoral epiphysis, septicarthritis of the hip, transient synovitis, and tumor.

Legg–Calve–Perthes occurs between the ages of 2 and 12 years (but between 4 and 8 years is most common) and may manifest as limp following activity, and hip, groin, or knee pain. The athlete has decreased hip range of motion, particularly abduction, flexion, and internal rotation. X-rays are usually diagnostic with osteopenia, necrosis, and collapse of the femoral epiphysis and neck. Bone scan may also aid with diagnosis. Treatment is aimed at "containment" of the femoral head and maintenance of hip range of motion. Slipped capital femoral epiphysis occurs in a slightly older patient population (11–16 years of age). Symptoms may be similar to Legg–Calve–Perthes, with some patients not able to bear weight on the affected extremity. Typically, the athlete with slipped capital femoral epiphysis is obese (although approximately 10% of cases are slender and in a growth spurt), and the hip goes into external rotation as it is flexed. Diagnosis is made by X-rays that show the femoral neck to be superiorly and anteriorly displaced and externally rotated from the epiphysis. The athlete should be referred to an orthopedic surgeon for surgical internal fixation of the slipped epiphysis.

If hip pain is associated with signs of infection such as fever, or elevated white blood cell count or sedimentation rate, infection must be considered. If suspected, an orthopedic surgeon should be consulted for a hip aspiration (usually done with fluoroscopic assistance), and, if a septic joint is confirmed, the joint is surgically drained.

In adult athletes, other causes of hip pain include osteonecrosis and osteoarthritis of the hip. Osteonecrosis is usually secondary to trauma, alcohol, or steroids, but many other possible etiologies exist. X-rays may show evidence of osteonecrosis, but MRI is the most useful test to detect this condition early in its course. If in its early stages, procedures such as core decompression may prevent disease progression.

TREATMENT OVERVIEW

Treatment of injuries to the spine and pelvis is diagnosis-specific. However, general guidelines can be applied. With back injuries, acute management usually involves a brief period of rest (generally not longer than 3 days), followed by rehabilitation. Further periods of bed rest may be detrimental, as this will lead to further weakness and stiffness. Rehabilitation is guided toward safely returning to sports. The use of ice, massage, and NSAIDs may be helpful during this process. Braces or corsets may help alleviate symptoms during therapy. The mainstays of rehabilitation involve improving muscle flexibility and strength. Muscle-stretching exercises may improve the pain-free range of motion and decrease the risk of future injury. The strengthening program should be based on the athlete's symptoms. Trunk strengthening will help the athlete maintain a neutral, pain-free position. Balance, proprioception, and coordination training are incorporated into the rehabilitation process. Cross-training, such as swimming, may be helpful. Sport-specific activities are then initiated, followed by return to full function. Maintenance of flexibility and strength are important factors in preventing re-injury. Correction of the athlete's technique and training regimens may also help prevent recurrent injury.

Time for recovery varies with the specific condition. Symptoms of soft-tissue injuries should improve significantly over 4–6 weeks. Herniated disks and spondylolytic stress fractures may take 6 months to resolve, but bracing may allow the athlete to become asymptomatic and return to play in the brace as early as 4–6 weeks after treatment begins. The team physician must know when to refer an athlete with a back problem to an orthopedic surgeon or neurosurgeon.

Spinal cord injury, caudaequina syndrome, or fracture warrants emergent referral. If the work-up reveals a massive herniated disk, progressive neuropathy, infection, or tumor, or if an athlete has back pain that has not resolved after 4–6 weeks, then this should also be referred. With pelvic injuries, stress fractures, particularly of the femoral neck, warrant a surgical referral. Most other conditions can be treated non-operatively. General guidelines include a course of relative rest, compression, NSAIDs, and therapeutic modalities such as ice, massage, and ultrasound. As acute symptoms subside, gentle stretching is followed by strengthening and gradual return to activities. When full range of motion and strength are achieved, the athlete may return to play. As with back injuries, however, treatment is individualized and diagnosis-specific.

ACKNOWLEDGMENT

The editors acknowledge the assistance of Grover Price, PT, of Boston Children's Hospital, for contributing to, and reviewing, the rehabilitation sections in this chapter.

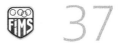

SUGGESTED READING

Bharam S. Labral tears, extra-articular injuries, and hip arthroscopy in the athlete. *Clin. Sports Med*. Apr. 2006; 25(2): 279–92.

Farber A.J., Wilckens J.H. Sports hernia: Diagnosis and therapeutic approach. *J. Am. Acad. Orthop. Surg*. Aug. 2007; 15(8): 507–14.

Flynn, J.M. *Orthopaedic Knowledge Update 10*. Rosemont, IL: American Academy of Orthopaedic Surgeons. 2011.

Gurd D.P. Back pain in the young athlete. *Sports Med. Arthrosc*. Mar. 2011; 19(1): 7–16.

Hiti C.J., Stevens K.J., Jamati M.K., Garza D., Matheson G.O. Athletic osteitis pubis. *Sports Med*. May 1, 2011; 41(5): 361–76.

Jacoby L., Yi-Meng, Kocher M.S. Hip problems and arthroscopy: Adolescent hip as it relates to sports. *Clin. Sports Med*. Apr. 2011; 30(2): 435–51.

Keoogh M.J., Batt M.E. A review of femoroacetabular impingement in athletes. *Sports Med*. 2008; 38(10): 863–78.

Kibler, W.B. *Orthopaedic Knowledge Update: Sports Medicine 4*. Rosemont, IL: American Academy of Orthopaedic Surgeons. 2009.

Kim H.J., Green D.W. Spondylolysis in the adolescent athlete. *Curr. Opin. Pediatr*. Feb. 2011; 23(1): 68–72.

Medniguchia J., Rughelli M. A return-to-sport algorithm for acute hamstring injuries. *Phys. Ther. Sport*. Feb. 2011; 12(1): 2–14.

Sakai T., Sairyo K., Suzue N., Kosaka H., Yasui N. Incidence and etiology of lumbar spondylolysis: Review of the literature. *J. Orthop. Sci*. May 2010; 15(3): 281–8.

Sierra R.J., Trousdale R.T., Ganz R., Leunig M. Hip disease in the young, active patient: Evaluation and nonarthroplasty surgical options. *J. Am. Acad. Orthop. Surg*. 2008; 16(12): 689–703.

Smith D.V., Bernhardt D.T. Hip injuries in young athletes. *Curr. Sports Med. Rep*. Sept.–Oct. 2010; 9(5): 278–83.

CHAPTER 17

KNEE INJURIES

Christer G. Rolf and Kai-Ming Chan

TRAUMATIC KNEE INJURIES

Anterior cruciate ligament (ACL) rupture

Fieldside assessment

The athlete suffers an acute knee sprain followed by swelling within hours (bleeding –hemarthrosis) and pain, disabling the athlete from continuing sport. A "popping sound" is often reported. This injury is common in pivoting sports such as soccer, rugby, and basketball. It can easily occur without substantial external forces from a tackle, but often involves a sudden change in direction while running. The mechanism of injury is often a combined valgus stress–external rotation injury with the foot fixed, or hyperextension of the knee. Associated injuries to the cartilage, menisci, or other ligaments are common.

Chronic ACL insufficiency

An athlete with chronic ACL insufficiency of the knee often presents with subjective instability, a "giving way" on pivoting or cutting activities. Typically, there is quadriceps atrophy and recurrent effusion of the knee. Associated injuries to the meniscus and cartilage occur frequently.

Diagnosis

The diagnosis of an ACL rupture is based on history and clinical examination. The ACL may rupture in its substance, partially or completely. Owing to frequent concomitant injuries, the symptoms and signs may vary. A skeletally immature athlete may instead have avulsed the distal insertion of the ACL (tibia spine fracture). In the majority of cases, hemarthrosis is present. Sometimes, an extension lag is caused by impingement of the ACL stump. Positive Lachman test and anterior drawer test are usually present, with the exception of a partial tear. The tests require the athlete to be relaxed, and both a substantial hemarthrosis and subjective pain and muscle response can blur the clinical tests. The Lachman test is most sensitive.

379

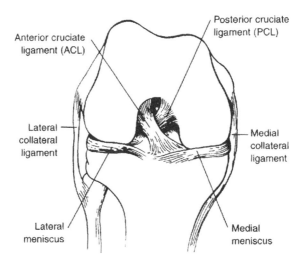

Figure 17.1 Knee anatomy demonstrating the location of frequently injured structures

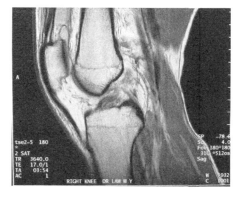

Figure 17.2 MRI of the knee is the gold standard to illustrate most of the structures of the knee in assessing injuries

In the chronic situation, the pivot shift test is often positive and defines the presence of pivoting. However, this test is difficult to elicit in the acute situation. Clinical examination is superior even to magnetic resonance imaging (MRI) for an ACL tear. However, as the ACL rupture often occurs in association with other injuries, MRI is often used. It must be stressed that the outcome of an MRI is dependent on a close collaboration between the clinician and radiologist, as the MRI technique used varies substantially when different structures are examined in detail. A clear clinical suspicion is therefore vital for the value of the MRI.

Figure 17.3
The ACL can rupture completely or partially in the mid substance, proximally or distally

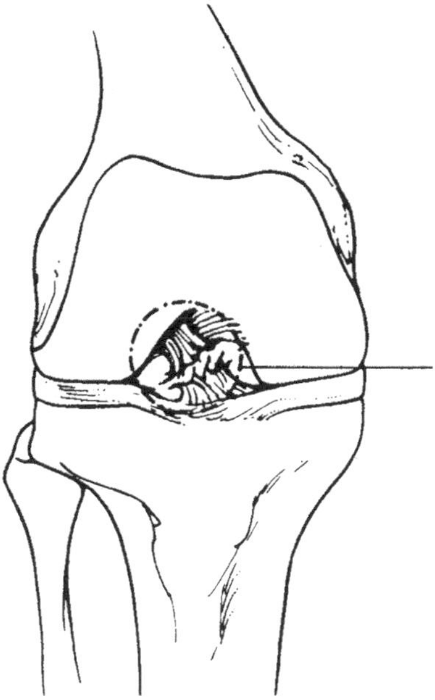

Anterior cruciate ligament sprain

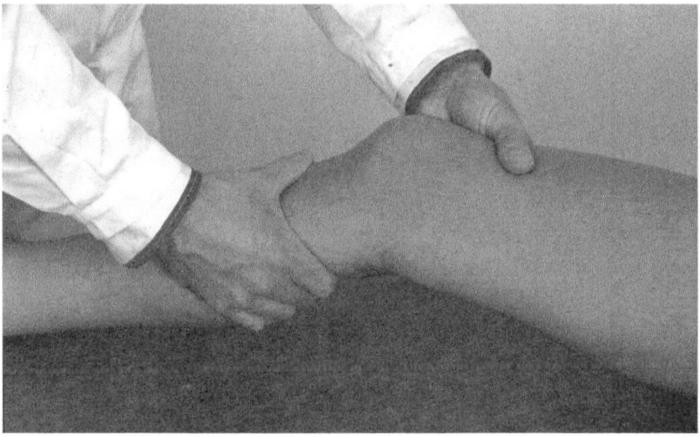

Figure 17.4 The Lachman test is the most sensitive

A patellar subluxation and dislocation may have similar history, so always examine the patellofemoral joint as well for pathologic laxity and suspicion of osteochondral fracture from patella.

The Lachman test is the most sensitive test for an ACL rupture. The injured athlete should be relaxed, in the supine position. Flex the knee 20–30°. The tibia is then gently translated anteriorly, with one hand holding the proximal tibia, while the distal thigh is stabilized with the other hand. The test is positive if (1) there is increased anterior laxity (compare with non-injured side) and (2) there is no distinct end point (Figure 17.4).

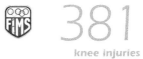

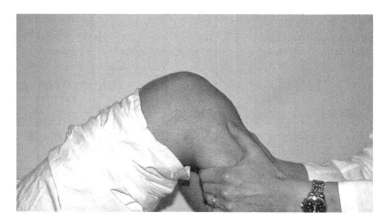

Figure 17.5 The anterior drawer test is also a valuable test

The anterior drawer sign is not as sensitive as the Lachman test, but is very valuable. It should be performed with the patient's foot in internal rotation, neutral, and external rotation. The knee is flexed 90°. The examiner sits gently on the athlete's foot and pulls the tibia anteriorly, keeping the hands just below the joint space. The test is positive if the tibia moves anteriorly without a distinct end point (Figure 17.5).

The pivot shift test aims to reduce an anterior subluxation of the tibia, which is caused by the absence of a functioning ACL. Again, the athlete must be relaxed, in supine position. The lower leg is internally rotated, and the knee is moved from full extension to flexion while a gentle valgus force and anterior push of the fibular head are applied. Initially, at full extension, the lateral tibia plateau is anteriorly subluxated. At 20–30° of flexion, the anterior subluxation is reduced as the tibia falls back into its normal position in relation to the femur. This "jerky feeling" or "shift" corresponds to the giving-way sensation reported by the athlete with an ACL-insufficient knee. An X-ray should be performed in immature and elderly athletes to rule out skeletal injuries. Again, an ACL rupture is often associated with injuries to the meniscus, cartilage medial collateral ligament (MCL), posterolateral or posteromedial structures, PCL, or other soft tissues, which makes a comprehensive diagnosis difficult. In unclear cases, MRI or arthroscopy is indicated early for a comprehensive diagnosis.

Treatment

Stop ongoing sports activities to avoid further damage until the diagnosis is clear. A compression–ice bandage should be applied to stop the bleeding (after clinical examination), followed by RICE therapy. The athlete should use crutches, avoid full weight-bearing, and seek medical advice from a specialist as soon as possible. Further management depends on a number of factors, and current ideas vary over the world. The most common recommendation for physically active athletes in pivoting sports is surgical ACL reconstruction within 8 weeks of injury, to decrease the risk of secondary injuries and to improve knee function, thus allowing return to sport, usually within 6–8 months. Many surgeons recommend delaying reconstruction until the athlete has full range of motion (ROM) and no more than mild swelling. Physiotherapy, including proprioceptive training, is initiated early. If there are multiple ligament injuries, acute open stabilization may be indicated. On suspicion of associated cartilage-meniscus tears, an early arthroscopy is indicated. If non-operative treatment is advocated for the ACL tear, the athlete's level of performance must be modified accordingly.

Rehabilitation

Early mobilization is the gold standard, with or without surgical intervention. Rehabilitation should focus on quadriceps strengthening, both concentrically (from 90° to 45° knee flexion) and eccentrically (from 0° knee extension to 90° flexion). As the ACL is responsible for limiting anterior translation of the tibia on the femur from 45° flexion to 0° knee extension, open chain-resisted knee extension is contraindicated in the ACL-deficient or post-surgical knee. Rehabilitation of 6–12 months, initially including closed-chain activities, is usually required. Cycling and other closed-chain strength training can be done from the start, but jumping and running/pivoting activities must be abandoned for around 3 months.

ANTERIOR CRUCIATE LIGAMENT RUPTURE

History
- Sudden deceleration and change of direction or valgus/rotational force.
- Athlete "heard a pop".
- Rapid onset of marked effusion/hemarthrosis.

Examination
- Positive Lachman test, anterior drawer and/or pivot shift test.

Treatment
- Compression and ice, crutches.
- Refer to specialist who may advocate X-ray, MRI, or arthroscopy.
- Surgical treatment recommended for athletes in pivoting sports.

Functional non-operative treatment for some athletes
- 6–12 months' rehabilitation before return to play.

Return to play
- Full ROM, strength, and proprioceptive function.
- At least 90% normal strength and endurance.

A trained physical therapist should guide the pre- and post-operative planning and rehabilitation program. Clinical follow-ups are continued until the athlete's knee shows no "giving way" symptoms, a negative Lachman test, full ROM, muscle strength, single-limb balance, single-limb squats, and plyometric testing, as compared with the uninjured leg.

Return to play

The injury may, despite treatment, result in 6–12 months' absence from competitive pivoting sports. However, regular participation in modified training (e.g., straight-line running and strength training with the club) should be encouraged to avoid other negative effects of being sidelined.

Medial collateral ligament (MCL) rupture

Fieldside assessment

The athlete presents with medial knee pain and a sensation of "giving way" after a valgus knee sprain, sometimes with concomitant effusion/hemathrosis or local medial swelling/bruising of the knee. After a brief clinical examination, a compression–ice bandage should be applied to stop the bleeding, followed by RICE therapy. Stop ongoing sports activities to avoid further damage to the joint, until the diagnosis is clear. The athlete should use crutches, avoid full weight-bearing, and seek medical advice from specialist.

Diagnosis

An MCL tear is a clinical diagnosis (Figures 17.6 and 17.7). The MCL tear may be partial or complete, with rupture of the outer (extra-articular) and/or inner (deep-distal part, which is intra-articular) portion of the MCL and adjacent capsule. There is typical tenderness on palpation of the ligament from the proximal to distal insertion or over the medial joint line of the knee. A valgus stress test should be used to evaluate the grade of injury. Suspect associated injuries to the medial meniscus, as the inner portion of the MCL is attached to the medial meniscus. Ultrasound or MRI may confirm the diagnosis.

The valgus stress test is performed with the athlete in a supine position. The athlete's foot is fixed under the examiner's shoulder to avoid rotation of the leg. The examiner applies a gentle valgus/varus stress to the knee. If the test is positive (valgus opening) in full extension, the entire ligament and probably at least part of the medial-posterior capsule is ruptured. If the test is positive at 15–25° of flexion but not at full extension, the inner portion of the ligament is ruptured.

Treatment

For an isolated MCL tear, non-operative treatment and early physical therapy are advocated. Bracing is usually not necessary. Full weight-bearing is allowed. Avoid knee abduction and pivoting activities.

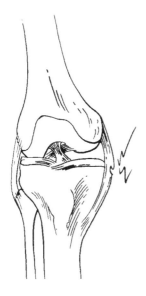

Figure 17.6
MCL injury

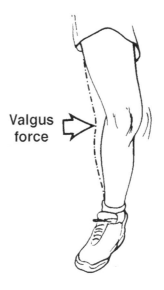

Valgus
force

Figure 17.7
Valgus force is usually responsible
for MCL sprains

MEDIAL COLLATERAL LIGAMENT RUPTURE

History

- Valgus force.
- Localized medial swelling/bruising or hemarthrosis.

Examination

- Local tenderness on palpation over MCL.
- Valgus stress test indicates severity.

Treatment

- For isolated MCL tear, protected mobilization, weight-bearing as tolerated.
- Ultrasound or MRI may be helpful if diagnosis is unclear.

Return to play

- Pain-free, full ROM, at least 90% strength, and good proprioception.

Note: A peripheral meniscus tear may be successfully stabilized in the early phase by arthroscopic surgery. Thus, if such is suspected, MRI and/or arthroscopy are indicated.

Rehabilitation

It is important to maintain leg-muscle function during the around 8-week healing period. Early closed-chain quadriceps/hamstring strength training and proprioceptive training are advocated. Open-chain vastus medialis obliquus (VMO)/quad and hip adductor strengthening can be useful to promote healing and stability. Avoid breaststroke if swimming, and avoid jumping activities and running for 6–8 weeks. Cycling, step-ups, cross-trainers, and closed-chain strength training are good alternatives.

Return to play

This injury requires 6–12 weeks absence from competitive pivoting sports. Clinical follow-up should be continued until the athlete is symptom free. If there is persistent pain or swelling, suspect an associated medial meniscus tear.

PCL rupture

Fieldside assessment

The athlete presents with sudden onset of pain and effusion/hemarthrosis after a knee sprain caused by forced hyperextension, hyperflexion, or a direct blow to the proximal tibia (dashboard injury). A compression–ice bandage is applied to stop the bleeding, followed by RICE therapy. Stop ongoing sports activities to avoid further damage to the joint until there is a clear diagnosis. The athlete should use crutches, avoid weight-bearing, and seek medical advice from a specialist.

Diagnosis

A proximal substance rupture of the PCL or an avulsion of the distal attachment to the posterolateral tibia may occur from hyperextension or flexion of the knee or from a dashboard injury to a flexed knee. This injury is often associated with concomitant injuries to cartilage or menisci. Injuries to the medial or lateral posterior structures must also be ruled out. A PCL tear is a clinical diagnosis. There is posterior sagging of the proximal tibia when the knee rests at 90° of flexion on the posterior drawer test. X-ray may show avulsion fragments from the distal tibia insertion. In such case, a CT scan may delineate the extent of the bone injury. MRI may provide additional, useful information.

Note: Sometimes the clinical findings are misinterpreted as an ACL rupture. When the PCL is ruptured, the tibia is anteriorly translated during an anterior drawer test because of the initial posterior sagging, but it stops in a neutral position with a firm end point (Figure 17.8).

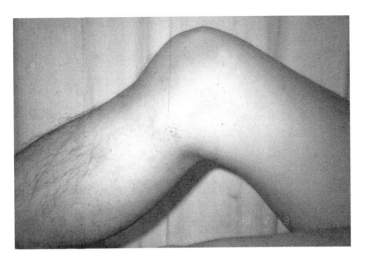

Figure 17.8 Posterior sagging of tibia indicating a PCL tear

Treatment

Open fixation of an avulsed bony fragment may be required. An orthopedic surgeon should be consulted, and MRI and/or an arthroscopy is often undertaken to delineate associated injuries. With proximal or mid-substance PCL ruptures, non-operative treatment is often preferred on isolated PCL tears, and delayed reconstruction of the ligament is undertaken only if function and performance are limited. A PCL brace may be used during the first weeks to hold the knee in a favorable position during healing. Multi-ligament injuries including PCL should be treated in specialized sports injury centres.

Rehabilitation

A physical therapist may guide a program of muscle strengthening, with the focus on quadriceps strengthening, ROM, and proprioception. Neuromuscular electrical stimulation can be helpful to the hamstrings to increase strength early on in the rehabilitation. Resistive open-chain hamstring strengthening is contraindicated in PCL-deficient patients, owing to the posterior movement of the tibia on the femur. Modified training with bicycling, water running, and closed-chain strength exercises is recommended until the effusion and acute inflammatory signs are gone. Long-term follow-up is recommended. Persistent pain is a sign of associated injuries. Subjective instability and a positive posterior drawer test despite a thorough training regime are indications for late reconstruction.

Return to play

Participation in pivoting sports is often possible with chronic isolated PCL injuries also without surgical intervention. If the athlete elects rehabilitation without surgery, 6–12 weeks may be needed to restore function before competitive pivoting sports are resumed. Rehabilitation after PCL reconstruction is similar to ACL reconstruction at around 6–9 months.

POSTERIOR CRUCIATE LIGAMENT RUPTURE

History

- Blow to proximal anterior tibia in flexion or forced hyperextension or hyperflexion of the knee.
- Extent of injury often not initially apparent.

Examination

- Hemarthrosis, positive posterior sag test, positive posterior drawer.
- Check for associated ligament/meniscus injury.

Treatment

- Individualized treatment, initial bracing may be valuable, operative or non-operative.

Return to action

- Full ROM and function compared with other leg.
- Strength, endurance, and proprioception to meet demands of sport.

Meniscus injuries

Fieldside assessment

This injury is very common in a number of contact, as well as individual, sports. Locking, sharp pain, and effusion of the knee may occur after a tackle/knee sprain in younger athletes, and sometimes after trivial trauma in elderly athletes. The meniscus can be injured in many ways and in different locations (flap tear, bucket handle tear, vertical tear, horizontal tear, radial tear), thus causing a variety of symptoms and signs. Following brief clinical examination, a compression–ice bandage should be applied to stop the bleeding, followed by RICE therapy. Stop ongoing sports activities to avoid further damage to the joint, until the diagnosis is clear. The athlete should use crutches, avoid weight-bearing, and seek medical advice from a specialist.

Diagnosis

A precise clinical diagnosis may be difficult from clinical examination only. The diagnosis may be particularly difficult in elderly athletes with underlying osteoarthritis (OA) and athletes with previous ACL or PCL rupture. With an isolated meniscus tear, the athlete typically has localized tenderness on palpation to the

christer g. rolf and kai-ming chan

affected joint line. Routine MRI frequently misses this diagnosis. Knee effusion after a day or two is typical. Hemarthrosis suggests bleeding from a peripheral tear (in the more vascular portion of the meniscus). There is often a positive compression and rotation test (Apley's test). There are several additional, specific tests for meniscal tear. These include forced knee flexion with the foot in external rotation, which may provoke pain from medial posterior horn tears. A medial flap tear often results in a snapping pain on knee extension with the foot in external rotation (McMurray's test). A bucket handle tear commonly locks the knee in a flexed position, causing painful extension and flexion. However, specialists may also fail to reach a comprehensive diagnosis after clinical examination only. The compression rotation test is a valuable screening test that aims to squeeze the injured meniscus between the femur condyle and the tibia plateau and should be done at varying degrees of flexion, but it can well be positive from a chondral injury as well.

Treatment
A specialist should be consulted for diagnosis and treatment. Arthroscopy should be done if there is locking, pseudo-locking, painful clicking, hemarthrosis, or recurrent effusion. The injured meniscus can be partially excised or repaired. A physical therapist should be consulted for restoration of leg muscle strength, ROM, and proprioception after surgery.

Rehabilitation
Avoid rotation/compression pivoting activities until there is a clear diagnosis and treatment plan. In the post-surgical meniscectomy or repair, ROM is usually

---

MENISCUS TEAR

History
- Twisting and/or flexion injury; suspect associated ligament rupture.
- Effusion may be sudden or occur over 24 hours.
- Clicking, clunking, locking, or extension lag.

Examination
- Focal joint line tenderness on palpation.
- Pain on compression/rotation test.

Treatment
- Arthroscopic surgery often indicated for specific diagnosis and treatment.

Return to action
- Timing dependent on whether meniscus repaired or partially excised.
- Full ROM and able to meet demands of sports.

---

restricted from 30–90° flexion to full knee extension allowed in the first 4–6 weeks. After that time frame, ROM is unrestricted per the physician. Neuromuscular electrical stimulation can be useful in improving quadriceps strength. The goals of rehabilitation are to gain full ROM, strength, and proprioception and to promote return to sport and full function.

Return to play

Arthroscopic meniscus repair often requires up to 12 weeks for sufficient healing to allow safe participation in sports. Athletes who undergo partial excision of a torn meniscus are typically ready to begin full training by 2–4 weeks after surgery. Clinical follow-up continues until the athlete is symptom-free and has full ROM and muscle strength compared with the uninjured side.

Osteochondral or chondral fracture

Fieldside assessment

The athlete with an acute osteochondral fracture (Figure 17.9) often presents with hemarthrosis and pain after a sprain or a direct blow to the knee. There may be pseudo-locking or an extension lag. A compression ice bandage should be applied to stop the bleeding, followed by RICE therapy. The athlete should stop ongoing sports activities to avoid further damage to the joint, until there is a clear diagnosis. The athlete should also use crutches, avoid weight-bearing, and seek medical advice from a specialist.

Diagnosis

A chondral or osteochondral fracture may occur in association with patellar dislocation, ligament injury, or a direct blow to the knee. A pre-existing and non-symptomatic osteochondritis dissecans (OCD) lesion may be torn free from its bed with relatively trivial trauma. There is no direct correlation between the grade of cartilage damage and severity of symptoms. Cartilage injuries are graded from

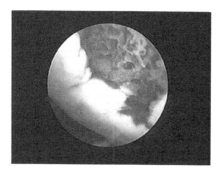

Figure 17.9 Osteochondral fracture of femoral condyle

I to IV, where grade I refers to frailed softening of the cartilage, and IV refers to a full-thickness tear. If the injury is localized to an important weight-bearing area (which may vary between different sports), exertional pain and swelling may be more severe. There is usually effusion, localized tenderness on palpation in the joint line, and a positive compression rotation test. A loose body may be palpable one moment, then disappear into the joint. X-rays, including a tunnel view, and/or MRI may be useful to demonstrate an OCD, but frequently miss localized superficial chondral fractures.

Treatment
Refer to a specialist. Arthroscopy is indicated if there is extension lag, locking, and/or effusion, even with a normal MRI. Arthroscopic excision of loose bodies, debridement, and microfracture of the affected bony area may be indicated.

Rehabilitation
Physical therapy includes training of muscle strength, ROM, and proprioception of leg muscles. The athlete should avoid jumping and running (pivoting activities), until there is a clear diagnosis. Closed-chain strength training, cycling, and water running may be recommended.

Return to play
This type of injury may cause minimal or severe short-term symptoms and long-term disability, depending on the size and location. Return to sport varies from 2 weeks after excision of a loose body to months after microfracturing or more extensive surgery. Clinical follow-up is required until the athlete is symptom-free and has full ROM proprioception and strength compared with the uninjured side.

Patellar dislocation

Fieldside assessment
The athlete presents with a sudden onset of anterior knee pain and effusion/hemarthrosis after a forceful "giving-way" sprain, typically from a valgus/external rotation force on an extended knee. The athlete may report the sensation of a double clicking pop (patella dislocates over the lateral femoral condyle and returns back again). If spontaneous repositioning of the patella does not occur, the knee remains "locked" in a 45° flexion. A compression–ice bandage should be applied to stop the bleeding, followed by RICE therapy. Stop ongoing sports activities to avoid further damage to the joint, until there is a clear diagnosis. The athlete should use crutches, avoid weight-bearing, and seek medical advice from a specialist if the dislocation cannot be repositioned on the field.

Diagnosis
This is usually a clinical diagnosis. If the patella is dislocated with the knee in a flexed position, it can be seen or palpated on the lateral aspect of the knee.

The dislocated patella is repositioned by gently extending the knee, initially maintaining outward rotation of the lower leg. Hemarthrosis is present, and there is pain on palpation of the proximal medial aspect of the patella (ruptured retinaculum). When the patella hits the lateral femoral condyle, a chondral or osteochondral fracture of either the patella or the lateral femoral condyle may occur, resulting in a loose body or flap tear. Remember that an ACL rupture and patellar dislocation may result from similar mechanisms of injury. X-ray may show the bony fragment. The small fragment visible on X-ray often underestimates the extent of the cartilaginous injury. MRI may be useful for further diagnosis.

Treatment

Early mobilization is advocated, with cycling, closed-chain strength training, and physical therapy modalities, until swelling has resolved and ROM is full. If there is locking and/or persistent effusion, an arthroscopic intervention is indicated. Consult a specialist if there are doubts in the diagnosis, locking, or hemarthrosis. Occasionally, open surgery with reinforcement of the torn medial retinaculum is indicated. If recurrent dislocations occur, other types of reconstructive surgery may be indicated later.

PATELLAR DISLOCATION

History

- Sudden giving-way sensation when kneecap dislocates; may reduce spontaneously or remain in dislocated position.

Examination

- Hemarthrosis.
- Patella may still be dislocated, usually laterally.
- Exquisite tenderness on palpation on medial retinaculum.
- Tenderness on palpation of anterior lateral femoral condyle.
- Associated ACL tear may occur.

Treatment

- Early mobilization, possible arthroscopic surgery for treatment of articular fracture and/or medial repair.

Return to play

- Full range of motion, strength, and proprioception compared with other leg.
- Medial vastus of quadriceps needs particular attention.
- When athlete can meet demands of sport.

Rehabilitation

Physical therapy is required using closed-chain strength exercises, stretching, and proprioceptive training, focusing on the quadriceps muscles. Taping or bracing may be used in the initial phase. Cycling, water running, and closed-chain strength training can be recommended.

Return to play

This injury can cause long-term, recurrent problems, and so proper rehabilitation of muscle strength and proprioception is essential before sports are resumed. Clinical follow-up continues until the athlete is symptom-free and has regained quadriceps muscle strength, ROM, and proprioception equal to the non-injured side.

Rupture of the quadriceps muscle

Fieldside assessment

The athlete presents with sudden, sharp pain in the anterior thigh, which may cause "giving way" of the knee. A sensation of tearing of the distal quadriceps muscle in conjunction with eccentric landing, jumping, or running is typical. A partial or complete rupture may occur at any portion of the muscle, but is more common in the proximal or distal insertion or musculotendinous junctions. A compression–ice bandage should be applied to stop the bleeding. Stop ongoing sports activities to avoid further injury, until there is a clear diagnosis. The athlete should use crutches, avoid weight-bearing, and seek acute medical advice from a specialist.

Diagnosis

This is a clinical diagnosis. The athlete is unable to stand, walk, or squat actively (the knee may give way). There is weakness or pain on knee extension against resistance, as well as local tenderness on palpation and localized swelling. A defect in the muscle may be palpable. X-ray may distinguish this injury from a patella fracture, if distal rupture is suspected. Ultrasound or MRI is often valuable to determine the exact location and extent of the rupture and the size/location of associated hematoma. It is important to distinguish between an intra- and intermuscular hematoma.

Treatment

A specialist should be consulted to evaluate whether surgical intervention is indicated. For a complete rupture, surgical repair is usually recommended, followed by rehabilitation over around 12 weeks or longer. For a partial tear, non-operative treatment includes physical therapy and strength training in closed-chain modes. Painful partial tears may be surgically repaired later if non-operative treatment fails. Intramuscular hematoma may need surgical evacuation.

Rehabilitation

Physical therapy is indicated to regain strength, ROM, and proprioception. Closed-chain exercises, including non-impact cycling and water exercises, are good alternatives. It is very important to regain full muscle function before going back to full sports activity. The risk of sustaining a recurrent rupture is otherwise very high. Clinical follow-up continues until the athlete is symptom-free and has full ROM and quadriceps strength compared with the other side.

Return to play

Depending on the severity of the injury, the athlete may require between 6 weeks and 6 months to return to full sporting activities with high eccentric impact, such as jumping and running.

Muscle contusion of the quadriceps muscle

Fieldside assessment

This injury occurs as a direct contusion to the thigh, often referred to as a "dead leg." The typical athlete finds it difficult to continue playing sports and refers to localized pain and swelling. A compression–ice bandage is applied to stop the bleeding, followed by RICE therapy. Stop ongoing sports activities to avoid further damage, until there is a clear diagnosis. The athlete should use crutches, avoid weight-bearing, and seek medical advice from a specialist.

Diagnosis

This is a clinical diagnosis, but the injury and bleeding may require further investigations. A direct contusion presses the muscle against the underlying femur, causing bleeding and damage, particularly to the deeper portions of the muscles. The bleeding may be substantial and localized intra- and/or intermuscularly. Weakness and localized pain with muscle contraction against resistance, with the knee held in extension, suggest injury to the rectus femoris muscle. Weakness and pain when the knee is extended from a flexed position suggests injury to the vastus medialis, lateralis and/or intermedius. Stretching of the muscle causes pain, and there is local tenderness on palpation. Ultrasound or MRI can determine the size and location of the hematoma.

Treatment

In the acute phase, a compression–ice bandage is the best treatment to stop the bleeding and thereby reduce the time to recovery. Maintaining the knee at 90°, or even in maximal flexion, is recommended by some for the first 12–24 hours to reduce bleeding and provide earlier return of full ROM. A compression bandage may be recurrently used for a few days to shorten the time for rehabilitation. A specialist should be consulted regarding the possible need for evacuation of an intramuscular hematoma. The hematoma may otherwise later ossify (myositis

394

ossificans), causing excessive scarring and a chronic pain condition that is difficult to treat.

Rehabilitation

A physical therapist should be consulted to provide local symptomatic treatment and to lead a progressive strength-training program using closed-chain exercises. In principle, immobilization should be avoided, and early mobilization is advocated. Continuation of compressive shorts can be useful in promoting healing and return to activity. The athlete should avoid eccentric jumping and running initially, especially on hard surfaces or downhill. Cycling, closed-chain strength training, and water running are recommended.

Return to play

This injury may cause an absence from competitive sports with high impact (jumping and running sports) for 3–12 weeks or longer, depending on the extent of the injury. Clinical follow-up is continued until the athlete is symptom-free and has normal strength, ROM, and proprioception compared with the uninjured side.

NON-ACUTE INJURIES

Anterior knee pain

On-field assessment

The athlete presents with activity-related anterior knee pain. Prolonged sitting aggravates the symptoms (positive "movie sign"), and squatting and downhill/stair walking are painful. Running also increases pain, in particular downhill.

Anterior knee pain is a "working diagnosis," comprising a number of entities with similar clinical presentations, which may include chondromalacia patella, OA, osteochondritis dissecans, patella maltracking syndrome, subluxating patella, dislocating patella, medial plica syndrome, meniscus injury, discoid meniscus injury, patella tendon disorders, prepatellar bursitis, functional disorders such as tight and/or weak quadriceps muscles, or referred pain from the back.

The key to successful management is to delineate the patho-anatomic cause of the pain.

Rule out intra-articular disorders (trauma, clinical symptoms, effusion, locking, instability), infections (no trauma, fever, local inflammatory signs, pain at rest, progressive symptoms), tumors (night pain, palpable lump), and referred pain from the lower back (examine back and neurology). Analyze muscle function (strength, muscle balance, range of motion, proprioception) and gait (foot/ankle bio-mechanical predisposing factors). X-ray may be indicated, including AP, lateral, tangential patella (such as the skyline or Merchant view), and tunnel view. MRI and/or 3D CT scans can be useful. Ultrasound may be useful for defining suspected soft-tissue disorders around the knee. Discuss your clinical suspicions with a radiologist. Arthroscopy is a useful diagnostic and therapeutic tool for specific indications. Discuss your clinical suspicions with a specialist.

Treatment

Treatment depends on the diagnosis. Non-operative treatment, with various physical therapy modalities and training alterations, is usually the first-line treatment, as long as anterior knee pain is the working diagnosis. NSAIDs may be useful to decrease pain. Consult a specialist (depending on your clinical suspicion), if symptoms do not respond to your initial treatment.

Rehabilitation

A physical therapist may evaluate ROM and muscle balance, strength and endurance of quadriceps/hamstrings, and gait/running pattern. Core stability should be evaluated. Closed-chain strength training, stretching, taping, and various local treatments are commonly used therapies. Modification of training is often motivated. With an emphasis on non-impact, cycling, water training, skiing, closed-chain strength training, stretching, and running on soft, even ground may be useful training alternatives. The athlete should avoid prolonged sitting.

ANTERIOR KNEE PAIN, NON-ACUTE

History
- Gradual onset of pain.
- Single, specific location, multiple locations, or diffuse.
- Effusion suggests intra-articular injury.
- Consider previous injuries to any portion of the limb.

Examination
- Determine specific locations of tenderness.
- A thorough clinical examination, including core stability, hip, knee, ankles, and back, is required.
- Muscle flexibility, strength, and proprioception should be evaluated; X-ray, MRI, US, or CT may be required.

Treatment
- Depends on the diagnosis.
- Physiotherapy to maintain function.
- Symptomatic treatment such as NSAIDs, RICE.

Return to play
- Full ROM, no effusions, and able to meet demands of sport.

Give practical advice such as "walk upstairs and take the elevator down." Clinical follow-up continues until there is proper diagnosis and adequate treatment in place.

Return to play
Try to keep the player in training and competition, if possible, during investigations.

Recurrent patellar instability

On-field assessment
The athlete presents with subjective instability and recurrent "giving way" of the knee. This condition may follow previous patella dislocation or may be due to patella dysfunction or malalignment. Often, it is seen in young athletes with general joint laxity. The patella generally subluxates in the range from full knee extension or hyperextension to 30° of flexion. Pain when the patella is moved laterally is considered a positive apprehension test. The patella may have decreased mobility on attempts to move it medially, and it may be tilted laterally as well as tethered. This is primarily a clinical diagnosis, but X-ray or other imaging studies may be useful. Consult with a radiologist. Arthroscopic dynamic assessment of the patellofemoral joint may show specific anatomic abnormalities that can be corrected surgically.

Apprehension test
Displace the patella with a manual, lateral push. In a positive test, the athlete experiences pain or becomes tense and apprehensive.

Treatment
Initial treatment includes quadriceps strengthening (in particular, the vastus medialis) and stretching (in particular, the vastus lateralis). Tight hamstrings and/or gastrocnemius muscles are stretched. A patellar-stabilizing knee brace may be useful. NSAIDs may be useful in the acute phase after a subluxation. Consult an orthopedic surgeon for consideration of surgical intervention if symptoms are severe, or there are frequent episodes of giving way.

Rehabilitation
A physical-therapy program, including alternative training, is essential. Do not advocate rest. Strengthening of VMO, quads, and hip adductors is especially important. Stretching of lateral retinaculum, ITB, hamstrings, and gastrocnemius is important. Education in, and monitoring of, avoidance of knee hyperextension in standing is important for both in and out of the clinic with exercises and functional activities. Cycling, skiing, skating, and careful running on soft, even ground (in particular, uphill) may be recommended. Clinical follow-up continues until the athlete is symptom-free and has regained full strength and ROM, equal to the asymptomatic knee.

Return to play

There is no need to stay away from sports, as long as the athlete can meet the demands of the sport safely.

Jumper's knee (patellar tendon injury)

On-field assessment

"Jumper's knee" is a working diagnosis for a number of conditions affecting the patellar tendon, including partial ruptures (acute onset), tendinosis (chronic condition, often proximal location), and Osgood–Schlatter's disease (location at tibial tuberosity in adolescents). The athlete presents with sudden or gradual onset of activity-related pain over the patellar tendon. This injury is particularly common in jumping sports, gymnastics, sprinting, dancing, and basketball. There is localized tenderness on palpation of the patellar tendon and on eccentric impact (such as landing from a jump on the forefoot). In acute cases of partial rupture, there is local swelling and ecchymosis. In chronic conditions, there is mainly localized pain. Ultrasound may delineate extra- or intratendinous abnormalities. MRI, with or without gadolinium contrast, may show typical intratendinous alterations. X-ray is useful. Note: A few cases of Ewing's sarcoma have been reported and mistaken for Osgood–Schlatter's disease.

Treatment

Progressive closed-chain quadriceps training is the first line of treatment. Local physical therapy and NSAID gel may be useful. In chronic (> 6 months) conditions, open excision of the degenerative areas of the tendon gives good, functional results. An orthopedic surgeon should be consulted for surgical treatment if there are persistent symptoms with failure of physical therapy. Occasionally, the apex of the patella impinges on the proximal patellar tendon during flexion of the knee, and arthroscopic excision may be useful. Osgood–Schlatter's disease should be treated with ice, closed-chain quadriceps strengthening (as pain has usually caused quadriceps atrophy), and stretching of any tight lower-extremity muscles.

Rehabilitation

Physical therapy includes eccentric quadriceps training and local modalities. Cycling, water training, closed-chain strength training, running on soft ground, and avoiding jumping on hard surfaces may be helpful. Objective measures of quadriceps strength and ROM compared with the uninjured side are important.

Return to play

Do not advocate rest. Clinical follow-up continues until the athlete is symptom-free (may be months or up to 2 years). After surgical treatment, the athlete is restricted from jumping sports for approximately 12 weeks.

Osgood–Schlatter's disease

On-field assessment

The young athlete presents with gradual onset of activity-related pain over the tibial tuberosity, most often affecting 12–16-year-old boys during their growth spurt. It is a local inflammation caused by excessive tension at the apophysis of the tibial tuberosity in growing adolescents, with secondary symptoms from the extensor (quadriceps) muscles and the patellar tendon. This is a clinical diagnosis, with local tenderness on palpation and local swelling over the tibial tuberosity (Figure 17.10). An X-ray is useful and can differentiate from skeletal tumors.

Treatment

Training advice and information given to the parents are the essential parts of treatment. Symptomatic local physical therapy and stretching of the quadriceps are useful.

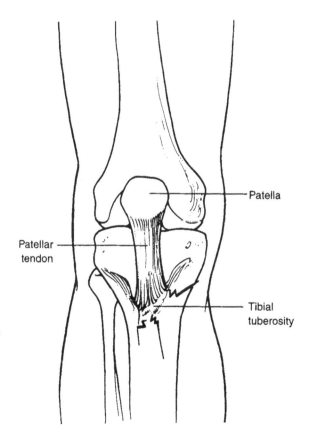

Figure 17.10 Osgood–Schlatter's disease

Rehabilitation

A physical therapist may perform objective tests of muscle function and local treatment. Quadriceps strengthening and lower-extremity muscle stretching are usually indicated. An orthopedic surgeon is consulted if there are atypical or progressing symptoms for differential diagnosis. Do not advocate rest. Jumping and sudden stops should be restricted temporarily. Cycling, mountain biking, swimming, strength training, and most other sports can be continued.

Return to play

There is no need to stay away from sports. A soft kneepad may be used to decrease symptoms.

Runner's knee (iliotibial band friction syndrome)

On-field assessment

The athlete presents with the gradual onset of localized lateral knee pain, aggravated by running, in particular downhill or on a slope. The pain may be caused by periostitis, or inflammation of the bursa between the iliotibial tract and the lateral femoral condyle, likely caused by repetitive friction (Figure 17.11). There is localized lateral knee pain on palpation. The athlete experiences pain when the examiner presses the distal iliotibial tract on to the femur and asks the athlete to flex/extend the knee. Without the compression, the pain with this maneuver

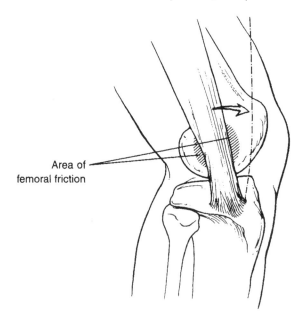

Area of femoral friction

Figure 17.11 Iliotibial band syndrome

decreases. X-ray may be of value to rule out underlying disorders or stress fractures (if suspected, consider a bone scan or MRI). Ultrasound examination may show a hypertrophied bursa.

Treatment
Stretching of the iliotibial tract and vastus lateralis and strength training of the hip abductors and quadriceps are advocated, combined with local symptomatic treatment. An orthopedic surgeon is consulted if pain persists, to evaluate the athlete for possible partial resection of the distal iliotibial band, with or without excision of local bursae.

Rehabilitation
A physical therapist may teach and perform stretching and plan strength training. Manual therapy, PNF stretching, and modalities may be helpful to jump-start flexibility. Do not advocate rest. Temporarily avoid running downhill, in particular on a slope.

Return to play
There are no strict contraindications to continuing sporting activities. Symptoms may be quite prolonged.

Prepatellar bursitis

On-field assessment
The athlete presents with local swelling and inflammatory signs over the mid portion of the patella (housemaid's knee). There is typical fluctuant localized swelling, without effusion of the knee joint. This finding can be caused by bleeding, infection, or inflammatory reaction to direct repetitive trauma. Rule out infection. An ultrasound examination and X-ray may be useful in doubtful cases.

Treatment
If there is no infection, NSAIDs can be used symptomatically, combined with a padded knee brace to protect against direct trauma. Bleeding (prepatellar hematoma) is treated similarly, with the addition of ice and compression. If an infection is present, acute surgical drainage and antibiotics may be indicated. Consult an orthopedic surgeon if septic bursitis is suspected.

Rehabilitation
There is a need for local physical therapy. Clinical follow-up is recommended until the symptoms are gone.

Return to play
Avoid any training with infection or large hematoma.

Osteochondritis dissecans (OCD)

On-field assessment

The athlete, often an adolescent, presents with gradual onset of activity-related knee pain, effusion, and occasional locking. The athlete may or may not report previous trauma. The etiology is unknown. The medial femoral condyle is most often affected, and lesions may be bilateral. The diagnosis may be difficult to establish clinically. There is effusion and localized pain on palpation. Wilson's test may be positive. An X-ray shows a typical radiolucent area and surrounding sclerosis (use the tunnel view). MRI is very useful in delineating the extent of the lesion (Figure 17.12). The injury is graded from I (undermined but intact cartilage) to grade IV (full-thickness tear and loose fragment in the joint).

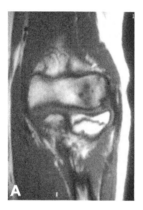 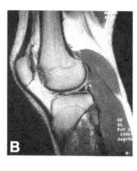

Figure 17.12 MRI showing OCD: (A) AP view; (B) lateral view

Wilson's test

The examiner rotates the athlete's tibia inward while extending the knee, causing impingement between the tibial spine and femoral condyle. Pain with the tibia rotated inward but not outward may suggest OCD of the femoral condyle.

Treatment

Advise activities appropriate to the location and stability of the lesion and severity of symptoms. Consult an orthopedic surgeon for further investigation and arthroscopic intervention, if indicated. Arthroscopic techniques can be used to debride the area of OCD, drill through the lesion to stimulate bony healing, microfracture, or refix the loose fragment.

Rehabilitation

A physical therapist may lead a modified training program and provide symptomatic treatment. The athlete should avoid pivoting activities and should partake in non-impact activities, such as cycling, elliptical training, skiing and/or Fitter or

Skier's Edge, free-style swimming, and aqua-jogging, and sometimes jogging on soft, even ground may be safely used. Clinical follow-up depends on symptoms and knee function. This may become a career-threatening injury.

Return to play
Return to play depends on the location and severity of the injury.

Popliteus tenosynovitis

On-field assessment
The athlete presents with gradual onset of activity-related pain in the posterior–lateral knee, with no preceding trauma. Symptoms are worse with downhill or slope running. This is a clinical diagnosis. There is tenderness on palpation of the posterolateral joint line, as well as a positive provocation test against resistance. There may even be partial rupture of the popliteus tendon, which passes intra-articularly through the posterolateral corner of the knee joint, from its origin on the tibia to its insertion on to the lateral femoral condyle. Arthroscopy or MRI may differentiate between a lateral meniscus tear and popliteus tenosynovitis.

Provocation test to the popliteus tendon
The athlete is in a prone position. Flex the knee approximately 45° and rotate the lower leg and foot internally. Ask the athlete to externally rotate the lower leg against your resistance, as you palpate the posterolateral joint line. Increased tenderness indicates a positive test.

Treatment
NSAIDs, modifications in training, and local physical therapy modalities are advocated. A local anesthetic injection may be used for diagnostic purposes. Arthroscopy may be indicated to differentiate popliteus tenosynovitis from a lateral meniscus tear.

Rehabilitation
A physical therapist should teach the athlete an appropriate stretching and strength-training program, based on individual impairments, and advise the athlete to consult an orthopedic surgeon if there is persistent pain despite physical therapy. Do not advocate rest. Avoid pivoting activities and downhill running, which often aggravate symptoms. Cycling is a good alternative. Clinical follow-up continues, depending on symptoms. Measure strength, ROM, and proprioception compared with the non-injured side.

Return to play
This disorder can cause several months of discomfort, but sports should be continued if possible.

Osteoarthritis

On-field assessment

OA is a soft-tissue disorder affecting structures around and in the knee joint. It may be primary, or secondary to previous injury. Cartilage degeneration and damage are an important part of this disease. The grade of cartilage damage is not directly correlated to the severity of symptoms. A previous ACL rupture or meniscus injury may predispose to a progression of the disease. The typical athlete presents with recurrent pain and effusion, stiffness, difficulty squatting, and occasional locking or pseudo-locking. Palpation typically causes tenderness over the joint lines. X-rays are graded from I to IV, depending on the severity of the OA, but early OA may well be present with a normal X-ray.

Treatment

NSAIDs can be useful to decrease swelling and relieve symptoms, but, owing to the chronicity and long-term need for treatment, side effects must be weighed against clinical effect. Hyaluron injections into the knee joint may relieve symptoms for a limited time in some athletes, but the documentation of long-term efficacy is poor. Cortisone injections may be useful for short-term relief. An orthopedic surgeon should be consulted for surgical intervention if the athlete with known OA experiences locking, recurrent effusions, severe pain, and failure of non-operative treatment. Note: A meniscus injury may hide in the osteoarthritic knee and actually be the cause of symptoms. Thus, a partial meniscectomy may relieve symptoms and restore function, even in an osteoarthritic knee, and may delay the need for a knee replacement. The combination of ACL insufficiency and OA is not uncommon among older athletes and should be treated by a specialist.

Rehabilitation

A physical therapist may design a strength-training program for the leg muscles, using closed-chain activities along with flexibility and proprioceptive training. Moist heat prior to exercise and/or a neoprene compression sleeve can assist the athlete in his/her chosen activity, providing warmth and proprioceptive input to the surrounding knee musculature. Also, custom foot orthotics can be helpful to dissipate forces at the knee. Do not advocate rest. Cycling is an excellent alternative training method (adjust the saddle height), as well as the elliptical trainer, swimming (avoid breast stroke), running on soft, even terrain, and most non-pivoting activities. Clinical follow-up depends on symptoms.

Return to play

This is a life-long disorder that leads to changes in activity level over time, but progression varies greatly between individuals. Remember to treat the athlete, not the X-ray. Many athletes with apparently severe OA on X-ray actually do very well following stretching and strengthening therapy.

Synovitis/reactive arthritis

On-field assessment

The athlete presents with gradual or acute onset of pain and knee effusion and local increased temperature, often without preceding injury. This is a multifactorial disorder. Synovitis can be caused by infection, a reactive response to mechanical injury, OA, or an ongoing general inflammatory disease. In septic arthritis, the knee is painful, with decreased motion. Fever is common. Joint aspiration and investigation of the synovial fluid are often useful: creamy, white fluid or thin, gray fluid usually indicates infection. Dark, thick fluid may be caused by infection or bleeding, or seen in pigmented villonodular synovitis. Brownish, thick fluid may be infectious or reactive. More than 5 ml of clear, thin fluid reflects a reactive, inflammatory arthritis. Clear viscous fluid within 5 ml is normal.

Treatment

Septic arthritis must be ruled out first. This is an emergency condition that requires immediate arthroscopic lavage and intravenous antibiotics, and the patient must be sent to a specialist on the spot. It can occur after previous surgery to the knee (typically 1–2 weeks after) or spread via blood or local cellulitis. Symptoms are usually severe, with fever and inability to move the knee, but can be initially mild and then deteriorate dramatically within hours. Treatment of reactive arthritis depends on the suspected diagnosis. Consult an orthopedic surgeon or rheumatologist for further investigation and diagnosis. Gout, rheumatic arthritis, psoriatic arthropathy, etc. are some of the many diagnostic alternatives.

Rehabilitation

During active infection, physical therapy is contraindicated and is only reinstated with physician clearance as appropriate, primarily to restore ROM and strength of likely atrophied quadriceps. Clinical follow-up should be continued until the athlete is symptom-free.

Return to play

Septic arthritis: no training and no weight-bearing over long periods. Reactive arthritis: avoid training until there is a clear diagnosis.

ACKNOWLEDGMENT

The editors acknowledge the assistance of Grover Price, PT, of Boston Children's Hospital, for contributing to, and reviewing, the rehabilitation sections in this chapter.

SUGGESTED READING

Andrish, J., 1996. Meniscal injuries in children and adolescents. *J. Am. Acad. Orthop. Surg.*, Volume 4, pp. 231–7.

Chan, K., et al., 1998. In: *Controversies in orthopedic sports medicine*, Sections 1–4. Hong Kong: William & Wilkins, pp. 3–285.

Cole, B. and Harner, C., 1999. Degenerative arthritis of the knee in active patients: Evaluation and management. *J. Am. Acad. Orthop. Surg.*, Volume 7, pp. 389–402.

Grelsamer, R., 2000. Current concepts review: Patellar malalignment. *J. Bone Joint Surg. (Am.)*, Volume 82, pp. 1639–50.

Mandelbaum, B., et al., 1998. Current concepts: Articular cartilage lesions of the knee. *Am. J. Sports Med.*, Volume 26, pp. 853–61.

Woo, S., Vogrin, T., & Abramowitch, S., 2001. Healing and repair of ligament injuries in the knee. *J. Am. Acad. Orthop. Surg.*, Volume 8, pp. 364–72.

CHAPTER 18

LOWER-LEG INJURIES

Angela D. Smith

ACUTE INJURIES OF THE LOWER LEG

Fractures

Fieldside assessment

The athlete presents with severe lower-leg pain, between the knee and the ankle, following a twisting injury or a direct blow. Deformity may be visible. Often, weight-bearing is not possible. Depending on the severity of the injury, the athlete is either assisted from the field, or a splint is applied to the limb before the athlete is moved. Further evaluation is carried out in a controlled environment.

Diagnosis

Tenderness and swelling are localized to the site of the injury, which may be extensive, particularly with a spiral fracture. Generally, both the tibia and fibula are fractured, but either one may be fractured individually. The fracture may be accompanied by ligament injury at the knee or ankle. Examine for signs of compartment syndrome. Usually, the first clinical sign of this is pain on passive stretch of the muscles within the compartment.

For example, with a tibia fracture, the anterior compartment is most likely to develop compartment syndrome owing to bleeding into the compartment: examine for this possibility by passively plantarflexing the athlete's toes. If severe pain is caused by this maneuver, not consistent with simple pain from the fracture, acute anterior compartment syndrome is likely. Loss of sensation suggests greater duration and severity of acute compartment syndrome. In the setting of suspected acute compartment syndrome, decreased sensation in the first dorsal web space, between the great toe and the second toe, strongly suggests severe acute anterior compartment syndrome. Loss of sensation in the plantar/medial aspect of the foot suggests posterior/deep posterior acute compartment syndrome.

Treatment

The athlete's limb is splinted, and appropriate X-ray studies are obtained. If the fracture severity is minimal, and deformity is minimal or absent, then closed treatment with an appropriate cast or brace may be appropriate (Figures 18.1 and 18.2). For athletes, intramedullary or other rigid internal surgical fixation with a rod should be considered, to allow the athlete to begin early motion and prevent much of the atrophy that would occur with cast immobilization. If there is evidence of acute compartment syndrome, emergency fasciotomy is required.

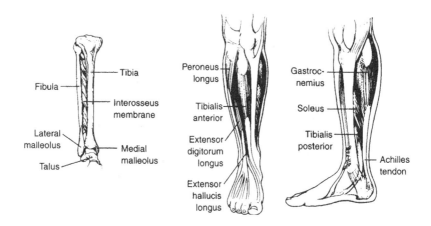

Figure 18.1 Lower-leg anatomy

Rehabilitation

As soon as fracture stability allows, the athlete begins range-of-motion exercises. Neuromuscular electrical stimulation (NMES) may be used to initiate muscle activity if muscle contractions are weak; once full muscle contractions are obtained, NMES is discontinued. With further stability, progressive strengthening exercises begin, followed by proprioception training exercises. During fracture healing, the athlete performs cross-training exercises to maintain general conditioning.

Return to play

The athlete gradually resumes training as fracture healing, flexibility, and strength allow. Return to full sport activity is also dependent on the demands of the sport. Protective bracing may be used in the early phases of a return to sport.

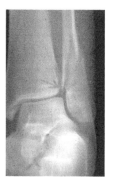

Figure 18.2
Fracture of the fibula

angela d. smith

NON-ACUTE INJURIES OF THE LOWER LEG

Stress fracture, posteromedial tibial syndrome, exertional compartment syndrome, tendinitis

Diagnosis

Virtually all of the overuse injuries of the lower leg are caused by one or more of the following factors: inadequate shock absorption, abnormal pronation, or training errors. Poor shock absorption may be caused by intrinsic or extrinsic factors. Intrinsic factors include cavus – high-arched feet – which are more rigid than average; weak intrinsic muscles of the foot; and poor calf-muscle flexibility. Extrinsic factors include inadequate footwear and running on excessively hard surfaces. Excessive pronation, here meaning too rapid movement of the hindfoot into an abnormal amount of valgus very rapidly after heelstrike during running, is also implicated in the development of some non-traumatic injuries of the lower leg. This pronation may be accompanied by sagging of the medial midfoot, seen as loss of the arch during weight-bearing. Training errors also cause such overuse injuries: errors such as increasing running distance or activity intensity too rapidly, changing to running on sloped surfaces or hills without a gradual progression, or changes in footwear that alter the athlete's biomechanics

Of course, as with any non-traumatic sports injuries, the athlete's nutritional status should be determined, and the regularity of menstrual periods of female athletes should be assessed.

Etiology

- Inadequate shock absorption.
- Abnormal pronation.
- Training errors.

The major diagnostic groups for non-traumatic lower-leg pain include stress fracture, posteromedial tibial syndrome, exertional compartment syndrome, and tendinitis (Figure 18.3). Other diagnoses, such as tumor, infection, and metabolic bone disease, must also be considered.

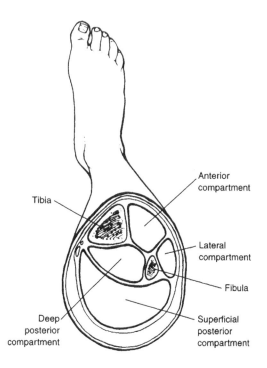

Figure 18.3 Compartments of the lower leg

The athlete with stress fracture of the tibia or fibula reports aching pain that con-tinues long after the activity stops.

Pain may even persist overnight and cause symptoms when the athlete rises in the morning. There may have been a prior period of diffuse tenderness along a greater extent of the bone. Generally, the pain and tenderness of a stress fracture are localized to a narrow area of the bone.

Diagnosis

The diagnosis with posteromedial tibial stress syndrome, often known as "shin splints," must be one of exclusion. All other diagnoses should be ruled out, including tibial stress fracture and posterior tibial tendinitis. Tenderness and, often, palpable swelling are present along much of the posteromedial border of the tibia. The athlete often has tight calf muscles and/or excessive pronation. The athlete with posterior tibial tendinitis typically has tenderness along the course of the tendon itself. Athletes often have symptoms of both these problems, which can be thought of as a spectrum. Similar biomechanical factors may lead to either or both of these diagnoses. The athlete with recurrent exertional compartment syndrome experiences aching pain with activity. The pain generally resolves within minutes after stopping activity. However, mild-to-moderate aching may persist for hours, the sensation being relatively similar to that of delayed-onset muscle soreness. Symptoms are often bilateral.

The athlete with severe exertional anterior compartment syndrome may notice gait changes during running after the pain begins. Once the tibialis anterior muscle ceases to function normally, because of the increased compartmental pressure and decreased circulation (and eventually decreased nerve function), the foot begins to slap as the athlete runs, as normal, controlled dorsiflexion is compromised. Athletes with posterior tibial exertional compartment syndrome often report decreased sensation on the plantar aspect of the foot as a major symptom, and may feel pain in the posterior medial calf. Lateral exertional compartment syndrome symptoms include decreased sensation in the distribution of the superficial peroneal nerve.

Tendinitis of the lower leg may be associated with excessive, recurrent tension on the tendon, or with compression of the tendon by a piece of equipment (Figure 18.4). For example, posterior tibial tendinitis is most frequently found in athletes who have tight calf muscles and/or increased pronation, causing increased tension on the posterior tibial tendon with each step. Tendons of the peroneal, anterior tibial, and long tendons to the toes are more likely to have been injured by compressive forces (such as the top of a ski boot or skate) if they are painful in the lower leg or ankle. The flexor hallucis longus tendon may become inflamed in dancers, who often have associated relative tightness of the tendon sheath that leads to compression and friction against the tendon.

411

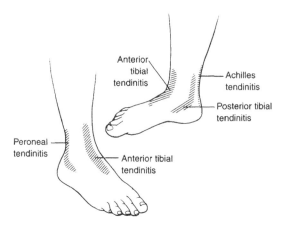

Anterior
tibial
tendinitis

Achilles
tendinitis

Posterior tibial
tendinitis

Peroneal
tendinitis

Anterior tibial
tendinitis

Figure 18.4 Potential sites of tendinitis in the lower leg

POSTERIOR TIBIAL TENDINITIS

- Nagging pain, occasionally burning, worse with activity.
- Tenderness along tendon itself.
- Often related to tight gastrocnemius.
- Same forces may cause subsequent distal tibial stress fracture.
- Treatment: RICE, arch support, remove causes.

PERONEAL TENDINITIS

- Etiology: boot-top pressure (skating, skiing); overuse in sports that use peroneals greatly (skating, ballet).
- Same forces may go on to cause subsequent fibular stress fracture.
- Treatment: RICE, remove causes, pad tender area.

ANTERIOR TIBIAL, EXTENSOR DIGITORUM, AND HALLUCIS LONGUS TENDINITIS

- Usually caused by pressure from equipment.
- Less often caused by repetitive tensile forces.
- Treatment: remove cause, pad tender area.

angela d. smith

Treatment

All non-traumatic injuries of the lower leg are initially treated by rest of the injured area until a specific diagnosis can be determined. Any factors that are likely causes of the injury should be determined and corrected. Athletes with excessive pronation often benefit from use of an over-the-counter arch support or a custom-made orthosis. Increased cushioning of running shoes may also be helpful. If the injury is caused by compression, such as from a piece of the athlete's equipment, then two possible methods of padding are very useful. Either a pad can be applied directly over the injured area, or pads may be placed immediately adjacent to the injured area to relieve the pressure from the injured area. Viscoelastic padding materials, such as silicone or closed-cell foam, are particularly useful.

Most stress fractures of the tibia in athletes can be treated initially by a very short period (generally a few days) of non-weight-bearing, with crutches, until the athlete is pain-free. As soon as the athlete is pain-free, weight-bearing, as tolerated, is allowed. Often, the use of a brace or a cast is necessary to allow the athlete to progress rapidly to full weight-bearing status. Established tibial stress fractures, especially those with a transverse black line on the tension cortex (usually the anterior medial aspect of the mid-shaft of the tibia), seen on plain X-rays, often require surgical intervention. A plastic stirrup-type brace that extends proximally almost to the knee can be very useful in treating stress fractures of the fibula (Figure 18.5).

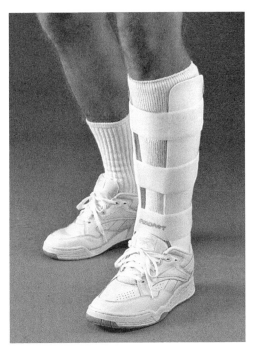

Figure 18.5
For stable lower-leg fractures, such as stress fractures of the mid-shaft to distal regions of the tibia or fibula, a long air-stirrup brace often provides sufficient immobilization and protection to allow the athlete to bear weight and perhaps even train, as long as the athlete remains pain-free

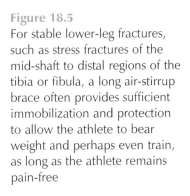

If exertional compartment syndrome symptoms do not respond to shoes and orthoses that improve the athlete's biomechanics, stretching of the calf muscles that decreases hindfoot pronation, and changes in training, then surgical release of all affected compartments may be indicated. If surgery is to be considered, then all compartments should be examined by monitoring intracompartmental pressure during or immediately after exercise that actually provokes the athlete's symptoms. Any compartments that show excessive pressure that does not rapidly drop to normal range within a few minutes after stopping the exercise should be released during the surgery. In the future, MRI with special exercise and scanner protocols, or near-infrared spectroscopy, may supplement or replace invasive intracompartmental pressure monitoring.

Rehabilitation

During treatment of a stress fracture, it is important that the athlete be able to monitor symptoms and remain pain-free during progression of activity, and so medications that may mask symptoms should not be used if they will still be active while the athlete is stressing the injured area. Generally, satisfactory healing progresses, even if the athlete has mild aching near the end of activity, but all pain resolves within 2 hours after finishing activity. However, if the athlete has pain at bedtime, then the amount and intensity of training the following day should be significantly decreased. If the athlete has pain in the injured area when rising in the morning, consideration should be given to not doing any training that stresses the injured area that day. Cross-training or lighter exercise to the injured area should be performed, as long as it is pain-free; this will help the athlete maintain overall endurance and continue recovery to the injured area. Once able to exercise at a high level without pain, the athlete should perform functional return to sport activities under the supervision of a rehabilitation specialist, to evaluate readiness and advance the athlete's return to the specific sport.

During treatment, the athlete works on flexibility and strengthening of all of the muscles of the limb. Activities that maintain cardiovascular endurance as well as maximum function of the other limbs should be performed.

COMPARTMENT SYNDROME

- Most frequently in anterior or deep posterior compartment of the lower leg.
- Generally resolves very quickly after cessation of activity.
- May be accompanied by numbness.
- Treatment: orthoses, technique changes, fasciotomy.

Return to play

The athlete gradually returns to activity as symptoms allow, as long as he/she can meet the demands of the sport without risking either recurrent injury to the same area or injury to another region.

ACKNOWLEDGMENT

The editors acknowledge the assistance of Grover Price, PT, of Boston Children's Hospital, for contributing to, and reviewing, the rehabilitation sections in this chapter.

SUGGESTED READING

Rome K., Handoll H.H., Ashford R. Interventions for preventing and treating stress fractures and stress reactions of bone of the lower limbs in young adults. *Cochrane Database Syst. Rev.* 2005.

Ryan M.B., MacLean C.L., Taunton J.E. A review of anthropometric, biomechanical, neuromuscular and training related factors associated with injury in runners. *Int. Sport Med. J.* 2006;7:2.

van den Brand J.G., Nelson T., et al. The diagnostic value of intracompartmental pressure measurement, magnetic resonance imaging, and near-infrared spectroscopy in chronic exertional compartment syndrome: A prospective study in 50 patients. *Am. J. Sports Med.* May 2005; 33(5):699–704. Epub. Feb. 16, 2005.

Yates B., White S. The incidence and risk factors in the development of medial tibial stress syndrome among naval recruits. *Am. J. Sports Med.* Apr.–May 2004; 32(3):772–80.

Yeung S.S., Yeung E.W., Gillespie L.D. Interventions for preventing lower limb soft-tissue running injuries. *Cochrane Database Syst. Rev.* July 2011; 6(7):CD001256.

CHAPTER 19

MUSCLE INJURIES

Emin Ergen

Skeletal muscle is the largest tissue in the body and makes up 40–45% of total body weight. Indirect (intrinsic) muscle injuries, also called strains or tears, and direct (extrinsic) injuries are quite common both in competitive and recreational physical activities. These injuries may also lead to complications such as myositis ossificans and muscle hernia. Delayed-onset muscle soreness (DOMS) is another frequently occurring muscle problem associated with strenuous exertions.

INDIRECT TRAUMA

Muscle activation produces force within the muscle. During a concentric contraction, the resisting load is less than the force generated by the muscle, and the muscle shortens. If the resisting force is greater than that generated by the muscle, the muscle lengthens, which is referred to as eccentric contraction. Most of the muscle activity in athletic activities occurs in an eccentric fashion. Eccentric contraction helps to absorb kinetic energy and protect joints, such as, in the case of landing from a jump, the quadriceps muscle contracts, protecting the knee. Eccentric muscle activation can generate a higher amount of force or tension within the muscle compared with concentric contraction, making it more susceptible to rupture or tear. Injuries can be seen either in the muscle belly or near the myotendinous junction. In younger individuals, the weakest point in the muscle–tendon–bone complex is the apophysis. Factors that contribute to muscle strain injury can be inadequate flexibility, inadequate strength or endurance, dys-synergistic muscle contraction, insufficient warm-up, or inadequate rehabilitation from previous injury.

CLASSIFICATION

Muscle strains are clinically classified as either complete or partial, according to severity. Complete tears are associated with total loss of function and strength in the affected muscle, whereas incomplete tears are associated with only partial or minimal loss of strength. Complete tears are easier to detect by physical

MUSCLE-INJURY CLASSIFICATION

First degree (mild)
- Tear of only a few muscle fibers.
- Mild swelling, pain, and disability.
- Can also be characterized by patient's ability to produce strong, but painful, muscle contraction.

Second degree (moderate)
- Disruption of a moderate number of fibers, but muscle–tendon unit is intact.
- Moderate amount of pain, swelling, and disability.
- Characterized by patient's weak and painful attempts at muscle contraction.

Third degree (severe)
- Complete rupture of muscle–tendon unit.
- May be at origin, muscular portion, musculotendinous junction, within tendon itself, or at tendon insertion.
- Characterized by patient's extremely weak but painless attempts at muscle contraction.
- May require surgical repair.

examination, but incomplete tears are much more common. Muscular strains usually occur in the lower extremities, with the rectus femoris and biceps femoris muscles being most commonly affected groups, followed by the semitendinosus, adductors, vastus medialis, and soleus. Indirect traumas may lead to inter- or intramuscular hematoma.

Predisposing factors can play a role in muscle strains. Restricted flexibility is one of the most important predisposing factors. There are three levels of muscular tightness:

1. *Normal physiological tightness*: Normal amount of resistance to the extremes of motion found in all individuals, which is more significant in athletes with tendency to tight muscles and joints.
2. *Excessive physiological tightness*: An exaggerated condition of normal physiological tightness seen in untrained or elderly individuals, athletes with normally tight muscles, or occasionally after prolonged rest period or injury. If there were a measurable restriction in range, it would be considered unacceptable for pre-season assessment and sufficient to increase the risk of injury.

417

3. *Pathological contracture*: Often seen after injury, surgery, or immobilization. The restriction is more significant if there is scar-tissue formation or muscle contracture.

Flexibility can either be static, such as the measured range of motion available in a joint or a series of joints, or dynamic flexibility, such as a measure of the resistance to active motion about a joint or a series of joints. Dynamic flexibility may be critical for maximizing human performance and efficiency, as well as minimizing the risk of injury, especially in high-velocity activities such as sprinting and gymnastics.

DIRECT TRAUMA (CONTUSIONS)

Traumatic injury to muscle due to direct force may produce superficial or deep-muscle contusion in contact sports. The quadriceps or brachialis muscles are two muscle groups generally involved in contact or collison sports. Myositis ossificans is a complication following direct (or sometimes indirect) trauma, and therefore a permanent loss of function may occur. Contusions (and some tears) may also be subdivided into intermuscular and intramuscular hematomas,

Intermuscular hematomas are localized near the large intermuscular septa or muscle fascial sheats. Their location facilitates early dispersal of the extravasated blood with the help of gravity, which minimizes the inflammation response and the potential scarring, allowing early resolution.

Intramuscular hematomas are seen secondary to muscle damage and usually take two to three times longer to recover compared with intermuscular lesions. The hemorrhage tends to be more confined, the mass is often palpable, and the inflammatory response is greater, posing a higher risk of myositis ossificans. There is also a chance of compartment syndrome after intramuscular hematoma in some locations. Owing to severe pain and limited function, restoration of the joint range of motion and subsequent muscle function is relatively slow. In some cases, surgical repair or open drainage of a large intramuscular hematoma is indicated. The risk of compartment syndrome with a large intramuscular hematoma is rare but must be excluded. It is a clinical diagnosis, including tenseness of the swelling as well as diminishing peripheral pulses, sensation, and function. Early surgical intervention, with release of the fascia and aspiration of the clot, is necessary.

Diagnosis

Generally, a sharp or stabbing pain is felt at the moment of injury and reproduced by contracting the muscles involved. In resting position, the pain is not very severe. Pain can inhibit muscle contraction. In total ruptures, the muscle is unable to contract, and no movement is available. A slight defect can be palpable in partial ruptures, whereas there is a significant gap in total ruptures. There is often

Table 19.1 Signs and symptoms of direct trauma (contusions)

Degree	Pain	Swelling and bruising	Structural defect	Loss of ROM	Loss of function
First (mild)	+	Minimal	0	Minimal	Minimal
Second (moderate)	+ +	Moderate	±	Significant	Significant
Third (severe)	<	Extensive	+	Severe	Complete

localized tenderness and swelling over the damaged area. Muscle spasm may accompany tenderness. After about 24–48 hours, bruising and discoloration may be seen, often below the site of injury.

Ultrasound and computed tomography (CT) are superior to plain radiography for imaging of soft tissues. Magnetic resonance imaging (MRI) has become the technique of choice for imaging muscles, tendons, and ligaments over the last two decades. Because the majority of muscle injuries are self-limiting, and the cost of MRI scans is rather high, specific indications for the use of MRI in patients suspected of having muscle tears should be taken into account. They include:

1. to delineate the extent of the muscle injury in high-performance athletes; this can be valuable for determining which patients will be treated surgically and which can be treated conservatively;
2. to evaluate patients who present with a soft mass, but no clear history of trauma; typically, these patients present with a soft-tissue mass to the tumor clinic rather than to the sports clinic;
3. to provide a prompt diagnosis when rapid initiation of proper therapy is crucial;
4. to evaluate obscure muscle pain, such as intermittent muscle herniation through a fascial rent;
5. to assess severe cases of DOMS.

MRI findings in muscle strains depend on whether the rupture is complete or partial. In the acute partial tear, blood and edema may infiltrate between the muscle bundles, especially in the region of the myotendinous junction. Blood and edema may also collect between the fascial planes. A mass is detected at the site of the injury in acute cases. This mass is usually associated with abnormal signals from bleeding and edema, as well as muscle retraction. In the chronic phase, a defect is detected at the site of rupture. Complete tears show total disruption of the muscle; muscle retraction, blood, and edema within the lesion and surrounding fascial planes can also be seen. Collection of blood or intramuscular hematoma is a frequent finding in patients with sports-related muscle injuries. Blood degrades in time, resulting in changed signal characteristics. Intramuscular hematomas and hemorrhages are often encountered on MRI examinations without a clear history

419

of trauma. Typically, an intramuscular hematoma resorbs spontaneously over a period of 6–8 weeks.

Treatment

Protection, rest, ice, compression, elevation, and support (PRICES) form the general approach after an acute strain or contusion, followed by progressive, symptom-guided rehabilitation.

Other treatment modalities are commenced within 24–36 hours by the physician and physiotherapist:

Oral anti-inflammatory medication
NSAIDs are commonly used in treating musculoskeletal sport injuries. Their use is based on physicians' empiric results rather than objective scientific studies. Choice should always be made according to known side effects (e.g., renal and gastrointestinal complications). NSAIDs are not recommended during the later phase of healing owing to their inhibiting effect on remodelling. Myorelaxants and analgesics can be prescribed if there is severe pain and spasm. Corticosteroid injection to the injured area is not indicated, owing to the risk of scar-tissue formation.

Physical modalities
Cold during the initial phase, heat, ultrasound, iontophoresis, and electrical muscle stimulation, along with the progression of healing, are commonly employed physical modalities.

Therapeutic exercises
Therapeutic exercises are very important, but most commonly under-utilized means of treating and rehabilitating musculoskeletal sport injuries. These exercises are not only important to correct the weakness resulting from injury, but also those that predispose to injury. Rehabilitation of muscle should be aimed at restoration of muscle strength, flexibility, and endurance to pre-injury level. High-speed motion, with rapid development of peak torque and sudden deceleration, has to be introduced with caution and certainly not until full range has been nearly restored. Active muscle exercises should adhere to specific principles and be carried out in the following order:

- static exercises without load;
- static exercises with load;
- limited dynamic muscle training with exercises within active range of movement, to the pain threshold;
- dynamic exercises with increasing load;
- strength exercises;

- proprioceptive training;
- protected load-bearing activities;
- sport-specific exercises.

Proliferative therapy

Regenerative injection therapy (RIT), also known as proliferative therapy, has been used for over 30 years in some countries in patients with muscular, peripheral joint, and ligamentous pathologies. It involves the injection of mildly irritating medications into muscles, ligaments, and tendons, most commonly at origins and insertions. These injections cause a mild inflammatory response that "triggers" the normal healing process and results in the regeneration of these structures.

Herbal substances

Herbal remedies have been reported to be effective in controlling inflammation for acute soft-tissue injuries.

Dry needling

Through puncturing with a dry (acupuncture) needle, a microinjury in the affected tissue is made that then leads to electrophysiological, biochemical, and metabolic changes. This limited tissue damage triggers the release of mediators (such as bradykinin) followed by vasodilation and increased cellular-membrane permeability. With the stimulation of nociceptive nerve endings, a pronounced pain inhibition may occur (gate control). Endorphin release is also increased with needle puncturing. Mast-cell migration due to needling of the affected area helps to enhance healing processes. Local trophic substances such as platelet-derived growth factor (PDGF) have also been speculated as acting as an additional element following needling. Dry needling can be a complementary modality in subacute cases.

Bandages, supports, and other devices

An elastic bandage is helpful for supporting the affected muscle groups during the acute phase of injury. In later phases, a thigh support for hamstring problems is recommended to help keep the muscle warm, and its use is advised until full recovery.

Hyperbaric oxygen therapy

There has recently been a growing interest in hyperbaric oxygen (HBO) treatment in sports therapy. Oxygen naturally plays an important role in recovery from injury. By administering HBO treatment, more oxygen is dissolved in the plasma of the pulmonary vein via the alveoli, increasing the oxygen reaching the peripheral tissues. HBO treatment is expected to promote recovery from injury and fatigue. HBO treatment has been reported to decrease swelling in animals and in humans following injury. Positive results have also been reported regarding tissue remodelling after injury, with injuries involving bones, muscles, and ligaments showing improved recovery. It should be remembered that HBO treatment is not risk-free. Elevated oxygen concentrations in tissues may cause a risk to DNA through oxidative damage, which can lead to pathological changes in the CNS and the lungs. Therefore, safe administration of HBO treatment is essential.

Evaluation techniques following, or prior to, muscle injuries

Certain musculoskeletal parameters are commonly measured in athletic injuries in order to evaluate the pre-injury level or outcome of treatment and rehabilitation.

Flexibility testing

In testing for flexibility, it should be considered whether the restriction is due to muscular tightness or other sources of restriction, such as lack of joint range of motion or pain.

1. *Heel cord flexibility*: The patient sits with knee extended and is asked to actively dorsiflex the ankle. A goniometer is used for measurement. A value of at least 10° beyond plantigrade value is considered normal. This may also be done with the knee flexed to assess tightness within the soleus (normal value should be at least 20° beyond plantigrade).
2. *Hamstring flexibility*: The patient lies supine, with the hip at 90° flexion position, and is asked to extend the knee actively without changing the hip position. A goniometer is used for the measurement. Less than 10° short of full flexion is considered to be normal.
3. *Quadriceps flexibility*: The patient lies prone, and the knee is flexed passively by the physician. A full knee flexion without tilting of the pelvis is considered to be normal.
4. *Iliotibial band flexibility (modified Ober test)*: The patient lies on the opposite side, near the edge of the examination table, facing away from the physician. The hip is slightly extended and passively adducted by gravity, on the side to be examined. The iliotibial band should not slip anterior or posterior to the greater trochanter or allow lateral tilting of the pelvis. If the knee drops level to or below the level of the table, it is considered normal.

Strength testing

Although there are many ways to assess strength, it is best evaluated using dynamometers (static or isokinetic), providing objective results. Manual testing can also be an alternative in case of unavailability of dynamometric evaluation. In case of athletes, each sport has its own normative data. Return to full training and competition presupposes that strength has been regained to within 10% of normal. The agonist/antagonist ratios must be restored for the entire limb, not only the involved side.

Myositis ossificans

Traumatic myositis ossificans is a heterotopic bone formation caused by deep-muscle contusion or strain, especially after marked hematoma formation. Common sites where myositis ossificans may occur are: quadriceps, biceps, triceps, brachialis, hip girdle, groin, and lower leg. Continuing to play after injury, massaging the injured area, early application of heat, passive, forceful stretching, aggressive and rapid rehabilitation, premature return to sport, reinjury of the same site, and individual proneness to heterotopic bone formation are some of the risk factors. A calcification area may occur following injury within a couple of months. Excision of myositis ossificans is rarely necessary. Only cases of residual weakness or limited range of motion may require surgical intervention, performed after the calcification matures. There is a high rate of recurrence if it is excised too early. It is important to prevent the formation of myositis ossificans rather than treat it. Therefore, athletes who have sustained severe muscular strains and are diagnosed as presenting hematoma should be re-evaluated frequently, initially after 10 days.

Muscle herniation

Blunt traumas can produce a defect in the fascia, allowing the underlying muscle to protrude over the skin. Herniation through a defect in the muscle fascia is usually seen in the leg, particularly over the anterior tibial compartment. Muscle herniation is a rare condition that is often diagnosed clinically, although occasionally the symptomatology is confusing, and MRI may offer an unequivocal diagnosis. It may be helpful to perform the MRI scan with the herniated muscle both relaxed and contracted, in order to demonstrate a change in size of the herniated portion. Usually, no surgical intervention is necessary for muscular herniation.

Delayed-onset muscle soreness

DOMS is a very common complaint and another form of muscle injury. Following unaccustomed muscular exertion, athletes develop DOMS and experience a sensation of discomfort and pain in their skeletal muscles. For example, after prolonged downhill running (eccentric muscle activity), athletes may experience pain in all the extensor and flexor muscle groups around the hip, thigh, and leg. Structural abnormalities in the Z band and a rise in the serum creatine kinase have been described. Pain may increase in intensity for the first 24 hours after exercise, peak between 24 and 72 hours, and then subside in 5–7 days. Temporary loss of strength, up to 50%, can be present. The diminished performance may be due to reduced voluntary effort due to pain, as well as reduced capacity of the muscle to produce force. The soreness is believed to be related to reversible structural damage at the cellular level. There is no associated long-term or residual damage, nor reduced function in the muscles. The syndrome of increasing pain, made worse by stretching the affected muscle groups and eventually sensory changes, should alert the physician. The compartment is usually tense and tender to palpation. There is a special form of exercise-induced muscle trauma that is related to viral infections. Viral myalgia is the aching and lethargic feeling in muscles accompanying acute viral illness. This short-lived phenomenon is associated with minimal muscle injury. In some cases, the virus-induced myalgia is parallel with inflammatory myopathy with limited muscle breakdown (rhabdomyolysis). Intense or even moderate exercise can worsen the effect of the muscle damage significantly, which prolongs the illness. It would be wise not to allow the athlete to train if he/she presents with signs and symptoms of significant bacterial or viral infection, particularly if associated with fever or myalgia.

Diagnosis

The diagnosis is mainly based on clinical findings. MRI of DOMS is very rarely required. Muscle strain and DOMS frequently have similar appearance, and the two clinical conditions are difficult to differentiate on the basis on the imaging findings alone. As DOMS is not associated with bleeding, it is assumed that the MRI findings are primarily due to edema. Muscle strain often appears less extensive or uniform in its distribution within muscle than DOMS by MRI.

Treatment

Treatment of DOMS is generally symptomatic. Modification of athletic activity from strenuous to low level, myorelaxants, intermittent pressure, massage, and jacuzzi baths are recommended.

Myofascial pain syndrome

Myofascial pain syndrome (MPS) is a painful disorder that affects the muscles and fascia. MPS is thought to be a pain syndrome caused and maintained by one or more active trigger points and their associated reflexes. The trigger point is the actual tissue causing the pain state. Many athletes under strenuous training may have myofascial pain. Trigger points are usually associated with a taut band, a ropey thickening of the muscle tissue. Typically, a trigger point, when pressed, will cause the pain to be felt elsewhere. This is considered to be "referred pain."

Myofascial trigger points (MTrPs) may be active or latent. An active MTrP is a focus of hyperirritability in a muscle or its fascia that causes pain and tenderness at rest or with motion that stretches or loads the muscle. It prevents full lengthening of the muscle, as well as causing fatigue and decreased strength. Pressure on an active MTrP induces/reproduces some of the patient's pain complaint and is recognized by the patient as being some or all of his or her pain. A latent MTrP does not cause pain during normal activities. It is locally tender, but causes pain only when palpated. It also refers pain on pressure. It can be associated with a weakened, shortened, and more easily fatigued muscle.

The following are factors that cause trigger points:

- trauma to musculoskeletal tissues (muscles, ligaments, tendons, bursae);
- injury to intervertebral disks;

- generalized fatigue (fibromyalgia is a perpetuating factor of MPS; perhaps chronic fatigue syndrome may produce trigger points as well);
- overuse conditions in sport, excessive exercise, and muscle strains;
- systemic conditions (e.g., gallbladder inflammation, heart attack, appendicitis, stomach irritation);
- lack of activity (e.g., immobilization in a sling or cast);
- nutritional deficiencies;
- hormonal changes (e.g., trigger point development during PMS or menopause);
- nervous tension or stress;
- chilling of areas of the body (e.g., sitting under an air-conditioning duct; sleeping in front of an air conditioner).

Diagnosis

The diagnosis is made by the history and physical examination. There is no laboratory test or imaging studies to confirm the diagnosis. A history of acute trauma or chronic overuse should be looked for. On examination, there is typically restricted motion with pain in the affected muscle. Other medical problems (e.g., low-back pain) need to be ruled out with imaging or other studies.

Differential diagnosis

To diagnose MPS accurately, other potential sources of myofascial and skeletal pain should be considered and eliminated. The presence of MTrPs does not preclude a tumor or other hidden cause of ongoing pain.

MPS is often confused with fibromyalgia. However, they are distinct entities. In 1990, the American College of Rheumatology established diagnostic criteria for fibromyalgia: 11 out of 18 specific points must be tender, and widespread pain must be present for at least 3 months. Like trigger points, the tender points of fibromyalgia are tender on palpation and may have taut bands of muscle fibers; however, they do not exhibit local twitch responses.

Fibromyalgia tends to be more global and is more prevalent in women than in men. MPS, in contrast, is more regional and affects men and women equally. In addition, unlike MPS, fibromyalgia has a poor prognosis. Certain neurologic conditions such as multiple sclerosis, entrapment neuropathies, and radiculopathies should also be considered in the differential diagnosis, as well as rheumatologic conditions such as rheumatoid arthritis and systemic lupus erythematosus.

Treatment

Treatment of MPS can only begin after an accurate diagnosis is obtained. Methods for managing this painful condition include:

- trigger-point therapy (myofascial release therapy, myotherapy, massotherapy (medical massage therapy));

- spray and stretch technique (stretching of the muscles involved with a vapo-coolant spray – a coolant is sprayed on the trigger point to lessen the pain, and then the muscle is stretched; this is often done by a physical therapist);
- trigger-point injections (local anesthetics, such as lidocaine, injected directly into the trigger points);
- dry needling (the use of an acupuncture needle without anything being injected) (TrP injections and dry needling mechanically disrupt the trigger point; the use of lidocaine is no more effective, but it reduces the soreness after injection; for MPS there is no role for injected steroids);
- chiropractic or osteopathic manipulation treatment;
- craniosacral therapy;
- physical therapy (hands-on);
- exercise;
- nutritional interventions (in case of inappropriate nutrition);
- changing sleeping habits;
- the use of tricyclic antidepressants in low doses;
- elimination of stress; biofeedback; counseling for depression, which may result from this painful condition.

SUGGESTED READING

El-Khoury G.Y., Brandser F.A., Kathol M.H., Tearse D.S., Callaghan J.J., Imaging of muscle injuries, *Skeletal Radiol.*, 25(1):3–11, 1996.

Fomby E.W., Mellion M.B., Identifying and treating myofascial pain syndrome, *The Physician and Sports Medicine*, 25(2): February 1997.

Malone T.R., Garrett W.E., Zachazewski J.E., Muscle: Deformation, injury, repair, in *Athletic Injuries and Rehabilitation*. Zachazewski J.E., Magee D.J., Quillen W.S. (Eds.), Philadelphia, Saunders, 1996.

Reid D.C., *Sports Injury Assessment and Rehabilitation*. New York, Churchill Livingstone, 1992.

Walsh W.M., Ronnie D.H., Peter L.E., Mellion M.B., Injury prevention, diagnosis and treatment, in *37: Musculoskeletal Injuries in Sport*. Mellion M.B., Walsh W.M., Shelton G.L. (Eds.), pp. 361–70.

CHAPTER 20

FOOT AND ANKLE INJURIES

Margaret L. Olmedo and Per A.F.H. Renström

ANKLE INJURIES

Ankle fracture/dislocation

Fieldside assessment

The athlete presents with severe ankle pain, usually on the lateral side of the ankle, following a twisting injury or a direct blow. Swelling is rapid. Marked deformity may be obvious. Weight-bearing may be possible, depending on the severity of the injury. If severe deformity is apparent, the limb may be moved into a more normal position (reduced) by applying longitudinal traction, pulling the foot distal as an assistant holds the athlete's knee in 90° of flexion. Emergent reduction of these severely deformed ankles is recommended to reduce tension on stretched neurovascular structures. The athlete is removed from play, the limb is splinted and elevated, and the athlete is transported for further evaluation and management.

Diagnosis

Observe and palpate the bone and soft-tissue structures for localized tenderness. Examine and monitor the neurovascular integrity. Anatomic diagnoses are confirmed by plain X-ray (Figures 20.1 and 20.2).

Treatment

Specific treatment depends on the structures injured. For an athlete, anatomic reduction is strongly recommended. Generally, surgical internal fixation is required to maintain reduction. Treatment of some specific fracture/dislocation types will be discussed later in the chapter.

Rehabilitation

As soon as ankle stability allows, the athlete begins to use a removable splint or brace and begins a non-weight-bearing range-of-motion exercises (Figure 20.3). When healing is sufficient, strengthening exercises begin, first non-weight-bearing,

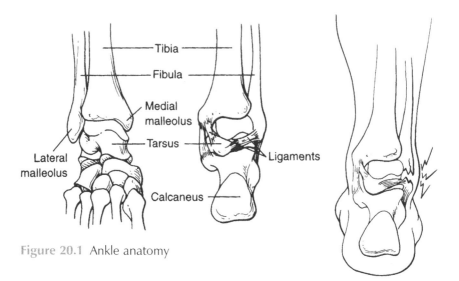

Figure 20.1 Ankle anatomy

Tibia
Fibula
Medial malleolus
Tarsus
Lateral malleolus
Ligaments
Calcaneus

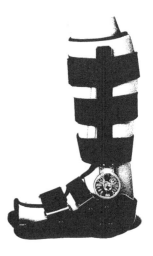

Figure 20.2
Ankle fracture

typically with resistance bands. When healing is sufficient, weight-bearing exercises are begun, with an emphasis on gastrocnemius and soleus strengthening and stretching, as well as proprioception training. The kinetic chain should also not be forgotten, and some time should be given to strengthening the ipsilateral knee and hip musculature, as walking in an immobilizing boot for several weeks can cause havoc for even the fittest athlete, causing muscle-timing issues and compensatory patterns.

Return to play

The athlete may return to limited training with a protective brace. The progression of return to training and to sport is highly dependent on the specific injury pattern and treatment.

Figure 20.3
A "walking boot" of the sort often prescribed for persons with stable ankle or lower-leg fractures

Ligament injuries of the ankle

Fieldside assessment

The athlete presents with severe ankle pain, usually on the lateral side of the ankle, following a twisting injury.

Weight-bearing may or may not be possible. Mild-to-severe swelling occurs over the next few hours. The athlete is removed from play until a careful evaluation can be completed.

Diagnosis

Ankle injuries make up 15% of all sports injuries. Sprains of the lateral ligaments of the ankle account for approximately 15% of all athletic injuries and are the most common injury in most sports. Eighty-five percent of lateral ankle sprains are caused by inversion of the hindfoot (Figures 20.4 and 20.5). The anterior talofibular (ATF) ligament is the most frequently injured ligament. Ankle sprains are typically classified according to the severity of the injury (Table 20.1).

An accurate diagnosis can be made from a good history of the mechanism of the injury, the site and time of onset of the swelling, the functional ability of the patient following the injury, and examination with fingertip palpation to localize the pain. These aspects have been shown to be almost as accurate as (and more cost-effective than) the numerous diagnostic studies that are available. A careful, accurate history will lead the examiner to an appropriately focused physical examination based on the mechanism of injury, looking for one of the common

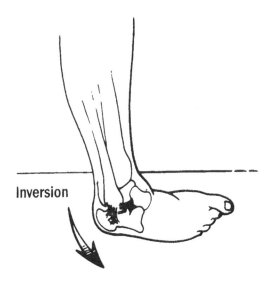

Inversion

Figure 20.4 Inversion is the most typical injury mechanism in ankle sprain

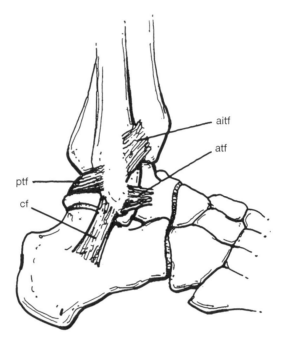

The lateral ligamentous complex of the ankle consists of the anterior talofibular (atf), calcaneofibular (cf), and posterior talofibular (ptf) ligaments. Aitf = anterior inferior tibiofibular ligament.

Figure 20.5 Lateral view of ankle ligaments

Table 20.1 Ankle sprains classified according to the severity of the injury

Grade		Swelling	Tenderness	Function	Stability
I.	Mild stretch	Minimal	Minimal	Normal/near normal	Normal
II.	Partial tear	Moderate	Moderate	Difficulty toe walking – Talar tilt	+ Anterior drawer
III.	Complete tear	Marked	Marked	Significant loss + Talar tilt	+ Anterior drawer

injury patterns shown in Table 20.2. Fracture may occur with these same mechanisms of injury, so examine the distal tibia and fibula, anterior process of the calcaneus, base of the fifth metatarsal, and proximal fibula particularly carefully. Remember that grade III sprains are associated with up to an 80% incidence of peroneal and posterior tibial nerve damage, usually subclinical.

Table 20.2 Common injury patterns

Position	Ligaments injured
Plantarflexion/inversion	ATF, then calcaneofibular
Dorsiflexion/inversion	ATF or subtalar ligaments
Dorsiflexion/external rotation	ATF and syndesmosis
Eversion/external rotation	Deltoid, then syndesmosis

Clinical tests for instability include the anterior drawer and the talar tilt. Comparison with the uninvolved side should always be made. The anterior drawer test is used to evaluate the ATF ligament (Figure 20.6A). Holding the ankle in 10–20° of plantar flexion (the position of greatest instability), the examiner stabilizes the tibia and attempts to pull the talus forward. Anterior translation indicates an ATF ligament tear. If the test appears to be positive without apparent anterior movement of the talus, the test may indicate instability at the subtalar joint.

The talar tilt (inversion stress) test is considered a test for the calcaneofibular ligament, but can also test the ATF ligament (Figure 20.6B). Holding the foot and ankle in a neutral position, the examiner inverts the hindfoot. If the calcaneofibular ligament and the ATF ligament are disrupted, the articular surfaces of the talus and tibia will separate, forming an angle referred to as a talar tilt. With plantarflexion, the ATF ligament is strained more, and the calcaneofibular ligament becomes more relaxed.

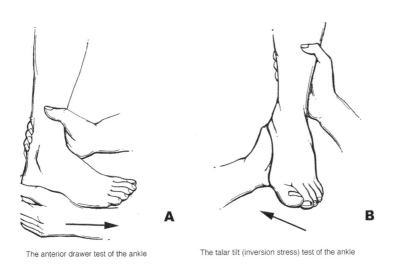

A The anterior drawer test of the ankle

B The talar tilt (inversion stress) test of the ankle

Figure 20.6 (A) Anterior drawer test. (B) Talar tilt test

The syndesmosis is examined by the squeeze test and external rotation test. The squeeze test is done by compressing the fibula and tibia together above the midpoint of the calf. The external rotation test is performed with knee flexed 90° and the ankle in neutral, the examiner rotating the foot outward. With both tests, pain in the syndesmosis area indicates injury (see later section on tibiofibular syndesmosis disruption).

X-rays are often not needed for athletes with ankle sprains, particularly if they are skeletally mature. The Ottawa Ankle Rules predict which adult athletes with ankle sprains should have X-rays. X-rays are needed for athletes with: (1) tenderness at the posterior edge or distal tip of the medial or lateral malleolus; (2) inability to bear weight for four steps; or (3) pain at the base of the fifth metatarsal. However, plain films are recommended with all significant ankle injuries. If the physical examination found areas of bone tenderness, they should be X-rayed.

Among skeletally immature athletes, inversion ankle injury often causes a non-displaced (Salter I) growth plate fracture of the distal fibula, a diagnosis made clinically. Occasionally, an adolescent athlete has surprisingly little tenderness even over a displaced distal tibial growth plate fracture, and so skeletally immature athletes with ankle swelling following an injury generally warrant X-ray examination. Stress tests and stress radiographs may be used to determine the extent of the injury but do not change the treatment protocol. Subtalar joint arthrography (injection of dye into the joint) may occasionally be considered to distinguish between simple sprains of the ATF ligament and more complex injuries of the hindfoot. It is most accurate if it is performed within 24 hours of the injury. Currently, few sports orthopedic surgeons recommend immediate surgical repair of ruptured lateral ankle ligaments, and so arthrography is rarely done. MRI is helpful in evaluating the ankle joint for osteochondral injuries. Ankle arthroscopy can be used for diagnosis and treatment of persistent post-traumatic ankle pain that is unresponsive to conservative treatment.

Treatment

The treatment of a severely sprained ankle is controversial, but protected mobilization is generally recommended for most ankle sprains. There are 20–40% of ankle sprains treated conservatively that have residual symptoms. Inadequate treatment can result in chronic ankle instability, with recurrent sprains and early degenerative arthrosis. The mainstays of treatment are protected mobilization, followed by muscle strengthening and proprioception training. Non-operative functional treatment is recommended for all grades of ankle sprain. Functional treatment of patients with little or no evidence of instability (grade I or II) consists of three phases. Phase I is RICE therapy. Phase II includes a short period of immobilization and protection of the ankle (1–3 weeks), with supportive bandaging, taping, or bracing in a neutral position and protected weight-bearing to control pain and swelling. Once the swelling and pain have subsided, the athlete may begin limited plantar flexion and dorsiflexion exercises with low resistance. The

432 FiMS

athlete may maintain aerobic conditioning by riding a stationary bike or swimming. Protection from inversion is important during this phase, to prevent overstretching of the healing ligaments. Protected mobilization follows, using a supportive bandage or brace that prevents inversion/eversion but allows gradually increasing dorsiflexion/plantarflexion as symptoms decrease. In Phase III, once weight-bearing and pain-free range of motion have been established, the athlete begins muscle-strengthening exercises. Particular attention is paid to strengthening the anterior tibial and the peroneal muscles. Assisted eversion exercises should be performed, with the foot dorsiflexed to strengthen the peroneus brevis and tertius, and plantarflexed to strengthen the peroneus longus muscle. The athlete may begin proprioceptive training with a balance board once muscle strength has improved sufficiently, typically 3–4 weeks after the injury. Proprioception training is continued for a minimum of 10 weeks.

The best treatment for grades II–III sprains remains controversial. The combination of a brace and elastic wrap is generally recommended as initial treatment. Once swelling has subsided, the brace may be worn alone. With this treatment alone, 10–30% of patients with a lateral ligament injury develop chronic symptoms. It is important to differentiate between mechanical (incompetent ligaments) and functional (poor muscle strength/proprioception) instability. Well-trained dynamic stabilizers (the supportive muscles) of the ankle can compensate for much mechanical instability.

Operative treatment is usually reserved for athletes with chronic, recurring ankle instability despite a well-supervised rehabilitation program. If surgery is needed, an anatomic delayed reconstruction of the ATF ligament and calcaneofibular ligament (Brostrom technique) is preferred. Rarely is surgical treatment for an acute sprain recommended. However, there are some cases where it is indicated: (1) a grade III sprain in a young competitive athlete whose stress radiographs demonstrate more than 15° of talar tilt and over 10 mm of anterior translation on the anterior drawer test; (2) an acute sprain in an athlete with a history of chronic instability; (3) a talar dislocation with complete ligamentous disruption; (4) a clinical anterior drawer sign; (5) over 15° of talar tilt with the inversion test; (6) the presence of an osteochondral fracture; or (7) widening of the ankle mortise. After surgery, the patient follows an intensive functional rehabilitation program.

Rehabilitation

During the first 6 weeks after injury, physical therapy modalities such as ice, ultrasound, hot–cold contrast baths, and electrical stimulation may speed recovery and allow earlier range-of-motion and strength training. Only ice (for acute swelling) and intermittent pneumatic compression (for chronic swelling) have proved effective in randomized studies. The calf muscles should be stretched if tight. Strengthening of the peroneal and anterior tibial muscles should be emphasized in functional activities, and proprioception must be addressed throughout rehabilitation. The use of orthotics should also be considered if the athlete has

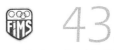

433

poor ankle alignment, such as pes planus; correction of alignment may improve patient ankle/forefoot proprioception.

Return to play

The injured ankle must have pain-free, full range of motion. The athlete must be able to walk and run without limping. The strength of the injured ankle must be at least 90% of that of the uninvolved side. If pre-injury results of running and functional tests are available, the athlete should show over 90% performance capabilities before returning to a normal practice schedule. The athlete must be able to reach his/her maximum speed in running and cutting before returning to competition. Athletes with previous ankle injuries have a two to three times greater risk for re-injury, and so continued bracing with a semi-rigid orthosis should be considered (Figure 20.7).

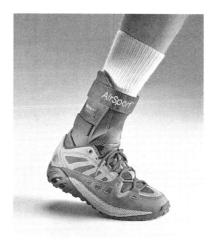

Figure 20.7 To prevent a recurrence of an ankle sprain, ankle braces such as these can be worn by athletes when playing and training

Acute deltoid ligament injuries

Fieldside assessment

The athlete presents with medial or global ankle pain following an injury. Pain and swelling are usually marked, and weight-bearing is not possible. The ankle may appear deformed. The athlete is removed from the field, has ice and a splint or compressive wrap applied, and is sent for further evaluation.

Diagnosis

Only about 3% of ankle ligament injuries occur on the medial side. Complete medial ankle ligament tears generally occur in combination with ankle fractures.

The most common mechanisms of injury of the deltoid ligament are pronation–abduction, pronation–external rotation, and supination–external rotation of the foot. The ligament may be avulsed from one of its attachment sites or torn interstitially. If there is a suspicion of a deltoid ligament injury, it is extremely important to rule out an ankle fracture or disruption of the syndesmosis.

Routine AP, lateral, and mortise view X-rays should be obtained. If clinically indicated, an X-ray of the proximal fibula should be obtained to rule out a Maisonneuve fracture.

Treatment

Partial deltoid ligament ruptures are treated non-operatively and usually have a good-to-excellent prognosis. However, partial tears occasionally result in longstanding problems, such as pain and tenderness over the anterior medial aspect of the deltoid ligament, where the fibers enter the capsule. Controversy still exists over the management of complete tears. The athlete with complete deltoid ligament rupture should be referred to a qualified specialist for treatment.

Tibiofibular syndesmosis disruption

Fieldside assessment

The athlete usually presents with severe ankle pain, typically following a forced dorsiflexion injury. Often, weight-bearing is not possible. The athlete is removed from competition, ice is applied, and weight-bearing is not allowed until the diagnosis is clear.

Diagnosis

The syndesmosis is made up of the anterior and posterior inferior tibiofibular ligaments and the interosseus membrane. Isolated complete ruptures of the syndesmosis without accompanying fractures are rare.

Syndesmosis tears mostly occur in soccer, skiing, motorcross, and skating. Partial tears of the anterior inferior tibiofibular ligament occur in soccer and football owing to violent external rotation and plantarflexion of the ankle.

In patients with complete tears of their syndesmosis, the tibiofibular diastasis may be so large that the diagnosis is clear by inspection. More typically, clinical diagnosis is by the squeeze test or the external rotation test. Routine AP, lateral, and mortise radiographs are needed to exclude fractures and osseous avulsions.

CT and MRI are helpful in ruling out associated osteochondral fractures of the talar dome (Figure 20.8).

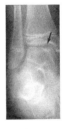

Figure 20.8 Osteochondritis of the talar dome

Treatment

Partial isolated tears of the syndesmosis without associated fracture are generally treated non-operatively, provided no widening of the distal tibiofibular joint is seen on X-rays. If syndesmosis rupture is complete, the athlete should be referred for consideration of surgical internal fixation.

Achilles tendon rupture

Fieldside assessment

The athlete presents with posterior ankle pain, reporting hearing a "pop" and feeling as if something hit the back of his/her calf. The athlete is removed from play and told to use crutches until further evaluation makes the diagnosis clear. Ice and a splint or compressive wrap are applied, and the ankle is elevated.

Diagnosis

There is often a palpable defect over the rupture site. Plantar flexion is weak. For Thompson's test, the athlete lies prone, and the examiner squeezes the calf muscles. Normally, the ankle should plantarflex with this maneuver. If the ankle does not plantarflex, Thompson's test is positive, indicating Achilles tendon rupture.

Treatment

Open repair with early range of motion is the treatment option of choice for athletes. The re-rupture rate after primary repair ranges 0–5%. After non-operative treatment the re-rupture rate is 8–39%.

Rehabilitation

Post-operatively, the athlete wears a protective brace, with the ankle in a neutral or slightly plantarflexed position.

With the more advanced repair techniques, supervised action movement from a neutral to a fully flexed position can start early. Protective bracing is discontinued 6 weeks following surgery, and active motion is allowed. With a 2-cm heel lift, the athlete may ride a bicycle and bear weight, as tolerated. Once the athlete has achieved full range of motion, strengthening can be added to the rehabilitation program. The athlete may begin a progressive running program when strength is 70% that of the uninvolved side.

Return to play

The athlete may return to sport when range of motion, strength, and endurance are normal. In most cases, the athlete can return to sports 3–4 months after surgery.

Osteochondral lesions of the talus

Diagnosis
Osteochondral lesions of the talus (OCLs) typically occur in younger athletes. This group of lesions includes osteochondritis dissecans of the talus, osteochondral fractures, and talar transchondral fractures.

Although osteochondral fractures result from an injury (usually one that was considered a simple ankle sprain at the time of the injury), most are not diagnosed until months or years after the injury. The most common locations for the lesions are posteromedial or anterolateral. The fragment may remain attached, or it may detach and move around in the joint, causing pain and further joint injury.

The athlete describes pain inside the ankle joint. Aching, stiffness, and mild-to-moderate swelling are common complaints. If the fragment is free floating, the athlete may report intermittent locking. On physical examination, the lesion can often be localized by direct palpation or by maneuvering the ankle into the position that causes painful impingement of the injured area against the tibia or fibula. Plain X-rays are often normal, but a plantar flexion mortise view may show the lesion. CT or MRI scans usually show the lesion well.

Treatment
Treatment depends on the athlete's symptoms. Complete immobilization of the ankle is not recommended, because motion of the joint provides nutrition to the cartilage for healing. Acute fractures are treated arthroscopically, with anatomical reduction and internal fixation of the fragment if it is large enough, or excision of the fragment if it is small.

When symptoms are relatively mild but chronic, and the fragment is stable rather than loose, the athlete may use crutches or a removable brace until pain-free, and then gradually resume range-of-motion, stretching, and strengthening exercises, as long as the ankle remains pain-free. For those symptomatic OCLs, arthroscopic debridement and cartilage resurfacing procedures may be considered.

Rehabilitation
The athlete treated with surgery is allowed only touchdown weight-bearing for 4–6 weeks, and then gradually returns to full weight-bearing over a 2–3-week period. Strengthening and proprioception training is performed. Strengthening is largely concentrated on the gastrocnemius and soleus muscles, as muscle atrophy is expected from lack of use.

Return to play
The results in athletes with non-displaced lesions are usually good, with most athletes returning to their sports after rehabilitation. Only 50–80% of athletes with displaced lesions will return to their sports. If surgery is not performed until more

than 1 year after injury, there is a less than 60% chance of a good result and return to sport.

The athlete may return to sports when pain-free, with full range of motion and strength. Proprioception should be normal or near normal. This is usually 3 months post-injury.

Insertional Achilles tendinopathy

Diagnosis

Insertional Achilles tendinitis can either be acute or chronic. It is common in runners and impact-loading athletes. Acute insertional Achilles tendinitis is associated with a recent history of an increase in the workload of the athlete, change in running surface, change in training environment, or change of footwear.

The athlete with acute insertional Achilles tendinitis usually complains of aching or burning pain in the posterior heel. The athlete has localized tenderness at the bony insertion or 1–3 cm above the insertion site. There may be an associated retrocalcaneal bursitis. On palpation, the athlete may have soft-tissue swelling, local tenderness, and crepitus.

Chronic insertional Achilles tendinosis occurs when the acute process does not resolve. The pain becomes recurrent and episodic. The pain is often worse after exercise and may become constant. The tendon becomes thickened, the pain localizes to the posterolateral heel, and the gastroc–soleus complex becomes tight. On palpation, the athlete may have a hard, nodular consistency to the tendon.

X-rays are usually negative, except for an occasional, prominent, posterior superior calcaneus (Haglund's) deformity. In the chronic situation, there may be calcific spurring at the bone–tendon interface.

Treatment

Acute insertional Achilles tendinitis usually responds to correcting the training error, stretching, using a heel lift, NSAIDs, ultrasound, and cross-training. If the athlete is limping, a short period of immobilization in a fracture boot is recommended in addition.

The non-operative treatment for chronic insertional Achilles tendinosis is similar to the acute treatment. The athlete may need an orthosis to correct excessive pronation.

Steroid injections around the Achilles tendon should be avoided, as they may increase the risk of tendon rupture. If non-operative treatment fails to relieve symptoms after 3–6 months, surgical intervention may be indicated. Post-operatively, the ankle is splinted in neutral for 2 weeks. Then, the athlete wears a cast boot for another 3–4 weeks, so that cross-training, early range of motion,

margaret l. olmedo and per a.f.h. renström

and gentle Achilles stretching can be started at 2–4 weeks, depending on the severity of the injury.

Rehabilitation
Physical therapy modalities or taping may be useful. Stretching of the gastro-cnemius–soleus and correcting any biomechanical or sports technique problems are important. If the athlete has poor rear-foot or forefoot positioning that may be contributing to the tendinopathy, over-the-counter orthotics or heel cups may be recommended.

Return to play
The athlete may need to return to sport with a heel lift and wean off it as tolerated. It is useful to warm up the Achilles tendon and stretch the gastroc–soleus–Achilles complex before training, and ice it for 10–15 minutes afterwards.

FOOT INJURIES

Metatarsal fractures/tarsometatarsal dislocations

Fieldside assessment
The athlete presents with severe foot pain following a twisting injury or a direct blow. Swelling is mild to severe. With the severest of these injuries, the foot rapidly swells to twice its normal size, and weight-bearing is impossible. The athlete is removed from play until further evaluation makes the diagnosis clear. Ice and a splint or compressive wrap are applied.

Diagnosis
There is tenderness localized to the injured areas. With a single metatarsal fracture, tenderness provides a very good indication of the specific injury. However, with much more severe injury, such as Lisfranc's fracture/dislocation of tarsometatarsal joints, combined with additional forefoot fracture and/or soft-tissue injury, the tenderness and swelling are nearly global over the midfoot and forefoot. X-rays are usually needed for specific diagnosis (Figures 20.9 and 20.10).

Treatment
Many stable metatarsal shaft fractures may be treated simply with a stiff-soled shoe, using crutches if needed for a few days. However, a transverse fracture of the shaft of the fifth metatarsal, near the base (Jones's fracture, at the junction of the diaphysis and metaphysis), requires at least 6 weeks of cast immobilization, with no weight-bearing. An additional 6 weeks of weight-bearing cast immobilization – or even surgical internal fixation – may be required for healing. An orthopedic surgeon should be consulted in this situation to individualize treatment, based on the athlete's needs, as early internal fixation may be the best solution. Internal

439

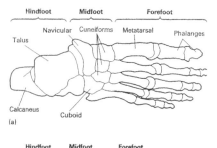

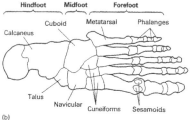

(a)

(b)

Figure 20.9
Foot anatomy

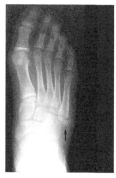

Figure 20.10
Fracture of the base of
the fifth metatarsal

fixation provides stability for reliable healing, allows accelerated rehabilitation, and decreases the time lost from sport.

Tuberosity fractures of the fifth metatarsal are treated with a removable fracture boot, early rehabilitation, and return to sports (wearing a stiff-soled shoe), when the athlete is asymptomatic. Supportive taping and a cuboid pad may be used to relieve pressure from the fracture site. An intra-articular fracture that has significant displacement (2–3 mm) usually indicates the need for open reduction and internal fixation with mini-fragment screws.

Spiral metatarsal fractures may shorten if adjacent soft tissues are significantly injured, and so these should be followed closely during the early phases of healing. Instability requiring surgical intervention is more likely if two or more metatarsals are fractured.

Lisfranc's fracture/dislocation requires emergency reduction and stabilization. Compartment syndrome of the foot occurs often with this injury and requires emergent decompression.

Rehabilitation

When fracture stability/healing is sufficient, weight-bearing activities begin, progressing as tolerated. Exercises to stretch the plantar fascia and toe flexors and strengthen the foot intrinsic muscles are particularly important. Strengthening and stretching of the ankle musculature should also be performed, as well as proprioception training. Orthotics for forefoot positioning correction and/or for comfort may also be appropriate.

margaret l. olmedo and per a.f.h. renström

Return to play

When fracture healing is complete, and strength and flexibility have returned to approximately 95% of the opposite, uninjured foot, the athlete is allowed full participation.

First metatarsophalangeal sprains (turf toe)

Diagnosis

Injuries to the first metatarsal phalangeal joint are common in athletes who participate on hard surfaces while wearing flexible shoes. Sprains of the first metatarsal phalangeal joint are caused by forced hyperextension, which causes tearing of the plantar portion of the capsule–ligament complex at its origin from the metatarsal head and neck. The initial pain and swelling can be minor, but then worsen over the next 24 hours.

In addition to the soft-tissue injury, there may be a fractured sesamoid, separated bipartite sesamoid, or metatarsal head impaction fracture.

Treatment

Non-operative treatment is the mainstay of treatment. With mild turf toe soft-tissue injuries, the athlete may wear a more supportive shoe, with a thin steel shank, to limit hyperextension of the first metatarsal phalangeal joint. The toe should be taped for sports. More severe injuries require temporary restriction from sports, or even protected weight-bearing with crutches for several days. Operative treatment is reserved for non-reducible dislocations or complete tear of the plantar structures with retraction of the sesamoids.

FOOT INJURIES: NON-TRAUMATIC

Hallux rigidus

Diagnosis

Hallux rigidus is a degenerative joint disease of the first metatarsophalangeal joint that may disable an athlete. It usually results from repeated dorsiflexion/jamming trauma. Degenerative changes of the first metatarsophalangeal joint may be associated with trauma, hyperpronation, osteochondritis dissecans, an unusually long first metatarsal, an elevated metatarsal, obesity, and/or poor footwear. Systemic arthropathies are also associated with hallux rigidus.

The athlete complains of pain in the great toe, and has pain, swelling, and decreased motion of the metatarsophalangeal joint. X-rays may show osteophytes, joint-space narrowing, and/or metatarsal head flattening. In late-stage hallux rigidus, ankylosis of the joint may occur.

441

Treatment

Footgear may need to be changed or modified, for example, with a steel or plastic plantar plate that limits first metatarsophalangeal joint motion. An extension to the tip of the great toe may be added to a typical functional orthosis in order to limit motion. For athletes with pain in the sesamoid area, weight can be shifted from the first metatarsophalangeal joint by cutting out (relieving) this area of the orthosis and leaving the remainder at full thickness.

An intra-articular injection of a short- or intermediate-acting steroid or oral NSAIDs may decrease the inflammation in the synovium and may be used as an adjuvant to correcting the biomechanics of the athlete's foot. When conservative treatment has failed, surgical treatment during the off-season may be considered. Surgical options include cheilectomy, decompression osteotomy, dorsiflexion osteotomy of the proximal phalanx, and arthrodesis. Cheilectomy (removal of the impinging dorsal bone and soft tissue) is the best option for most athletes who fail non-operative treatment.

Rehabilitation

Non-operative rehabilitation includes restoration of the best range of motion possible and strengthening of the intrinsic muscles of the foot. After surgery, the athlete wears a rigid post-operative shoe. Running activities may begin about 10 weeks after surgery, but footgear must be able to accommodate any post-operative swelling. Swelling may persist for 6–9 months after surgery.

Sesamoid dysfunction

Diagnosis

Athletes with cavus feet and associated plantarflexed first metatarsal head are most prone to sesamoid dysfunction. There is usually a history of repetitive minor trauma. Pain in the sesamoid area may be caused by bursitis, fracture, sesamoiditis, medial digital nerve compression, intractable plantar keratoses, or osteochondritis. Stress fractures of the sesamoid are usually caused by training errors. Sesamoiditis is inflammation and swelling of the peritendinous structures around the sesamoids (Figure 20.11).

The athlete presents with pain and tenderness plantar to the first metatarsal head. Dorsiflexion of the first metatarsophalangeal joint causes pain. Tenderness of the sesamoid may be difficult to distinguish from inflammation of the adjacent flexor hallucis longus tendon. Tendinitis pain can be exacerbated by active plantar flexion of the interphalangeal joint against resistance.

Sesamoid X-rays or a bone scan may be helpful in clarifying the diagnosis. Bipartite sesamoids are common, and differentiation of a normal bipartite sesamoid from a fracture can sometimes be difficult. A fracture typically appears as a straight radiolucent line on radiographs, and a congenital bipartite sesamoid will have irregular lines.

margaret l. olmedo and per a.f.h. renström

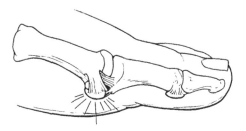

Figure 20.11 Sesamoiditis

Treatment

Treatment depends on the cause of the sesamoid dysfunction. Sesamoiditis can be treated non-operatively with padding, shoe modification or a custom orthosis, and NSAIDs. Corticosteroid injections should be used judiciously. Rarely is there a need for sesamoid excision in an athlete suffering with sesamoiditis. Bursitis pain and swelling will usually resolve when a functional orthosis is used to relieve pressure under the first metatarsal head. These orthoses are described in the hallux rigidus section. If the first metatarsal is plantarflexed, then surgical elevation of the first metatarsal may be considered in recalcitrant cases, but this is rarely recommended for athletes. Non-displaced sesamoid fractures are generally treated with a below-knee walking boot or cast for 4–6 weeks, followed by a pressure-relieving functional orthosis. If the athlete fails 6 months of conservative management, and there is clinical and radiographic evidence of a nonunion, surgery may be indicated. Both bone grafting and excision of the sesamoid have yielded satisfactory results.

Total sesamoidectomy should not be taken lightly, because removal of the sesamoid can cause significant biomechanical abnormality.

Stress fractures

Diagnosis

Stress fractures of the foot are caused by repetitive cyclical loading, usually occurring after an athlete suddenly increases the frequency, intensity, or duration of training. The athlete usually presents with pain, swelling, and well-localized tenderness. AP, lateral, and oblique X-rays of the foot may be diagnostic. A negative X-ray does not rule out a stress fracture, and a bone scan may be needed for a definitive diagnosis. Several foot stress fractures are notoriously slow and difficult to heal. These include the tarsal navicular, the talar neck, and the Jones's fifth metatarsal stress fracture. Initial treatment for non-displaced stress fractures of these bones may be non-weight-bearing-cast or removable-boot immobilization, but healing is often prolonged, and surgical fixation may be needed. For displaced

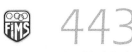

fractures of these bones, rigid internal fixation (with or without bone grafting, drilling, or electrical stimulation) is generally recommended, followed by weeks or even months of severely restricted weight-bearing (Figure 20.12).

Return to play

Return to sport after a complete fracture with surgical intervention is usually 6–9 months. The athlete with an incomplete fracture may return to sports after 6 weeks, if asymptomatic, using appropriate protective orthoses such as a steel shank and arch support for up to 6 additional months. Following any stress fracture, biomechanical abnormalities should be corrected/ compensated, and improved shoe cushioning should be used where possible.

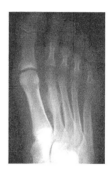

Figure 20.12
Healing stress of the second metatarsal

Plantar fasciitis

Diagnosis

Plantar fasciitis is the most common cause of heel pain in an athlete (Figure 20.13). Plantar fasciitis is chronic inflammation with its origin at the plantar medial calcaneal tuberosity on the anteromedial aspect of the heel. In the chronic setting, entrapment of the first branch of the lateral plantar nerve can contribute to the pain. Among children, the analogous injury is calcaneal apophysitis (Sever's disorder).

The affected athlete usually reports that the pain is worse after rest and with the first steps in the morning. The pain lessens with activity, but recurs again after rest.

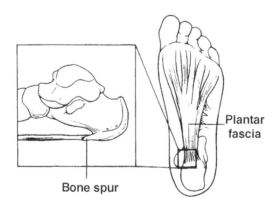

Bone spur

Plantar fascia

Figure 20.13 Plantar fasciitis

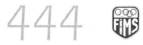

margaret I. olmedo and per a.f.h. renström

Swelling in the lateral side of the heel suggests stress fracture of the calcaneus, and radicular symptoms suggest discogenic pain. Bony spurs of the calcaneus can develop, but it is most often microscopic tears and inflammation of the plantar fascia that produce the symptoms. In addition to local tenderness, a frequently associated finding is a tight Achilles tendon. There is usually no associated malalignment abnormality, but hindfoot valgus with pronation increases the stress on the medial plantar fascia.

Treatment

Plantar fasciitis, even in the chronic setting (up to 9 months), is treated non-operatively. Aggressive Achilles tendon stretching consists of 2–4 minutes of passive stretching, three or four times per day. NSAIDs, soft heel pads, and arch taping help decrease symptoms during athletic activities. Occasionally, a custom orthosis, with a medial heel wedge and first metatarsal lift to relieve stress on the medial fascia and correct the pronation deformity, is prescribed for an in-season athlete. Judicious use of a long-acting steroid (no more than three treatments per year) may benefit the in-season athlete. Too many steroid injections may cause atrophy of the fat pad and make the heel pain worse. Shockwave therapy has been shown to be useful in cases that are refractory to conventional conservative treatment. Operative treatment is reserved for athletes who have failed 9–12 months of supervised non-operative treatment. Post-operatively, the ankle is splinted with a molded arch for 2 weeks. Then, a mild stretching program is started, and ambulation with crutches and a walking boot is allowed. Crutches are discontinued at 3–4 weeks. Biking in the boot and running in the pool are allowed at 3 weeks, with a gradual increase in impact activities over a 3–4-week period. Running and jumping are allowed at 8–12 weeks, depending on the symptoms. Return to sports is in 3–4 months.

Rehabilitation

The athlete should continue a rigorous stretching program, as initial treatment, following surgery, and throughout the athlete's subsequent career.

Return to play

The athlete may return to activity as symptoms allow.

SUGGESTED READING

Amendola A., Najibi S., Wasserman L., "Athletic ankle injuries," *Orthopaedic Knowledge Update: Sports Medicine 3*. Rosemont, IL: American Academy of Orthopaedic Surgeons, 2004.

Anderson R.B., James W.C., Lee S., "Athletic foot disorders," *Orthopaedic Knowledge Update: Sports Medicine 3*. Rosemont, IL: American Academy of Orthopaedic Surgeons, 2004.

Barker H.B., Beynnon B.D., Renström P.A., "Ankle injury risk factors in sports," *Sports Medicine*. 23(2):69–74, Feb. 1997.

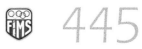

Beynnon B.D., Renström P.A., Alosa D.M., Baumhauer J.F., Vacek P.M., "Ankle ligament injury risk factors: A prospective study of college athletes," *Journal of Orthopaedic Research*. 19(2):213–20, Mar. 2001.

Beynnon B.D., Renström P.A., Haugh L., Uh B.S., Barker H., "A prospective, randomized clinical investigation of the treatment of first-time ankle sprains," *American Journal of Sports Medicine*. 34(9):1401–12, Sep. 2006.

Bring D.K., Kreicbergs A., Renström P.A., Ackermann P.W., "Physical activity modulates nerve plasticity and stimulates repair after Achilles tendon rupture," *Journal of Orthopaedic Research*. 25(2):164–72, Feb. 2007.

Carcia C.R., Martin R.L., Houck J., Wukich D.K., "Achilles tendinopathy: Clinical practice guidelines," *Journal of Orthopaedic and Sports Physical Therapy*. 40(9), Sep. 2010.

Chan K.M., Karlsson J., *ISAKOS-FIMS World Consensus Conference on Ankle instability*, 2005.

DeLee J.C., Drez D., Miller M., "Foot and ankle," *Orthopaedic Sports Medicine*. Philadelphia: WB Saunders Elsevier, 2010, 1865–2171.

Jelinek J.A., Porter D.A., "Management of unstable ankle fractures and syndesmosis injuries in athletes," *Foot and Ankle Clinics* 14(2):277–98, Jun. 2009.

Lynch S.A., Renström P.A., "Treatment of acute lateral ankle ligament rupture in the athlete. Conservative versus surgical treatment," *Sports Medicine*. 27(1):61–71, Jan. 1999.

McPoil T.G., Martin R.L., Cornwall M.W., Wukich D.K., Irrgang J.J., Godges J.J., "Heel pain-plantar fasciitis: Clinical practice guidelines," *Journal of Orthopaedic and Sports Physical Therapy*. 38(4), Apr. 2008.

Rammelt S., Zwipp H., Grass R., "Injuries to the distal tibiofibular syndesmosis: An evidence-based approach to acute and chronic lesions," *Foot and Ankle Clinics* 13(4):611–33, vii–viii, Dec. 2008.

Roos E.M., Engstrom M., Lagerquist A., Soderberg B., "Clinical improvement after 6 weeks of eccentric exercise in patients with mid-portion Achilles tendinopathy – a randomized trial with 1-year follow-up," *Scandinavian Journal of Medicine & Science in Sports*. 14(5):286–95, Oct. 2004.

Schenck R.C. Jr, Coughlin M.J., "Lateral ankle instability and revision surgery alternatives in the athlete," *Foot and Ankle Clinics* 14(2):205–14, Jun. 2009.

CHAPTER 21

HEAD AND NECK INJURIES

Anthony C. Luke

Head and neck injuries are among the few life-threatening emergencies in sports medicine. Injuries of the head and cervical spine can be serious because they may involve the brain, spinal cord, and peripheral nerves. Furthermore, the adjacent eyes, nose, throat, and ears may be injured, which can affect vision, breathing, speech, and hearing. Consequently, the team physician must be able to evaluate and initiate treatment for injuries to the head, neck, and sensory organs, which can result in death or permanent disability. The approach to management of head and neck injuries should be consistent: (1) identify the injury; (2) stabilize the athlete; and (3) transport the athlete for definitive treatment if necessary.

SERIOUS HEAD AND NECK INJURIES

■ Serious head and neck injuries can result in permanent disability.
■ Manage with a consistent approach: identify the injury, stabilize the athlete, and transport the athlete for definitive care if necessary.

SERIOUS NECK INJURIES

Fieldside assessment

A serious neck injury involves trauma to the cervical spine (C-spine), which may result in spinal cord injury. Serious head and neck injuries are most often seen in athletes participating in contact sports, or sports with a risk of falling from a height, such as diving or gymnastics. The mechanisms of neck injuries are usually an impact to the head, with axial load on the cervical spine from a collision, fall, or a blow, or forceful flexion or extension of the head, with or without rotation. A fracture of a cervical vertebra can directly injure the spinal cord and nerve roots, or can cause instability of the spine, leading to potential damage of the neural structures. Neck trauma can also cause contusions of the spinal cord and injury to the surrounding nerve roots without a fracture, known as cervical cord neuropraxia, especially if the neck has existing narrowing or stenosis of the spinal canal.

The identification of head and neck injuries should be part of the initial primary survey of an injured athlete on the field. It is important to begin with a consistent approach, "C–ABCDE", as neck trauma may be associated with a life-threatening airway injury (see Chapter 6). In the event of a serious head and neck injury, the initial management is always the same: (1) identify the injury; (2) stabilize the athlete; and (3) transport the athlete for definitive treatment.

If the history, mechanism of injury, or symptom pattern suggests a serious neck injury, the cervical spine should be immediately protected by maintaining in-line immobilization of the neck, either with two hands or a rigid cervical spine collar (see Chapter 6, Figures 6.2 and 6.7). All unconscious athletes are assumed to have an associated neck injury. Until adequate radiological evaluation has been completed, unnecessary movement of the athlete's neck should be avoided. Emergency services should be immediately informed of the injury, and a means of transfer to a medical center should be arranged.

On the field, the physician must clinically assess the severity of the injury. An athlete with a cervical spine injury may complain of immediate neck pain or neurological symptoms, such as radiating pain, numbness, tingling, weakness, or paralysis in any or all limbs. The neck can initially be palpated gently for any signs of tenderness along the cervical spine, from the occiput to the T1 vertebra, without moving the neck. If there are minimal complaints of neck pain, it is possible carefully to test the stability of the neck by asking the athlete actively to rotate the head 45° to each side and then flex the chin to the chest. An athlete with a significant neck injury usually will not want to move the neck. If there are any symptoms or signs suggesting a serious neck injury, the athlete's cervical spine should be stabilized with a rigid C-spine collar, and the player should be transferred for further evaluation on a spine board (see Chapter 6).

If an unstable neck or other emergent injury is not suspected, the athlete may be moved off the field to a controlled area for a more detailed examination of the neck and head. A thorough neurological exam should be performed to identify any subtle neurological or cognitive deficit (Table 21.1). If there is any uncertainty about the severity of injury, it is always advisable to transfer the athlete to an appropriate medical facility, using the appropriate stabilizing equipment, such as a cervical spine collar, spine board, and stretcher.

Diagnosis
Initially, C-spine radiographs are typically indicated, especially if there is a dangerous mechanism of injury such as a fall or axial load to the head, or if the individual has an altered level of consciousness. C-spine X-rays should include, at minimum, an anteroposterior (AP) view, a lateral view, and an open-mouth odontoid view. To properly interpret the lateral C-spine film, it is important to

Table 21.1 Neurological exam maneuvers*

	Test
Cranial nerves	
II (optic nerve)	Visual acuity
III, IV, VI (extraocular nerves)	Extraocular movements
V	Sensation to the forehead, cheek, and lower jaw (check both sides)
VII	Facial muscles (look for symmetry with raising eyebrows, showing teeth)
VIII	Hearing
IX, X	Soft-palate elevation (open mouth and say "Aah")
XI	Trapezius elevation (test shoulder shrug strength)
XII	Tongue movement (stick out tongue – look for deviation)
Nerve root level tested/sensory dermatome	
C5	Lateral shoulder (deltoid area)
C6	Thumb
C7	Middle finger (3rd finger)
C8	Little finger (5th finger)
T4	Nipple line
T8	Lower border of the sternum
T10	Umbilicus
T12	Symphysis pubis
L4	Medial aspect of the lower leg
L5	Webspace between 1st and 2nd toes
S1	Lateral aspect of the foot
S3, S4, S5	Perianal area
Motor strength testing (nerve roots involved)†	
Axillary nerve (C5, C6)	Resisted shoulder abduction (deltoid)
Radial nerve (C5, C6)	Resisted wrist extension (extensor carpi radialis)
Median nerve (C6, C7, C8)	Resisted elbow extension (triceps) or thumb to little finger (opponens)
Ulnar nerve (C8, T1)	Resisted abduction or adduction of fingers (interossei)
Femoral nerve (L2, L3, L4)	Resisted knee extension (quadriceps)
Deep peroneal nerve (L4, L5)	Resisted ankle dorsiflexion (anterior tibialis)
Tibial nerve (S1, S2)	Resisted ankle plantarflexion (gastrocnemius, soleus)
Sciatic nerve (L5, S1, S2)	Resisted knee flexion (hamstrings)
Reflexes	
Upper extremity	Triceps, biceps, brachioradialis
Lower extremity	Knee, ankle, babinski (soles of the feet)
Balance	
Romberg test	Have athlete stand with eyes closed, look for loss of balance
Coordination	
Finger–nose testing	Have athlete touch own nose, then the examiner's fingers, repeatedly
Tandem gait	Heel-to-toe walking in a straight line

Notes: * These are some suggested maneuvers; however, the neurological examination will vary as clinically appropriate. † Motor testing is graded: 5 = normal strength; 4 = active movement against resistance; 3 = active movement against gravity only; 2 = able to move limb with gravity eliminated; 1 = flicker of muscle contraction only; 0 = no contractions

449

head and neck injuries

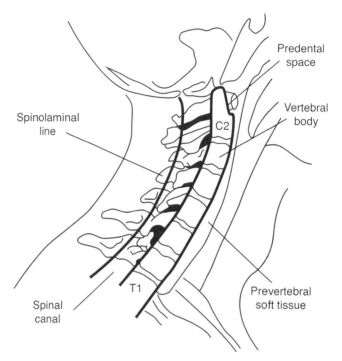

Predental space

Vertebral body

Spinolaminal line

C2

Prevertebral soft tissue

Spinal canal

T1

Figure 21.1 Contours of the cervical spine on lateral X-ray. The anterior and posterior vertebral lines, the spinolaminal line, and the tips of the spinous processes should make smooth contours. The prevertebral tissue in front of the C3 vertebrae should be less than 5 mm and should not be wider than the corresponding vertebral body at each level. Prevertebral tissue swelling or irregular contours suggest injury in the cervical spine

Source: Chuck d'Hemecourt

visualize all seven cervical vertebrae and the superior portion of the first thoracic vertebra. If the seventh cervical vertebra is not visible, a lateral swimmer's view of the neck can be performed, with one arm placed in an overhead position. The C-spine X-rays should be carefully examined for fractures. Other signs of injury or instability include prevertebral soft-tissue swelling, asymmetry of the bony architecture, and disruption of the normal contours of the vertebrae (Figure 21.1).

If the initial views are normal, but a C-spine injury is still suspected, more advanced imaging techniques can be performed. A computed tomography (CT) scan is useful in detecting injury, in particular bone pathology and fractures. Magnetic resonance imaging (MRI) may identify potential injury to the brain, spinal cord, and nerves. Flexion and extension lateral X-ray views can be performed under physician supervision to rule out any ligamentous injury resulting in vertebral instability.

anthony c. luke

A radionuclide bone scan can be used, if advanced testing is unavailable, to rule out any bone injury.

Treatment
Neck fractures may require immobilization or surgical stabilization. If there is compromise to the stability of the neck and risk of injury to the spinal cord, a neurosurgeon or orthopedic surgeon should direct treatment.

Rehabilitation
Depending on the severity of the injury and any residual disability, rehabilitation can be extensive and prolonged to recover appropriate neurologic function, especially if the spinal cord is involved.

CERVICAL SPINE INJURIES

History
- Blow to the head or forceful bending/twisting of the neck.
- Athlete complains of neck pain.
- Athlete may experience weakness or sensory changes in the extremities.

Examination
- Maintain in-line immobilization of the neck throughout the initial assessment.
- Always assume an unconscious athlete has a neck injury.
- Do not move the athlete or remove equipment unless necessary to address life-threatening problems (see Chapter 6).
- To clear the C-spine from injury, gently palpate for tenderness, deformity, without moving the neck (see Chapter 6).
- If the athlete is unwilling to move the neck, assume a serious neck injury.
- Perform a focused neurologic exam.

Treatment
- If suspicion of serious neck injury, immobilize the C-spine and transport athlete for further evaluation/treatment.
- Most minor soft-tissue injuries to the neck improve with symptomatic treatment and physical therapy.

Return to play
- When range of motion in the neck and neurologic exam is normal.
- When athlete is asymptomatic and can meet normal demands of sport.
- If any spinal cord injury has occurred, consider referral to specialist for return-to-play recommendations.

Return to play

Consultation with a specialist will help determine prognosis and return-to-play recommendations. Changing activities to avoid contact or collision sports may be required after a serious injury. In general, before returning to participation in a sport, the athlete should recover full, pain-free range of motion and adequate strength to avoid re-injury. The athlete's neurological exam should be normal, and the C-spine must be stable.

Education for athletes, parents, and coaches is important to raise their awareness of the potential for head and neck trauma, to prevent acute injuries. Athletes should avoid inappropriate or reckless physical contact with other players. Coaches must reinforce proper sports technique, such as tackling with the head up and heading the ball in soccer with the body positioned appropriately. A carefully supervised training program can develop strength and flexibility in the neck. Finally, the rules in sports should reflect principles of safe play and avoid unnecessary contact or dangerous activities that put the athlete at risk.

HEAD INJURIES

Fieldside assessment

Trauma to the head may result in contusion, bleeding, and swelling in the brain tissues. Direct impact to the head may cause a brain injury at the point of contact or on the side opposite to where the blow occurred. Skull fractures can have associated intracranial injuries. Bleeding or pooling of blood can form a hematoma between the tissue layers covering the brain or within the cerebral tissues (Table 21.2). Increased intracranial pressure as a result of bleeding and swelling in the head can potentially affect respiratory control in the brain stem. Consequently, death can occur from a head injury within minutes or hours, depending on the location of bleeding. Skull fractures, intracranial hemorrhages, and cerebral edema are potentially life-threatening injuries. More commonly, head injuries in sports result in a sport-related concussion, which is discussed in the next section.

A head injury should be suspected from the mechanism of trauma. Although most head injuries result from a direct blow to the head, they can also result from acceleration and/or deceleration of the head or neck when a blow is sustained by another part of the body. Any decreased level of consciousness following an impact to the head suggests the patient has sustained a head injury and possibly other neck injuries. A declining level of consciousness, prolonged confusion, post-traumatic seizure, skull fracture, or breathing irregularity may suggest a rapidly progressing intracranial lesion.

The primary survey, or "C–ABCDE" approach, of the acutely injured athlete should be followed (see Chapter 6). The Glasgow coma scale can be calculated by examining the athlete's speech, eye, and motor responses to verbal command or pain (see Chapter 6, Table 6.1). This scale is a useful method of assessing and

Table 21.2 Types of important intracranial injury

Injury	Description	Course	Treatment
Epidural hematoma	Bleeding from rupture of an artery, usually the middle meningeal artery, following a temporal skull fracture	Rapid progression within 2 hours; patient may have a lucid interval	Requires emergency surgical evacuation
Subdural hematoma	Bleeding between the brain surface and the dura, usually from a ruptured vein	Variable progression from 24 hours to several weeks; high fatality if rapidly progressing	Requires emergency surgical evacuation
Subarachnoid hemorrhage	Usually bleeding over the surface of the brain from small vessels or congenital vascular abnormality	Presents with severe headache; "worst headache ever"	Can be monitored unless congenital vascular abnormality present
Intracerebral hematoma	Usually bleeding into the brain tissue from an injured artery or congenital vascular abnormality	May be rapidly progressive	May require surgery

following an athlete's level of consciousness. Glasgow coma scale scores reflect the acute severity of the head injury and facilitate communication with other health professionals who are familiar with the scale.

Simple questions that the athlete should know the answers to, such as "What is your name?", may be asked to initially assess speech, mental status, and cognitive function.

During the eye exam, the pupils should be checked for symmetry. Assess the pupil reactivity to a penlight, by shining the light into one eye while observing the other. Have the athlete follow the penlight in all directions to test the movements of the eyes for symmetry. Unequal pupil size, asymmetric response of the pupils to light, and inappropriate movement of the eyes suggest underlying pressure effects in the head due to bleeding or swelling. Asymmetric movement of the eyes may suggest a cranial nerve palsy, orbital fracture, or an intracranial head injury.

Motor testing of the hands and feet should be performed. Asking the athlete to squeeze the examiner's fingers and move the feet grossly assesses limb motor function and the player's ability to follow commands. Sensation in the fingers and feet can be quickly checked at this time.

If there are any signs of an intracranial injury, the athlete should be stabilized and immediately transferred to a medical facility capable of providing neurosurgical

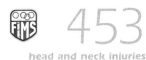

care. The athlete should be transported with C-spine immobilization. Consideration should be given to securing an airway prior to transport, especially if there is a depressed level of consciousness.

During the evaluation for neurological disability, the head is examined for signs of external swelling and trauma. Bleeding behind the tympanic membrane or from the ear canals suggests a skull fracture. Although often not present immediately after injury, bruising around the orbits of the eyes or the base of the skull also suggests a skull fracture. Clear fluid flowing from the ears or nose may indicate a leak of cerebrospinal fluid, which also suggests a skull fracture.

If, ultimately, there are no signs or symptoms concerning for skull fracture, structural intracranial injury, cerebral edema, or cervical spine injury, the patient may be taken off the playing surface and examined more thoroughly (Table 21.1), with particular attention to assessing for concussion (Figure 21.2).

Diagnosis

A CT scan or MRI is required to visualize intracranial bleeding, edema, or shifting of structures in the brain known as mass effect. Skull X-rays are unnecessary unless a skull fracture is suspected and advanced imaging tests such as CT are unavailable.

Treatment

Skull fractures and intracranial injuries are emergencies and should be treated at an appropriate medical facility by a qualified specialist, usually a neurosurgeon. Surgery may be required to evacuate the bleeding, in order to prevent further brain damage. Otherwise, athletes in serious condition are usually monitored closely in hospital until their neurological function recovers.

Athletes who appear stable acutely should be carefully monitored over the next 48 hours. In cases where a head injury is suspected but imaging is not available, precautionary monitoring of the neurological status can be practiced, including waking the athlete up every 2–4 hours during sleep. Early and frequent follow-ups with a physician are recommended. Symptoms may develop over days if slow bleeding is occurring in the head, such as from a subdural hematoma.

Rehabilitation

Rehabilitation depends on the extent of the injury and the residual disability. Serious injury may require physical, neuropsychological, and occupational therapy for cognitive and physical function to be recovered.

Return to play

Return to sports should be considered only when there is complete neurological recovery. A major concern is returning the athlete to sports too quickly. The basic principles are that the athlete may return when full motor and cognitive function have been recovered, and the player has had sufficient time for a brain injury to heal. If an operation such as a craniotomy has been performed, return to play is

anthony c. luke

HEAD INJURIES INCLUDING CONCUSSIONS

History

- Direct impact to the head, or acceleration of the head from a blow elsewhere on the body.
- Loss of consciousness may or may not occur.
- Concussive symptoms include headache, amnesia, dizziness, difficulty concentrating, confusion, sensitivity to light, blurred vision, nausea, increased irritability, emotional lability, sleep disturbance, and/or ringing in the ears.
- Declining level of consciousness, prolonged confusion, post-traumatic seizure, or breathing irregularity suggest a serious head injury.

Examination

- Always assume an unconscious athlete has a potential cervical spine injury.
- Assess eye, motor, and verbal responses to assess level of consciousness (Glasgow coma scale).
- Clear fluid discharge (cerebrospinal fluid) from nose or ear canals, bleeding behind the ear drum or in the ear canals, and/or bruising around the orbits or occiput suggest skull fracture.
- Detailed neurological exam should be performed, including mental-status exam.

Treatment

- For serious head injury, immediately transport athlete for evaluation and treatment.
- For concussions, management is individualized and guided by resolution of symptoms.
- Physical and cognitive rest is recommended while the athlete is symptomatic.
- Early, frequent follow-ups are recommended.
- Adequate time to permit the brain to recover should be allowed.

Return to play

- For simple concussions, the athlete should have no post-concussive symptoms at rest or with exercise and a normal neurological exam.
- Neuropsychological or neurocognitive testing should have returned to baseline, if available.
- The decision to return to play should be made by a physician familiar with sports-related concussion.
- For prolonged recoveries, severe symptoms, or severe cognitive dysfunction, a specialist should be consulted.

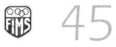

SCAT2

Sport Concussion Assessment Tool 2

FIFA®

Name _____

Sport/team _____

Date/time of injury _____

Date/time of assessment _____

Age _____ Gender ☐ M ☐ F

Years of education completed _____

Examiner _____

What is the SCAT2?[1]

This tool represents a standardized method of evaluating injured athletes for concussion and can be used in athletes aged from 10 years and older. It supersedes the original SCAT published in 2005[2]. This tool also enables the calculation of the Standardized Assessment of Concussion (SAC)[3,4] score and the Maddocks questions[5] for sideline concussion assessment.

Instructions for using the SCAT2

The SCAT2 is designed for the use of medical and health professionals. Preseason baseline testing with the SCAT2 can be helpful for interpreting post-injury test scores. Words in Italics throughout the SCAT2 are the instructions given to the athlete by the tester.

This tool may be freely copied for distribtion to individuals, teams, groups and organizations.

What is a concussion?

A concussion is a disturbance in brain function caused by a direct or indirect force to the head. It results in a variety of non-specific symptoms (like those listed below) and often does not involve loss of consciousness. Concussion should be suspected in the presence of **any one or more** of the following:

- Symptoms (such as headache), or
- Physical signs (such as unsteadiness), or
- Impaired brain function (e.g. confusion) or
- Abnormal behaviour.

Any athlete with a suspected concussion should be REMOVED FROM PLAY, medically assessed, monitored for deterioration (i.e., should not be left alone) and should not drive a motor vehicle.

Symptom Evaluation

How do you feel?

You should score yourself on the following symptoms, based on how you feel now.

	none	mild		moderate		severe	
Headache	0	1	2	3	4	5	6
"Pressure in head"	0	1	2	3	4	5	6
Neck Pain	0	1	2	3	4	5	6
Nausea or vomiting	0	1	2	3	4	5	6
Dizziness	0	1	2	3	4	5	6
Blurred vision	0	1	2	3	4	5	6
Balance problems	0	1	2	3	4	5	6
Sensitivity to light	0	1	2	3	4	5	6
Sensitivity to noise	0	1	2	3	4	5	6
Feeling slowed down	0	1	2	3	4	5	6
Feeling like "in a fog"	0	1	2	3	4	5	6
"Don't feel right"	0	1	2	3	4	5	6
Difficulty concentrating	0	1	2	3	4	5	6
Difficulty remembering	0	1	2	3	4	5	6
Fatigue or low energy	0	1	2	3	4	5	6
Confusion	0	1	2	3	4	5	6
Drowsiness	0	1	2	3	4	5	6
Trouble falling asleep (if applicable)	0	1	2	3	4	5	6
More emotional	0	1	2	3	4	5	6
Irritability	0	1	2	3	4	5	6
Sadness	0	1	2	3	4	5	6
Nervous or Anxious	0	1	2	3	4	5	6

Total number of symptoms (Maximum possible 22)

Symptom severity score
(Add all scores in table, maximum possible: 22 x 6 = 132)

Do the symptoms get worse with physical activity? ☐ Y ☐ N
Do the symptoms get worse with mental activity? ☐ Y ☐ N

Overall rating
If you know the athlete well prior to the injury, how different is the athlete acting compared to his / her usual self? Please circle one response.

no different   very different   unsure

Figure 21.2 Sport Concussion Assessment Tool (sides 1 and 2)

Source: Reproduced with permission from the BMJ Publishing Group; *Br. J. Sports Med.*, 2005; 39:196–204.

anthony c. luke

Cognitive & Physical Evaluation

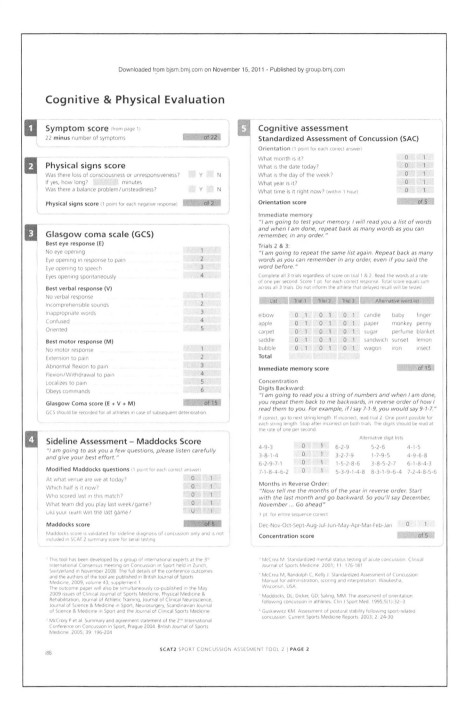

1

Symptom score (from page 1)
22 **minus** number of symptoms .... ▨ of 22

2

Physical signs score
Was there loss of consciousness or unresponsiveness? ▨ Y ▨ N
If yes, how long? ▨ minutes
Was there a balance problem/unsteadiness? ▨ Y ▨ N

Physical signs score (1 point for each negative response) ▨ of 2

3

Glasgow coma scale (GCS)
Best eye response (E)
No eye opening 1
Eye opening in response to pain 2
Eye opening to speech 3
Eyes opening spontaneously 4

Best verbal response (V)
No verbal response 1
Incomprehensible sounds 2
Inappropriate words 3
Confused 4
Oriented 5

Best motor response (M)
No motor response 1
Extension to pain 2
Abnormal flexion to pain 3
Flexion/Withdrawal to pain 4
Localizes to pain 5
Obeys commands 6

Glasgow Coma score (E + V + M) ▨ of 15

GCS should be recorded for all athletes in case of subsequent deterioration.

4

Sideline Assessment – Maddocks Score
"I am going to ask you a few questions, please listen carefully and give your best effort."

Modified Maddocks questions (1 point for each correct answer)
At what venue are we at today? .... 0 ▨ 1
Which half is it now? .... 0 ▨ 1
Who scored last in this match? .... 0 ▨ 1
What team did you play last week/game? .... 0 ▨ 1
Did your team win the last game? .... 0 ▨ 1

Maddocks score ▨ of 5

Maddocks score is validated for sideline diagnosis of concussion only and is not included in SCAT2 summary score for serial testing.

5

Cognitive assessment
Standardized Assessment of Concussion (SAC)
Orientation (1 point for each correct answer)
What month is it? .... 0 ▨ 1
What is the date today? .... 0 ▨ 1
What is the day of the week? .... 0 ▨ 1
What year is it? .... 0 ▨ 1
What time is it right now? (within 1 hour) .... 0 ▨ 1

Orientation score ▨ of 5

Immediate memory
"I am going to test your memory. I will read you a list of words and when I am done, repeat back as many words as you can remember, in any order."

Trials 2 & 3:
"I am going to repeat the same list again. Repeat back as many words as you can remember in any order, even if you said the word before."

Complete all 3 trials regardless of score on trial 1 & 2. Read the words at a rate of one per second. Score 1 pt. for each correct response. Total score equals sum across all 3 trials. Do not inform the athlete that delayed recall will be tested.

List	Trial 1	Trial 2	Trial 3	Alternative word list		
elbow	0 1	0 1	0 1	candle	baby	finger
apple	0 1	0 1	0 1	paper	monkey	penny
carpet	0 1	0 1	0 1	sugar	perfume	blanket
saddle	0 1	0 1	0 1	sandwich	sunset	lemon
bubble	0 1	0 1	0 1	wagon	iron	insect
Total						

Immediate memory score ▨ of 15

Concentration
Digits Backward:
"I am going to read you a string of numbers and when I am done, you repeat them back to me backwards, in reverse order of how I read them to you. For example, if I say 7-1-9, you would say 9-1-7."

If correct, go to next string length. If incorrect, read trial 2. One point possible for each string length. Stop after incorrect on both trials. The digits should be read at the rate of one per second.

		Alternative digit lists	
4-9-3	0 1	6-2-9	5-2-6	4-1-5
3-8-1-4	0 1	3-2-7-9	1-7-9-5	4-9-6-8
6-2-9-7-1	0 1	1-5-2-8-6	3-8-5-2-7	6-1-8-4-3
7-1-8-4-6-2	0 1	5-3-9-1-4-8	8-3-1-9-6-4	7-2-4-8-5-6

Months in Reverse Order:
"Now tell me the months of the year in reverse order. Start with the last month and go backward. So you'll say December, November ... Go ahead"

1 pt. for entire sequence correct

Dec-Nov-Oct-Sept-Aug-Jul-Jun-May-Apr-Mar-Feb-Jan   0 ▨ 1

Concentration score ▨ of 5

---

[1] This tool has been developed by a group of international experts at the 3rd International Consensus meeting on Concussion in Sport held in Zurich, Switzerland in November 2008. The full details of the conference outcomes and the authors of the tool are published in British Journal of Sports Medicine, 2009, volume 43, supplement 1.
The outcome paper will also be simultaneously co-published in the May 2009 issues of Clinical Journal of Sports Medicine, Physical Medicine & Rehabilitation, Journal of Athletic Training, Journal of Clinical Neuroscience, Journal of Science & Medicine in Sport, Neurosurgery, Scandinavian Journal of Science & Medicine in Sport and the Journal of Clinical Sports Medicine.

[2] McCrory P et al. Summary and agreement statement of the 2nd International Conference on Concussion in Sport, Prague 2004. British Journal of Sports Medicine. 2005; 39: 196-204

[3] McCrea M. Standardized mental status testing of acute concussion. Clinical Journal of Sports Medicine. 2001; 11: 176-181

[4] McCrea M, Randolph C, Kelly J. Standardized Assessment of Concussion: Manual for administration, scoring and interpretation. Waukesha, Wisconsin, USA.

[5] Maddocks, DL; Dicker, GD; Saling, MM. The assessment of orientation following concussion in athletes. Clin J Sport Med. 1995;5(1):32-3

[6] Guskiewicz KM. Assessment of postural stability following sport-related concussion. Current Sports Medicine Reports. 2003; 2: 24-30

Figure 21.2 continued

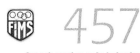

457

head and neck injuries

controversial. Many experts feel a craniotomy is a contraindication to return to play, especially to contact sports. Such athletes should be handled on a case-by-case basis. Some athletes may be advised to participate in non-contact sports with minimal risk of head injury. An experienced specialist may be required to provide these return-to-play recommendations.

CONCUSSIONS

Fieldside assessment

The International Conference on Concussion in Sport defined concussion as "a complex pathophysiological process affecting the brain, induced by traumatic biomechanical forces" (McCrory et al. 2009). Concussion is caused by an acceleration of the brain, either from a direct blow to the head, or from a blow elsewhere on the body with an impulsive force transmitted to the head. A concussion characteristically involves a rapid onset of symptoms, as a consequence of impaired neurological function, that resolves spontaneously. As it is a disturbance of brain function, as opposed to a structural injury, current neuro-imaging studies cannot detect a concussion.

A concussion can present in many different ways (Figure 21.2). The athlete may complain of headache, dizziness, ringing in the ears, nausea, and/or blurred vision. More dramatic symptoms include loss of consciousness, persistent memory loss, slurred speech, convulsions, and breathing irregularities. More subtle symptoms include cognitive impairment, for example, difficulty concentrating or feeling sluggish; feeling more emotions than usual; feeling irritable; or sleep disturbances, such as drowsiness or difficulty sleeping. Symptoms may appear immediately after the injury or may take several minutes to evolve. The acute concern for the team physician is to determine if there is an underlying, structural injury to the brain, or if the athlete has sustained a concussion alone. Although most concussions will resolve spontaneously, recurrent concussions may be cumulative (additive) in nature, and can lead to long-term issues with cognition, depression, and even frank dementia. Some athletes will sustain pathological changes to the brain known as chronic traumatic encephalopathy.

The initial assessment of an apparent concussion should follow the same "C–ABCDE" approach that was described earlier for assessing serious head and neck injuries. If the athlete does not have a condition that requires emergency transfer, the physician may then perform a systematic fieldside assessment. A careful history and neurologic exam (Table 21.1) should be performed to assess for cognitive deficits or abnormal neurologic signs.

The Sport Concussion Assessment Tool Version 2, or SCAT 2 (Figure 21.2), outlines suggested screening procedures to assess the athlete's mental status and cognitive function. Comprehension, memory, concentration, and attention are tested by having the athlete answer a series of questions, follow commands, memorize a list of words, and complete various cognitive tasks.

Exacerbation of post-concussive symptoms may occur after extraocular motion testing. The SCAT 2 includes a standardized balance assessment known as the balance error scoring system (BESS). Balance has been found to be compromised in concussed athletes. Ideally, athletes will have a baseline balance assessment prior to the injury with which post-injury scores can be compared. Any athlete with a suspected concussion should *not* be allowed to return to play on the same day.

Diagnosis

Concussion is a clinical diagnosis; modern neuroimaging studies cannot detect a concussion. The use of previous traditional systems for grading concussions by severity (grade 1, 2, or 3 (worst)) have been discouraged, owing to poor correlation between grading symptoms and clinical recovery. As the management of concussion is still evolving, it is recommended that the medical team and coaching staff should decide on a consistent protocol to manage concussion before the season starts.

Although modern imaging techniques cannot detect concussive brain injury, they may be needed to rule out other injuries, such as intracranial hemorrhages, cerebral edema, and skull fracture. Imaging is recommended particularly if there are signs of extracranial injury, an abnormal level of consciousness (abnormal Glasgow coma scale), or prolonged loss of consciousness (more than 1 minute).

Ideally, each player undergoes baseline balance and neurocognitive assessments before the season to aid the assessment of concussion. The BESS is available for free online and is part of the SCAT 2. In brief, athletes perform double-leg, single-leg, and tandem stances with their eyes closed and hands on their hips. The number of balance "errors" committed during a 20-second trail in each stance is recorded, with the maximum number of recorded errors for any given stance being ten.

Neurocognitive assessments may be recorded by licensed neuropsychologists using standard neuropsychological paradigms, or by a health professional trained in the administration and interpretation of computerized neurocognitive paradigms. Owing to their availability, convenience, and accuracy, computerized assessments have become the preferred method of neurocognitive testing for athletes at risk for concussion. Computerized neurocognitive assessments use specific tasks, often based on traditional neuropsychological tests, to measure verbal memory, visual design memory, concentration, visual processing speed, and reaction time. These tools are sensitive for the detection of sport-related concussion when used in conjunction with symptom reporting and clinical assessment, compared with symptom reporting alone. Baseline scores are then used for comparison after a concussion has been sustained, to determine the presence of clinically significant changes in brain functioning. The tests can be repeated to monitor recovery and help make return to play decisions.

Treatment

Athletes who sustain a sport-related concussion should be removed from play immediately and placed on physical and cognitive rest. Physical rest is well understood in most athletes and involves avoiding physical exertion. Athletes are instructed to refrain from any vigorous exercise, including running, cycling, swimming, and weight lifting, until their symptoms resolve. During cognitive rest, athletes avoid intellectually stimulating activities, tasks that require memory, concentration, and focus. During this stage of recovery, athletes should limit the amount of time they spend reading, playing video games, working online, doing schoolwork, and playing games that demand concentration, such as chess. As most athletes will recover quickly from their concussion, in a matter of a few days or a few weeks, often no further treatment is required. For those athletes who experience severe symptoms, pronounced cognitive dysfunction, or symptoms that persist beyond the first few weeks despite physical and cognitive rest, referral to a specialist in the management of concussion should be considered.

Rehabilitation

Usually, no rehabilitation is required, unless the athlete experiences cognitive or neurologic deficits. If such deficits exist, and there is a need for cognitive, vestibular, or other types of rehabilitation, referral to a specialist should be considered.

Return to play

No athletes should be returned to play until their symptoms have resolved, and never on the same day of the concussion. Athletes should be symptom-free both at rest and with exertion before following a graded return-to-play protocol. They should remain symptom-free after discontinuing any medications started to treat the symptoms of their concussion. In addition, when baseline balance and neurocognitive assessments are available, athletes should have returned to their original levels. Once symptom-free at rest, athletes should begin a graded, stepwise return to play such as that endorsed by the International Consensus on Concussion in Sport and outlined in the SCAT 2. Adults with concussion often recover within 7–10 days. However, younger athletes appear to take longer to recover from concussions, and more conservative management seems warranted. Many experts recommend a longer symptom-free waiting period prior to clearing younger athletes to return to contact sports. During this time, athletes can be encouraged to participate in the non-contact aspects of training and conditioning, if asymptomatic. In addition to age, many other factors may prompt clinicians to increase the symptom-free waiting period before returning an athlete to play, or to consider retiring an athlete from collision sports.

The cornerstone of concussion management is rest until all symptoms resolve, followed by a graded program of exertion before returning to sport. During the period of recovery in the first few days after an injury, it is important to emphasize

CONCUSSION CONSIDERATIONS

- *Age*: Pre-adolescent, adolescent, and elderly may be vulnerable to head injuries. Young athletes do take longer to recover than adults and should be held out longer, often approximately 2 weeks.
- *Number of lifetime concussions*: Although there is no absolute number of concussions after which athletes should be treated more conservatively, the overall number of concussions athletes have sustained should be taken into consideration when determining the timing of return to contact and game play. In general, the more concussions athletes have sustained, the more a conservative approach is warranted.
- *Duration of recovery time*: Athletes who experience prolonged recoveries should be held out of contact and game play for longer periods of time than those who recover more quickly. Likewise, if recovery periods seem to be increasing with successive concussions, a more conservative approach is warranted.
- *Severity of signs and symptoms*: Athletes who suffer severe symptoms, balance problems, or cognitive dysfunction after their concussions should be held out of contact and game play for longer periods of time than those with milder symptoms.
- *Amount of force producing injury*: If athletes seem to be sustaining concussions from collisions involving decreasing amounts of force, they should be held out of contact and game play for longer periods of time.
- *Learning disabilities/attention deficit disorder*: Patients with these conditions may have diminished abilities to compensate for changes in cognitive function while suffering from a concussion. Therefore, more detailed academic accommodations are often warranted, and longer recovery periods are often recommended prior to returning to contact and game play.

to athletes that physical and cognitive rest is required. Activities that require concentration and attention, such as reading or computer work, can exacerbate symptoms and delay recovery. In students, limits may be needed on scholastic activities while symptoms persist.

Many organized contact sports, such as American football, hockey, and rugby, have mandated guidelines for return to play after concussion. In addition, some localities have legislated return-to-play guidelines for athletes who have sustained sport-related concussions. The sports physician should be aware of the pertinent regulations in the particular sport and be prepared to follow them as a minimum requirement.

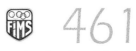

ACUTE CERVICAL SPRAIN/STRAIN

Fieldside assessment

The structure and mobility of the neck make it vulnerable to injury in sport. Ligament sprains and musculotendinous strains occur when neck structures are overstretched and fibers tear. Shearing can occur at the facet joints and the intervertebral disks. Significant muscle spasm can result, limiting range of motion.

Acute cervical sprains and strains can occur from impact to the head or neck, or from forceful rotation, hyperflexion, or hyperextension. A "whiplash" injury can occur when a single violent impact forces the neck into an extreme position, usually extension. Acute torticollis occurs when there are persistent spasms of the neck muscles on one side. The athlete with torticollis presents holding the neck in an unusual position for a prolonged period.

Remember that the initial approach is the same for any head and neck injury. Reluctance to move the neck may suggest a serious neck injury. Palpation of the C-spine should identify any areas of bony tenderness. An athlete with neck strain is usually tender over the soft tissues and muscle, as opposed to the spine itself. If there is tenderness over the spine itself, and the athlete is unwilling to move the neck, the cervical spine should be immobilized, and the athlete should be transferred to a facility capable of obtaining images of the cervical spine. If there is no spinal tenderness, the range of motion of the athlete's cervical spine may be assessed. Muscle spasm may limit movement, and passive stretching of the injured muscles may reproduce pain. It is important to examine the neurological status in the upper and lower extremities. Motor and sensory testing of the muscles in the arm and hand are useful for assessing injury to the brachial plexus and nerve roots (Table 21.1). Athletes with acute uncomplicated cervical sprains or strains will have a normal neurologic exam.

Diagnosis

The diagnosis of neck sprain or muscle strain is made only after more serious spinal injury has been excluded. A complete series of X-rays of the neck, including lateral flexion and extension views, may be necessary to assess bony or cervical disk pathology.

Treatment

Cervical sprains and strains are treated with conservative measures. Icing the affected area is beneficial in the first 48 hours. A short course of oral NSAIDs or other analgesic medications is helpful for pain control. Muscle relaxants are useful only if there is an obvious degree of muscle spasm. A soft cervical collar helps provide support, reducing neck symptoms, and is helpful, especially in the first 2 or 3 days following injury (Figure 21.3).

anthony c. luke

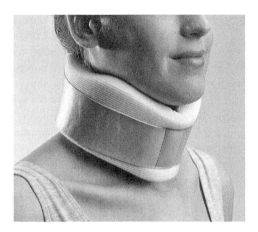

Figure 21.3 Neck collar

Rehabilitation

Early physical therapy is useful. Modalities, such as ice and ultrasound, and manual therapy may reduce discomfort. The goals of therapy are to reduce symptoms, improve range of motion, and ultimately improve the strength of the neck muscles.

Range-of-motion and stretching exercises should be started early to restore mobility to the neck. Isometric exercises are helpful early in therapy to strengthen the neck, to prevent recurrence of injury.

Return to play

The athlete may return to sports once full, pain-free motion is recovered and there are no neurologic symptoms. While doing therapy, athletes may modify training and activities in order to avoid painful activities and re-injury. Most neck sprains and soft tissue injuries resolve within 12 weeks, although some cases can cause prolonged symptoms over even longer than 6 months.

BRACHIAL PLEXUS NEUROPRAXIA

Fieldside assessment

Injury to the brachial plexus or cervical nerve roots result in radicular-type pain, or brachial plexus neuropraxia. These injuries are commonly referred to as "burners" or "stingers." There are three main injury mechanisms described: (1) nerve compression, usually due to narrowing of the neural foramina when the neck is extended and laterally bent; (2) nerve traction; or (3) a direct blow to the brachial plexus. Traction injuries are more common in children and adolescents, whereas compression injuries usually occur in adults. Rarely, permanent nerve damage can result from recurrent brachial plexus injuries.

At fieldside, it is most important to distinguish brachial plexus injury from spinal cord injury before moving the athlete. An athlete with a burner usually complains of a traumatic episode with transient numbness, weakness, and/or electrical pain that shoots down the arm to the hand, often in a specific nerve distribution, lasting from seconds to minutes. Athletes with burners may come off the field shaking their affected arm and hand. The most common pattern of symptoms is over the lateral aspect of the arm, along the radial-nerve distribution (C5–C6). Complaints are almost always unilateral, and the athlete will complain more of arm pain than neck pain. The cervical spine itself should be non-tender. A Tinel's sign may be elicited by tapping in the region of Erb's point (superior and deep to the medial clavicle, just lateral to the sternocleidomastoid muscle). A careful examination of sensation and motor strength should be performed on the upper extremities (Table 21.1). Neurologic testing of the lower extremities should also be performed as part of the examination to rule out spinal cord injury. If the cervical spine is non-tender, Spurling's maneuver may be performed by extending and laterally bending the neck toward the symptomatic side, with gentle downward pressure applied to the head and neck. Reproduction of symptoms down the arm is a positive Spurling's test. In cases of traction injury, lateral bending of the neck away from the symptomatic side may cause stretching of the brachial plexus, reproducing symptoms. The athlete with no sign of C-spine injury can be removed from play and observed on the sidelines.

Bilateral symptoms and cervical spinal tenderness suggest injury to the spinal cord. An athlete with either bilateral symptoms or cervical spinal tenderness should be immobilized and transferred to a facility with imaging capabilities and neurosurgical consultation.

Diagnosis
In cases with persistent radiculopathy after initial injury, or those with recurrent "burners," a complete evaluation, including appropriate imaging, is indicated. Nerve-conduction studies and electromyography can assess the degree and extent of injury, if the athlete experiences chronic neurological deficits of 2 weeks or more. C-spine X-rays and MRI can identify disk disease or cervical spinal stenosis (narrowing of the cervical canal) if these are suspected.

Treatment
Symptoms are usually self-limited. Modification of activities and anti-inflammatory medications help reduce symptoms. A soft neck collar may be used in order to restrict painful neck movement (Figure 21.3).

Rehabilitation
Range-of-motion exercises, including gentle neck stretches, should start as soon as pain diminishes, usually within 48–72 hours. Once the pain improves, the athlete can focus on strengthening the muscles around the neck to help prevent

recurrence of the injury. Any upper-extremity weakness resulting from the temporary neuropraxia should be addressed with appropriate strengthening exercises. Education on proper sports techniques, such as correct tackling in football or rugby, can help avoid these injuries.

Return to play

The symptoms of this condition are usually temporary. Practically, if the player has resolution of symptoms within 15 minutes, a normal neurologic exam, full strength, and pain-free range of motion in the neck, return to play may be considered. If symptoms last longer than 15 minutes, the athlete should be withheld from further sport, and early follow-up should be arranged. When the neurologic symptoms resolve, the athlete may resume some activity. Conditioning training can begin, provided the activities do not exacerbate the problem. After recovery of strength and full, pain-free range of motion in the neck, the athlete can return to full sports. Symptoms can prevent return to many activities even up to 2 weeks in some cases. A protective neck roll or collar is used in some cases to prevent recurrence.

BRACHIAL PLEXUS NEUROPRAXIA

History

- Burning pain or tingling sensation down the arm following lateral bending of the neck.
- Symptoms are unilateral (bilateral symptoms are concerning for spinal cord injury).

Examination

- May have decreased sensation and/or strength in the upper extremity.
- Examine for evidence of C-spine injury.

Treatment

- Symptoms usually self-limited.
- May need to strengthen weakened muscle groups.

Return to action

- When strength, range of motion, and neurologic exam are normal.
- May return to contest if symptoms completely resolve within 15 minutes.

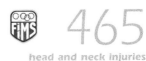

ACUTE CERVICAL DISK DISEASE, CERVICAL SPONDYLOSIS, AND CERVICAL RADICULITIS

Fieldside assessment

The intervertebral spinal disk has a fibrous envelope called the annulus fibrosus, which surrounds a gelatinous center known as the nucleus pulposus. With age and activity, the disks lose height and water content. Weakening of the fibers of the annulus may occur from repetitive movement, axial loading, or trauma involving the neck. Cervical spondylosis occurs when the space between the vertebrae narrows owing to disk degeneration. As the intervertebral spaces narrow, particularly in athletes who participate in contact sports, osteophytes (bone spurs) may develop, both about the disks and posteriorly at the facet joints adjacent to the neural foramina. Although the process of spondylosis may progress slowly over years, with a sudden neck hyperflexion or hyperextension injury, there may be an acute herniation of the nucleus through the fibers of the annulus. Bulging disk contents may encroach on neurologic structures in the spinal canal or neural foramina. In severe cases, fragments of the nucleus pulposus may rupture through the annulus and dislodge. A disk herniation or bone spur can impinge on nerve roots of the brachial plexus, resulting in cervical radiculitis and symptoms radiating to the upper extremity. If the compression of the nerve root is prolonged, permanent arm weakness may result.

The athlete may present with pain and limited neck motion. Pain may radiate from the neck to the top of the shoulder, over the scapula, or down the arm. Usually, radicular pain occurs only on one side, but symptoms may be bilateral. The athlete may report numbness and weakness in the arm and fingers. The physician should always be on alert for other causes for arm and neck pain, such as cardiac causes.

Signs of a serious neck injury should be ruled out. Discogenic neck pain, with or without associated nerve impingement, can usually be diagnosed clinically. The athlete's range of motion in the neck should be noted. Discogenic pain is often worse on flexion. Reflexes, muscle strength, and skin sensation should be examined (Table 21.1). Spurling's maneuver may cause discomfort in some cases.

On occasion, the athlete with cervical radiculopathy may complain of shoulder pain only, and an incorrect diagnosis and management plan may be instituted if the C-spine is not examined.

Diagnosis

Imaging may be required in athletes with severe, persistent symptoms to assess the bony architecture of the C-spine and rule out other problems. X-rays of the neck may reveal decreased disk spaces. Loss of the normal lordotic curve of the spine and marked degenerative osteoarthritis may be signs of "speartackler's spine". This is a more serious condition resulting from repetitive axial loading of the C-spine from impact. Athletes with speartackler's spine are advised to avoid contact sports.

An MRI scan is useful to show the level of the disk herniation or bone abnormality (osteophyte) and confirm the diagnosis. A CT scan is an alternative test, with contrast (myelography) helping to identify compression of neural structures. Electromyography and nerve-conduction studies may demonstrate chronic nerve deficits and help estimate prognosis for recovery.

Treatment

Treatment for these conditions is usually non-surgical. Uncomplicated episodes are usually self-limited, resolving within 2–6 weeks, although they can recur. For pain relief, anti-inflammatory or analgesic medications may be necessary. A heat pad or ice pack can be useful to reduce symptoms. Muscle relaxants are used specifically if there is significant muscle spasm. A soft cervical collar can reduce symptoms during a painful exacerbation. An orthopedic pillow can support the neck during sleep.

In cases of severe pain or persistent neurologic deficit, surgery may be required. Referral to a neurosurgeon or orthopedic spine surgeon is appropriate.

Rehabilitation

Early physical therapy is useful. Stretching and strengthening exercises are important to recover adequate mobility and maintain good support in the neck. Range-of-motion exercises may be performed, with the aim of centralizing any peripheral symptoms toward the neck. Manual therapy and traction are often helpful for reducing symptoms.

Return to play

The athlete can return to sports when full, pain-free range of motion and strength in the neck are recovered. The player may participate in conditioning, as long as symptoms are minimal and not exacerbated. Episodes of this condition can be recurrent, usually months apart. The athlete should learn to recognize the early symptoms of an episode, to modify activities, and to avoid exacerbation of the condition.

LACERATIONS TO THE HEAD AND NECK

Fieldside assessment

Lacerations to the head and neck may be dramatic. It is important not to be distracted by the bleeding and to be consistent with the initial "ABCDE" assessment, as injuries to the airway and C-spine may have occurred.

Consider the location of the laceration to determine the underlying structures that may have been injured. For example, lacerations to the anterior aspect of the neck may injure major blood vessels.

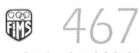

Do not disturb the wound by probing it. If the wound is suspected to be deep, apply firm but gentle pressure to slow bleeding, and transfer the athlete immediately to an appropriate facility. The injury should be evaluated in a controlled environment, with surgical support available. If there is possibility of a fracture underlying a laceration, the patient should also be sent immediately to the hospital. Lacerations involving the eye, lacrimal duct, and ear are often complicated and require repair by a specialist.

Diagnosis

When examining a laceration, first determine the size and depth of the laceration. Gentle pressure can be applied over the edges to decrease bleeding, so that the laceration can be examined. If you suspect that the laceration is very deep, for example a puncture wound, defer the examination until the athlete is at a medical center. If the laceration involves nerve or sensory-organ damage, extensive muscular injury, or a difficult cosmetic repair, the athlete should be sent urgently for care from a qualified specialist.

Treatment

If the injury is superficial, and the appropriate equipment is available, a laceration may be repaired. The laceration should be recent, preferably less than 12 hours old, and relatively clean. If the wound is dirty, it should be irrigated with large amounts of sterile saline solution. Remove all dirt and foreign bodies from the wound before closure. Local anesthetic can be used to infiltrate the wound edges or to perform a nerve block.

A laceration is usually closed with non-absorbable sutures, commonly made of nylon or silk. Deep stitches with absorbable sutures may be necessary in order to close muscle layers or to provide a strong closure. Surgical tape or adhesive skin glue may be used for very superficial wounds. Scalp lacerations can be closed with staples or sutures. Intraoral lacerations can be left without repair if small.

Lacerations involving the eyebrow and mouth should be repaired with particular care to restore the proper alignment of tissue borders. Cosmetic results are important, especially when they involve the face.

If the laceration has been left open for an extended period, the area should be irrigated, cleaned, debrided, and covered with an antibiotic ointment and a sterile dressing. If the wound is gaping, a few sutures may be used to oppose the wound edges; however, the laceration should be closed loosely in order to avoid infection.

Remember to check the athlete's tetanus status and arrange tetanus immunization if he/she is not up to date. If there is a risk of tetanus infection, tetanus prophylaxis may be required. The athlete should be counseled on signs of infection, instructions for wound care, and follow-up for suture removal. Sutures on the face can usually be removed within 5 days to avoid unnecessary scarring.

Rehabilitation

Usually, no rehabilitation is required.

Return to play

Return-to-play decisions are made on an individual basis. The athlete may return to sport if bleeding has stopped, there is no other significant underlying injury, and the area is protected from further damage. Wound dehiscence is a concern, if the area of the repair is located over a mobile joint or subject to excessive contact with equipment or an opponent.

EPISTAXIS (NOSEBLEED)

Fieldside assessment

Most nosebleeds are caused by trauma. Athletes may be predisposed to nosebleeds if they have allergies, a recent upper respiratory infection or previous trauma, or the environment is dry. Epistaxis most commonly involves a plexus of blood vessels on the inner aspect of each nostril along the septum, resulting in an anterior nosebleed. Less commonly, a posterior bleed can occur.

Diagnosis

A nasal speculum exam with a penlight is useful to visualize the site of bleeding. A posterior bleed is suspected if there is heavy blood flow along the oropharynx, with less bleeding anteriorly through the nostrils. Check for injuries to the nasal bones and cartilage.

Treatment

To treat an anterior nosebleed, have the athlete sit up, with the head tilted forward. The player can pinch the nose under the nasal bones, applying firm pressure with the thumb and index finger for approximately 10 minutes. Ice may also be applied. The athlete should not check repeatedly to see if the bleeding has stopped. If bleeding continues, a phenylephrine nasal spray, followed by application of pressure, can be useful. Otherwise, cauterization with application of silver nitrate over the areas of bleeding may be attempted. If bleeding is persistent, the nose requires anterior packing, ideally with petroleum-soaked ribbon gauze or other nasal packing material.

Steady bleeding into the oropharynx suggests a posterior nosebleed. Posterior nosebleeds are complicated to treat, and the athlete should be transferred to a medical facility for possible placement of a posterior pack and subsequent observation. At fieldside, a Foley catheter can be placed through the nose into the oropharynx, inflated, and pulled back, in order to tamponade the blood vessels in the nasopharynx.

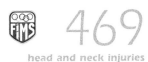

Rehabilitation

Usually, no rehabilitation is required.

Return to play

Players with anterior nosebleeds can return to play once bleeding has stopped. Application of petroleum gel or moisturizer in each nostril helps reduce dryness and irritation in the nose. If the athlete is using NSAID medication or aspirin, alternative medications, including anti-prostaglandin agents with platelet-sparing effects, may be recommended.

EPISTAXIS (NOSEBLEED)

History

- Direct blow to the nose.

Examination

- Nose deformity or pain on palpation of the nasal bones suggest possible fracture.
- Identify bleeding anteriorly from the nostrils or posteriorly along the oropharynx.

Treatment

- Anterior nosebleed: Sit athlete forward, while pinching nose under the nasal bones, applying pressure for at least 10 minutes; if bleeding continues, consider vasoconstrictor spray, cauterization, or anterior packing of nostrils.
- Posterior nosebleed: transport to medical facility for posterior packing.

Return to action

- When bleeding stops.

NASAL FRACTURES

Fieldside assessment

Nasal fractures are caused by direct trauma. Check the nose for bleeding, discoloration, and deformity. The nasal bones may be palpated lightly for tenderness and crepitus. Intranasal examination may show a septal hematoma, which presents as a large, bluish swelling on the inner aspect of the nostril along the nasal septum. The patency of the nasal passages can be evaluated by having the athlete very gently blow out through each nostril. The orbits, maxilla, and teeth should be palpated carefully to rule out any injury to the surrounding structures.

Diagnosis

The nose is usually extremely tender and may be deformed. X-rays of the nasal bones can identify fractures. X-rays of the facial bones should be obtained if there is suspicion of fractures of any other bony structures.

Treatment

Early treatment includes controlling any epistaxis with packing, and application of ice to the nasal area. Non-displaced fractures heal without treatment. The team physician may reduce a nasal bone fracture, as long as there are no worrisome associated injuries and the team physician is experienced. Displaced nasal bones can usually be reset relatively easily within the first 2 hours, before swelling becomes too significant. Otherwise, reduction of the fracture may be delayed for 3–5 days, until the swelling decreases. If a closed reduction cannot be performed within 7–10 days, the nasal fracture may require open reduction, which is typically delayed more than 1 month following the injury. If a septal hematoma is present, prompt drainage or aspiration of the hematoma, using a scalpel or needle, should be performed, followed by anterior packing of the nose. Close follow-up is needed to avoid septal abscess formation and/or permanent deformity of the cartilage in the nasal septum. A specialist should be consulted if available.

Rehabilitation

Usually, no rehabilitation is required.

Return to play

The healing period is approximately 4–6 weeks. Athletes with uncomplicated nasal fractures can return to sports that are associated with low risk for re-injury. However, if the activity involves contact or potential trauma, the athlete should not return to sports unless proper protection is available, such as a protective splint, a face shield, or a helmet with a face guard.

FACIAL FRACTURES

Fieldside assessment

Fractures of the facial bones occur from direct trauma. The bones most frequently involved are the zygoma (cheekbone), the maxilla (midface), the mandible (jaw), or the frontal bone (supraorbital rim of eye orbit). Any significant airway compromise, neck trauma, or intracranial injury should be identified first during the primary "ABCDE" survey.

When an athlete with facial fractures is assessed, the face is examined for swelling, lacerations, and areas of external trauma. Always examine the eyes, nose, and throat for associated injury. The facial bones should be palpated for irregularities, pain, and crepitus. Feel over the orbit and the zygoma for step-off deformities. Check the extraocular movements of the eye and the sensation over the inferior rim of the orbit, because the extraocular muscles and infraorbital nerve can be injured in an orbital fracture. Assess for a significant maxillary fracture by gently pulling forward on the upper front teeth to check for any movement of the midface.

The typical areas for fractures in the jaw are over the articulating joints (condyles), the angle of the jaw (corner of the jaw), and the chin. Look closely at the teeth and gums for signs of bleeding. Ask the patient to bite down, and look for asymmetry or unevenness of the teeth, referred to as "malocclusion." The athlete may describe pain or a feeling that the teeth are uneven. Palpate the temporomandibular joint as the athlete opens and closes the mouth, feeling for uneven motion of the jaw. The athlete may report pain with this maneuver. If any of these signs are present, a mandible fracture is suspected.

If there is a significant risk of respiratory compromise or aspiration due to facial trauma, the physician must secure the airway (see Chapter 6). A nasopharyngeal airway should not be placed if there is a midface fracture.

Intubation may be required to obtain a definitive airway, if the physician is experienced. The athlete should be immediately transferred to a medical facility with surgical capabilities.

Diagnosis

A CT scan is useful for defining the fractures and ruling out any intracranial injuries. A 3D image of any fractures may be reconstructed from the CT scan to help plan the specific management. Alternatively, special X-ray views may be necessary to visualize facial bone fractures well, depending on the bones of concern. Air–fluid levels in the sinuses suggest the presence of fractures.

Treatment

Displaced fractures are often treated with reconstructive surgery of the facial bones. Some repairs can be extensive and require the jaw to be wired shut. A qualified surgeon should direct treatment.

Rehabilitation

Rehabilitation may be extensive to restore movement and function, particularly in the jaw. Treatment includes modalities to the temperomandibular joint, manual therapy, and range-of-motion and coordination exercises.

Return to play

Return to sports can occur when the athlete is fully recovered and at minimal risk of re-injury. Recommendations are best provided by an appropriate specialist. Some athletes may return to sport earlier during the healing process with appropriate protective devices, depending on the extent of the injury. Preventive equipment such as a face shield or a helmet with full-face protection can be used in some sports to avoid re-injury.

anthony c. luke

DENTAL INJURIES

Fieldside assessment

A tooth may be cracked, chipped, loosened, or completely displaced by a collision with another athlete, or a direct blow from a piece of equipment. The front teeth in the upper row are usually affected. In approximately half of all cases, more than one tooth is damaged. Injuries to the teeth are more common in children than in adults. In children, tooth injuries that are not properly managed may lead to long-term dental deformity. The athlete with a dental injury should be sent to a facility that is able to provide appropriate dental care.

Signs of dental trauma include bleeding or swelling around a tooth or gum, or irregular appearance of the teeth. Check for malocclusion of the athlete's bite and for any intraoral lacerations. Carefully examine the teeth that are adjacent to obviously injured teeth. Apply gentle pressure to the teeth to check for discomfort and subtle loosening. If there is some bleeding around the gums, the athlete may apply light pressure by biting down on a saline-soaked gauze or cotton roll.

If an acute avulsion of a tooth occurs and its socket is clean, the tooth can be rinsed with water and repositioned in the socket immediately. The athlete is removed from play. If the socket is not clean, the tooth should be stored in a medium that will preserve the periodontal cells to optimize recovery. Exposure of the raw tooth to the air for more than 30 minutes can cause tooth death and make it impossible to rescue. There are commercially available solutions for storing avulsed teeth. Otherwise, pasteurized milk is a good medium that is relatively free from bacteria and can keep the periodontal cells viable for around 6 hours.

If this is not available, the tooth can be kept in the athlete's own mouth under the tongue if he/she is compliant. Water is used if there is no alternative.

Athletes complaining of severe pain and sensitivity to heat, cold, or pressure may have injuries to the root and the pulp. Fractures affecting the dentin and pulp may predispose the tooth to infection and tooth death.

Diagnosis

Almost all dental injuries should be assessed by a dentist or qualified physician. X-rays can help identify any injuries to the root, as well as fractures in the alveolar bone. Pulp testing is performed to check for viability of the nerve root.

Treatment

Dental injuries are best assessed by a dentist within 24 hours of the injury, depending on the severity. Some cases may require root canal, if necrosis of the pulp occurs.

Rehabilitation

Usually, no rehabilitation is necessary, unless there is injury to the tempero-mandibular joint.

Return to play

After initial treatment has been completed, the athlete should be able to continue training, as long as there is no risk of re-injury to the teeth. Dental injuries may take several weeks to heal, if there is significant dental or alveolar trauma. With serious injuries, the dentist should make the recommendations concerning return to contact sports. A protective mouth guard should be used if the athlete participates in a contact sport. Mouth guards may be custom-made by a dentist, or bought and molded by the athletes themselves.

DENTAL INJURIES

History
- Direct impact to the mouth/teeth.

Examination
- Bleeding or swelling around a tooth or gum.
- Cracked, chipped, or missing tooth.
- Check the teeth that are adjacent to obviously injured teeth for loosening.

Treatment
- Dentist should evaluate within 24 hours if severe injury.
- For tooth avulsion, immediately reposition tooth, after rinsing in water, in clean socket and transport athlete to medical/dental facility.
- If socket is not clean, store tooth immediately in an appropriate medium.

Return to action
- When there is no risk of further damage to tooth.
- Consult dentist for recommendations.
- Mouthguards can reduce the risk of injury to teeth.

EYE INJURIES

Fieldside assessment

Although eyes are naturally well protected from trauma, ocular injuries still occur during sports. Contact, ball, and racket sports are activities with high risk for eye injuries, particularly baseball and basketball. Eye injuries are usually caused by blunt or penetrating trauma to the eye. When an object hits the eye, bleeding can occur.

anthony c. luke

Bruising, swelling, and discoloration of the soft tissues around the eye are known as an orbital hematoma or "black eye." A "hyphema" is caused by bleeding into the anterior chamber of the eye, between the lens and the cornea. The posterior segment of the eye may also be disrupted, leading to retinal tears or detachment. Traumatic rupture of the globe, laceration of the eye, dislocation of the intraocular lens, penetrating injury, chemical exposure, and orbital fractures are other serious ocular injuries.

The athlete may complain of eye pain and blurred vision. Floating spots, flashes of light, partial or complete loss of sight, or decreased quality of vision are warning symptoms of internal injury to the eye. The physician should determine whether the athlete uses any corrective glasses or contact lenses. The athlete's past medical history, including previous eye injuries or eye surgeries, should be elicited. The eye exam should begin with visual acuity testing, using a small eye chart and any corrective lenses that the athlete wears. The eyes and lids should be inspected for swelling or lacerations. Both pupils should be examined with a penlight, looking for symmetry and constriction response to light. Extraocular movements can be tested by having the player track the examiner's finger or penlight in all directions. Evaluate peripheral vision in each eye by covering the athlete's non-test eye and asking him/her to identify objects, such as a small red pin or a finger, brought into the field of vision by the examiner. The athlete should fix his/her eye on the examiner's eye, directly positioned 2 feet in front, during peripheral-field testing. Palpate around the orbit for any deformity, crepitus, or pain. An ophthalmoscopic examination may identify corneal injury, bleeding in the anterior chamber, and injuries to the retina. However, this exam is often not practical on the field.

All eye injuries need to be taken seriously, because of the potential for long-term damage to the athlete's sight. If there is any evidence of decreased visual acuity, bleeding, or internal injury to the eye, the athlete should be transferred immediately to a hospital to be assessed by an ophthalmologist. A plastic or metal eye shield can be used to cover the affected eye until the athlete is evaluated by the specialist. If there is no eye shield available, the bottom of a clean, disposable cup can be cut out and used. If an internal injury to the eye is suspected, the athlete should sit up to avoid increasing intraocular pressure and should avoid any Valsalva-type maneuvers.

Diagnosis
A slit lamp examination is useful to examine the corneal surface and the internal structures of the eye. Medicated eye drops are used in some cases to anesthetize the eye and dilate the pupil for proper examination. Pressure tonometry may be performed if elevated pressure in the eye, referred to as "glaucoma," is suspected.

Treatment
Treatment may be complicated, depending on the nature of the injury, and should be directed by an ophthalmologist.

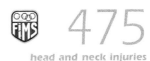

Rehabilitation

Usually, no rehabilitation is required.

Return to play

If the athlete has an acute soft-tissue injury with no visual disturbance, removal from play and observation are appropriate. Ice may be applied to the affected area, without putting pressure on the eye. If the athlete regains pre-injury levels of visual acuity and has normal peripheral vision, no eye pain, no headache, a normal eye exam, and a normal neurological exam, the player may return to competition.

If the athlete suffers a more serious eye injury, sufficient rest time should be allowed for the eye to heal, and an ophthalmologist should make the return-to-play recommendations. Typically, the athlete may return to play when visual acuity

---

EYE INJURIES

History

- Direct contact with the eye.
- Athlete often complains of eye pain, blurred vision, tearing.
- Floating spots, flashes of light, partial or complete loss of sight, and decreased quality of vision suggest internal eye injury.

Examination

- Check visual acuity.
- Examine pupils, extraocular movements, and peripheral-field vision.
- Perform fundoscopy with an ophthalmoscope if possible.
- Apply fluorescein to the eye to identify corneal abrasion with a cobalt blue light.

Treatment

- Transfer the athlete, sitting if possible, to a medical facility for immediate evaluation if there is decreased visual acuity, bleeding, or internal injury to the eye.
- Protect the eye with an eye shield and avoid any direct pressure to the eye.

Return to play

- When pre-injury visual acuity is recovered, the athlete is asymptomatic, and adequate time has passed to let the eye injury heal.
- Polycarbonate, protective eyewear can prevent eye injuries.
- An ophthalmologist can make return-to-play recommendations in complicated cases.

---

has returned to baseline levels, and there is no evidence of pain or internal injury to the eye. Proper protective eyewear should be worn. Glasses with polycarbonate lenses are commonly recommended for protection from injury. A visor or cage may be added to an athlete's helmet to protect the eyes and face.

A functionally one-eyed athlete is an individual with best-corrected visual acuity less than 20/40 (able to see at 20 feet what an average individual is expected to see at 40 feet). Such an athlete should be encouraged to participate in sports with low risks for eye injuries, such as track and field, swimming, or gymnastics, as damage to the good eye may result in severe handicap.

CORNEAL ABRASIONS AND FOREIGN BODIES

Fieldside assessment

A corneal abrasion occurs when the surface of the eye is scratched by an object such as a finger, stick, or foreign body. Symptoms may include pain, burning, tearing, blurred vision, sensitivity to light, or a foreign body sensation in the affected eye.

The eye will typically be red and injected. The athlete's visual acuity should be tested. An examination of the surface of the eye with a penlight or ophthalmoscope may identify a foreign body or a scratch on the cornea. The eyelids should be retracted and examined for foreign bodies.

Diagnosis

A corneal abrasion is best identified by placing fluorescein eye drops in the affected eye and examining the cornea with a cobalt blue light. An abrasion usually appears as a fluorescent green mark. Multiple vertical streaks over the cornea suggest a foreign body trapped under the eyelid.

Treatment

Corneal abrasions are treated symptomatically and often require pain medication. Antibiotic drops, such as erythromycin or gentamicin, are suggested to avoid infection. Abrasions should heal, regardless of treatment, without an eye patch, as long as there is no further injury to the eye. The athlete should be re-examined within 48 hours.

Any foreign bodies should be removed by an experienced physician. The upper eyelid can be retracted using a cotton-tipped applicator placed at the base of the eyelid. With the athlete looking down, the physician grasps the eyelashes and folds the eyelid over the applicator. Holding the lid inverted with one thumb, the examiner removes the foreign body from under the lid, using the applicator. If a foreign body is embedded in the cornea, such as a small piece of metal, a slit lamp can visualize the object clearly for safe removal. Experienced clinicians may consider removing the object with a small-gauge needle, after anesthetizing the

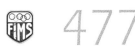

head and neck injuries

eye with drops. Follow-up should be arranged within 48 hours to identify any signs of corneal ulcers or rust ring formation, which require further management.

Rehabilitation

Usually, no rehabilitation is required. The epithelial layer of the cornea heals in 48–72 hours.

Return to play

Symptoms usually resolve in 3–5 days. The athlete may return to sports if visual acuity is normal and pain is tolerable. The eye can be protected from further injury with protective eyewear until the abrasion heals.

EAR INJURIES

Fieldside assessment

Ear injuries may be classified as outer-, middle-, or inner-ear injuries. External ear injuries in sports are usually due to trauma. The outer ear may be struck or grabbed, resulting in lacerations, contusions, and partial avulsions of the auricle. An auricular hematoma may form from subcutaneous bleeding and may involve the entire ear.

Trauma to the middle or inner ear can result from blasts, direct impact to the unprotected ear, or pressure changes. Middle- and inner-ear injuries may present with hearing loss, dizziness, vertigo, pain, or ringing in the ears (tinnitus). An athlete who complains of severe ear pain, bleeding from the ear canal, or impaired hearing after a blow to the side of the head should be sent to a facility for immediate medical evaluation.

Air-pressure injuries of the ear, known as "otic barotrauma," occur when the individual cannot equalize the air pressure between the middle ear and the external environment. This can occur during activities involving altitude or pressure changes, such as skydiving or scuba diving. Athletes with congestion of the nasal passages from a viral illness, allergy, or other infection are at increased risk of barotrauma. Pressure changes can cause bleeding in the middle ear and even burst the tympanic membrane (ear drum).

Infections can occur in the external and middle ear. Infections of the external ear canal often cause pain, itchiness, swelling, and discharge. This usually occurs in swimmers. Otitis media is an infection of the middle ear. Athletes may complain of pain and pressure inside the ear and often have an associated upper respiratory tract infection.

External injuries to the ear are usually easily seen. Examine the ear canal and the middle ear carefully with an otoscope. Bleeding behind the tympanic membrane (hemotypanum), bleeding from the ear canal, or leaking of clear cerebrospinal fluid suggest a possible skull fracture and intracranial injury. Check the extraocular movements for evidence of nystagmus, which are small, rapid, abnormal eye movements. Nystagmus suggests that the vestibular system in the inner ear is affected.

Hearing should always be carefully evaluated. The physician can grossly assess hearing by whispering three numbers in the athlete's ear while distracting the other ear by rubbing tissue paper outside the ear canal. The athlete should be able to repeat the numbers. More specifically, hearing can be checked by placing a tuning fork over the base of the skull, and then positioning the tines over the ear. An athlete with a conductive hearing loss, due to a middle- or external-ear problem, will hear the tuning fork over the base of the skull well, but will have more difficulty hearing the tuning fork over the ear. A sensorineural hearing loss, which suggests an inner-ear problem, will present with difficulty hearing the tuning fork in both locations. An appropriate specialist, usually an otolaryngologist, should be involved in cases that involve hearing loss.

Diagnosis
An audiogram should be performed to determine if there is a conductive or sensorineural hearing loss. A CT scan or MRI may be required, if there is any suspected trauma to the skull or inner ear.

Treatment
External injuries to the ear are usually treated conservatively. A soft-tissue injury to the external ear may be treated with brief application of ice. A preauricular hematoma should be aspirated with a needle or removed surgically near its inferior aspect. A firm compression bandage should then be applied over the ear to prevent reoccurrence of the hematoma. An experienced physician may repair simple lacerations or partial avulsions, although any anesthetic used should not include epinephrine. External ear infections are usually treated with antibiotic and corticosteroid eardrops.

Middle-ear problems should be followed carefully, while management for inner-ear injuries requires consultation. A ruptured tympanic membrane usually heals spontaneously within 8 weeks. Middle-ear infections are often treated with an appropriate course of antibiotics.

Rehabilitation
Usually, no rehabilitation is required.

Return to play
Athletes who have sustained an ear injury may return to sports, when they are at little risk of re-injury. The player should have adequate hearing function to participate safely and effectively. Protective headgear may be used to prevent further trauma to the ear. Athletes involved in sports with loud noises, such as shooting sports, should wear proper hearing protection. Water sports should be avoided in athletes who have a ruptured tympanic membrane, until it heals. During

activities at high altitude or underwater, athletes should frequently compensate for pressure changes by swallowing, chewing, or blowing through the nose while pinching the nostrils shut with the thumb and forefinger. Athletes with nasal-passage congestion should take precautions when flying and avoid sports with dramatic air-pressure changes to prevent barotrauma. An appropriate specialist may help make recommendations for participation in sports for athletes with specific hearing disabilities.

EAR INJURIES

History

- Usually due to direct trauma, pressure change, or infection.
- Middle- and inner-ear injuries may present with hearing loss, dizziness, vertigo, pain, or ringing in the ears.
- External ear problems present with pain and swelling.
- Check hearing in both ears.
- Examine the external and middle ear with an otoscope.
- Nystagmus suggests an inner-ear problem.

Treatment

- Acute hearing loss, sudden severe ear pain, and/or bleeding or cerebrospinal fluid leak from the ear canal should be evaluated immediately.
- A ruptured tympanic membrane usually heals spontaneously.
- Antibiotics can resolve external- and middle-ear infections.

Return to action

- When the athlete has adequate hearing to participate safely and effectively in sport.
- Avoid water sports until a ruptured tympanic membrane heals.
- Avoid activities involving altitude/pressure changes, while experiencing nasal congestion.
- Proper headgear and hearing protection can prevent ear trauma.

SUGGESTED READING

Cantu R.C. Intracranial hematoma. In: Cantu R.C. (Ed.), *Neurologic Athletic Head and Spine Injuries*. Philadelphia: WB Saunders; 2000:124–31.

Dailey A., Harron J.S., France J.C. High-energy contact sports and cervical spine neuropraxia injuries: What are the criteria for return to participation? *Spine*, 2010; 35(21 Suppl.): S193–201.

Emerich K., Kaczmarek J. First aid for dental trauma caused by sports activities: State of knowledge, treatment and prevention. *Sports Med.*, 2010; 40(5): 361–6.

Lovell M., Collins M., Bradley J. Return to play following sports-related concussion. *Clin. Sports Med.*, 2004; 23: 421–41.

McCrory P., Meeuwisse W., et al. Consensus Statement on Concussion in Sport. 3rd International Conference on Concussion in Sport, Held in Zurich, November 2008. *Clin. J. Sport Med.*, 2009; 19: 185–200.

Safran M.R., Nerve injury about the shoulder in athletes, part 2: Long thoracic nerve, spinal accessory nerve, burners/stingers, thoracic outlet syndrome. *Am. J. Sports Med.*, 2004; 32: 1063–76.

Stiell I.G., Clement C.M., McKnight R.D., et al. The Canadian C-spine rule versus the NEXUS low-risk criteria in patients with trauma. *N. Engl. J. Med.*, 2003; 349(26): 2510–18.

Weber T.S., MD. Training room management of eye conditions. *Clin. Sports Med.* 2005; 24: 681–93.

PART III

OTHER SPORTS INJURIES AND MANAGEMENT

CHAPTER 22

TAPING AND BRACING IN SPORTS

Jaspal S. Sandhu and Shweta Shenoy

INTRODUCTION

Taping is the application of adhesive tape around a joint to provide a semi-rigid, and sometimes rigid, splint. Bracing refers to application of orthoses over an injured joint or bone for immobilization while allowing functional range of motion in the required planes.

The oldest methods of preventing injuries in sports involve the application of external devices, be it bracing or taping. As early as the mid 1940s, Quigley et al. (1946) reported that there was a marked reduction in the risk of ankle sprains following usage of tape, to an extent of 50%. Taping has been used as a standard method of treatment and prevention of various injuries in healing tissues for the last 40 years. Healing tissue is susceptible to re-injury following premature or over-enthusiastic training, and it was standard practice to advise complete immobilization until the tissues healed completely. However, it is now known that immobilization increases the risk of complications such as stiffness and poor tensile strength in the healing tissue. Protected range of motion is now advised as a standard treatment, as it promotes alignment of collagen along the lines of stress. It is from this knowledge that the concept of taping and bracing has evolved. The idea is to support and protect healing and healed tissues until they have gained adequate strength, while allowing athletes to return to functional and sporting activity. This is important in reducing time to refrain from such activity to prevent deterioration. Taping and bracing are thus beneficial, if not absolutely necessary, in the subacute and chronic stages of healing. However, a proper anatomical and pathological diagnosis of injury is a requirement for providing appropriate external support. Equally important is the site and degree of injury. The basic aim of external support is to allow function and to prevent re-injury, allowing rehabilitation in athletes requiring surgery or otherwise. External support provides stability and support to injured structures that allow athletes to return to play before they have returned to their pre-injury status anatomically, but it is not a replacement for proper and adequate rehabilitation. External support can be an adjunct to various rehabilitation protocols followed. It is not a method to forestall adequate, appropriate, and complete

rehabilitation, which includes drug therapy, flexibility, strengthening, proprioception, endurance, etc. It also acts as a preventive barrier by reducing the velocity of
deformation, to limit the degree of injury and thus reduce its severity.

REVIEW OF LITERATURE

There have been several studies comparing taping with bracing as a preferred
procedure, keeping under consideration the capabilities of each procedure to
prevent injury, allowance of movement, and other neuromuscular factors, but it
has been clearly demonstrated that both taping and bracing have a positive role
in preventing injuries, while allowing adequate movement in the required planes.
Myburgh et al. (1984) observed that tapes provided a significant support before
and after 10 minutes of exercise, but lost their efficacy after 1 hour of exercise.
Non-elastic (zinc oxide) tape was proven to be restrictive, and the range of motion
was decreased between 30 and 50%. Löfvenberg and Kärrholm (1993) made
similar observations for semi-rigid orthoses especially to protect ligament reconstructions. Anderson et al. (1995) found that braces reduced the maximum
calcaneal inversion angle, lengthened the inversion time, and reduced the inversion
velocity, thus protecting the joint from substantial injury.

The stabilizing function of tape in the weight-bearing portions tends to decrease
after about 15 minutes of activity, whereas taping in the upper limbs seems to
maintain its protective function much longer. However, because of allergic skin
reactions and the necessity for the reapplication of tape, braces are preferred by
others. Tropp et al. (1985) suggested that orthosis was an alternative to taping in
the rehabilitation period after injury. Greene and Hillman (1990) found semi-rigid
orthoses to be more effective than taping in guarding against ligamentous
re-injury. Shapiro et al. (1994) opined that the advantage of bracing lay in the fact
that it could be re-adjusted to restore effectiveness, whereas taping deteriorated
with usage. Verbrugge (1996) noted that both air-stirrup brace and conventional
tape were effective in the prophylaxis of ankle injuries. Both ankle support systems
of taping and bracing are equally effective, and Gross et al. (1994) advocated
personal choice in selecting a system.

Besides limiting extremes of motion beyond the physiological limits, both systems
have a major role in providing afferent feedback. Indeed Rarick et al. (1962) noted
that, although tape lost its stabilizing effect after some time, it continued to have
a beneficial effect on reducing re-injury by enhancing proprioceptive feedback.
Feuerbach and Grabiner (1994) noted that orthoses increased the afferent feedback of cutaneous receptors, leading to improved ankle-joint position. Robbins et
al. (1995) proved that ankle taping improved proprioception before and after
exercise and corrected impaired proprioception partly caused by faulty athletic
footwear. Lohrer and Gollhofer (1999) observed that taping increased the proprioceptive amplification ratio, which was explained by physiological neuromuscular
regeneration and mechanical stabilization of the tape.

The increased neuron excitability following ankle bracing can be used for the purpose of rehabilitation (Alt et al., 1999). Karlsson and Andréasson (1992) observed shortening of the reaction time of peroneal muscles, as well as restriction of movement at the extremes, due to ankle taping. The findings of Ebig et al. (1997) were similar: they observed a diminished response time for both peroneal and tibialis anterior muscles. Cordova et al. (1998) noted that ankle bracing reduced the strain on the peroneus longus muscle during peak impact force.

Although there have been certain reports that these stabilizing devices may affect the athletes' performance, the benefits seem to outweigh this. Burks et al. (1991) and Gross et al. (1994) noted a minor decrease in performance following use of prophylactic ankle braces; however, this performance decrement was not significant enough to prevent the usage of tapes or braces. On the contrary, other investigators, such as Wiley and Nigg (1996) and Pienkowski et al. (1995), observed that ankle-joint orthoses restricted joint motion without affecting performance. This observation was also substantiated by the findings of Macpherson et al. (1995) on Aircast support stirrups and DonJoy RocketSoc, who found no adverse effects on performance. The effects of tape and bracing on improving postural control have also been documented. Feuerbach and Grabiner (1994) found a better postural control following usage of Aircast stirrups in their study on ankle injuries. Bennell and Goldie (1994) observed that tape or bracing made the athletes steadier during rehabilitation. Thus, bracing and taping help in rehabilitation and in reducing the risk of further injury (Goldie et al., 1994).

The efficacy of tape depends on the procedure and the skill of the practitioner. It is a common saying among the taping fraternity that, "Tape is the medicine, tension is the dose." When to tape or brace depends upon the accurate diagnosis and clinical acumen of the sports medicine consultant.

TAPING PROCEDURES

The application of adhesive tape – elastic (stretch) or non-elastic (rigid) – in order to provide support and protection to soft tissues and joints to minimize swelling and pain after injury is referred to as taping or strapping.

Figure 22.1
Anchors: The first strips of tape applied above and below the injury site, to which subsequent strips are attached. Anchors minimize the traction on the skin

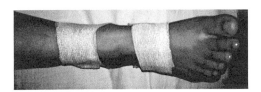

Figure 22.2
(A) Support strips or stirrups, to restrict unwanted sideways movement

(B) Horizontal strips/spurs, to add stability to the joint

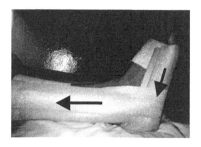

Figure 22.3
Basketweave: Stirrups or spurs in half overlapping layers to build a pattern

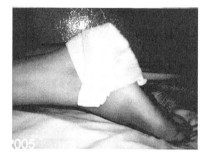

Figure 22.4
Locking straps: Short circular tapes to cover all exposed skin and lock down the tape job

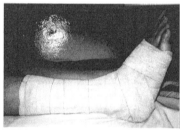

Figure 22.5
Foam padding: To fill in hollows, compress swelling, and pad sensitive areas

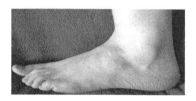

Figure 22.6
Figure of six: To support and reinforce one side of the ankle, start as a stirrup, and cross to form a six

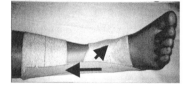

Figure 22.7

Half heel lock: The tape makes a U to lock one side of the heel. Full heel locks can also be used, which cover both sides of the heel

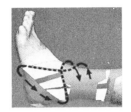

Figure 22.8

Bandage: Used as a compression bandage, as in PRICE

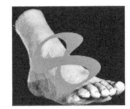

Figure 22.9

(A) Spica: Thumb spica is repeated figure 8. (B) Use check reins to restrict range of motion. (C) Use lock strips to secure cut end of stretch tape so that it does not roll back

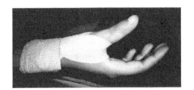

Table 22.1 Taping terminology

Guidelines	Application	Removal	Avoid
Wash, dry, and shave the area	Apply tape at room temperature	Tape, if left too long, leads to skin breakdown	Excessive traction
Remove oils	Position yourself and athlete so that there is minimal fatigue	Tape should not be left for more than 24 hours	Continuous circumferential strips and excessive layering, as they impair circulation and neural transmission
Cover broken lesions	Use correct type, width, and amount of tape	Peel tape carefully	
Use underwrap for sensitive skin	Overlap successive strips by half	Apply lotion	
	Apply it with even pressure	Check the skin for damage	
	Apply with comfort	Push the skin away from the tape while pulling the tape	

Table 22.2 Taping material

Non-stretch tape	Stretch/elastic tape	Hypoallergic
Non-yielding cloth backing used: • to support inert structures • to limit joint movement • to protect against re-injury • to reinforce stretch tape • to secure end of stretch tape	Stretch/elastic tape used: • to compress and support soft tissues, e.g. muscles • to provide anchors for muscles when applied without tension *Caution*: Allow lateral 2 cm to recoil before sticking down	1 Non-stretch 2 Stretch

Taping for injuries on lateral aspect of ankle

▓ Position: neutral.
▓ Indication: ankle inversion sprain, strain to peroneus tendons.

Method of application

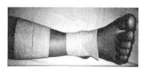

Figure 22.10 Anchors should be placed 5 cm distal to the belly of gastrocnemius

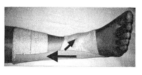

Figure 22.11 First support should start just proximal to the lateral malleolus

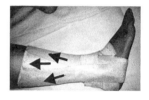

Figure 22.12 The second support starts proximal to the first support, creating a "V" with the first support. The third support is in the center of the first two

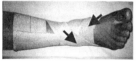

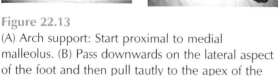

Figure 22.13
(A) Arch support: Start proximal to medial malleolus. (B) Pass downwards on the lateral aspect of the foot and then pull tautly to the apex of the medial arch

jaspal s. sandhu and shweta shenoy

Ligament and tendon support to the foot

- Position: neutral.
- Indication: eliminate posteromedial pain, posterior tibiotalar ligament pain.

Method of application

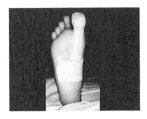

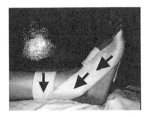

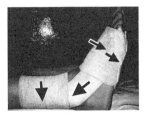

Figure 22.14
Apply tape from the plantar and distal aspect of great toe to the mid portion of the arch. Anchor the tape at the sole and phalanges of toe

Figure 22.15
Place a piece of 7.5-cm tape on the lateral aspect of the foot

Figure 22.16
Use 7.5-cm tape and anchor the tape around the foot and lower leg

Achilles tendon support: Method I

- Position: patient sitting with knee bent and foot relaxed.
- Indication: Achilles tendon strain.

Method of application

Figure 22.17
Cut 30-cm strip of 7.5-cm stretch tape, split it into four tails, 10 cm deep

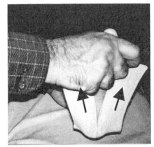

Figure 22.18
Wrap the front tails around mid foot, and other two tails above the Achilles tendon, pulling the foot in plantarflexion. Apply anchors at the edge

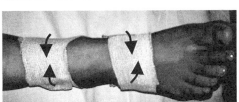

Achilles tendon support: Method II

- Position: patient lying prone, leg over the end of the bed.
- Indication: active sport.

Method of application

Figure 22.19 Apply two anchors, one around the foot, another around the proximal end of the calf

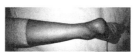
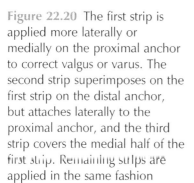

Figure 22.20 The first strip is applied more laterally or medially on the proximal anchor to correct valgus or varus. The second strip superimposes on the first strip on the distal anchor, but attaches laterally to the proximal anchor, and the third strip covers the medial half of the first strip. Remaining strips are applied in the same fashion

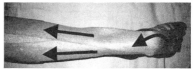

Figure 22.21 Spread the strips apart – no wrinkles

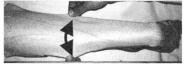

Figure 22.22 Lock the strips proximally and distally with half circles of tape

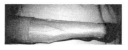

Figure 22.23 For lateral stabilization, apply 2–3 strips from medial to lateral, attaching to the proximal anchor

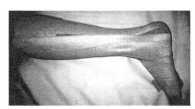

492

Heel bruise taping

- Position: patient prone, foot over the edge of the bed.
- Indication: reduce pressure on heel.

Method of application

Figure 22.24 Stick heel pad. Place the first strip around the calcaneus at the level of the Achilles tendon and the second strip passing under the heel and upwards to the medial aspect

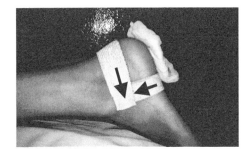

Figure 22.25 Continue basket weave, each strip should be overlapping with the others. Apply anchors for fixation

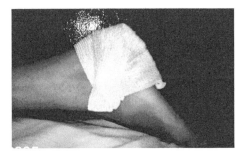

Medial fasciitis support

- Position: patient with leg prone, foot over the end of the bed.
- Indication: relieve medial longitudinal arch pain or over-pronation; lift and support the medial arch.

Method of application

Figure 22.26
Using 5-cm tape, start proximal to the head of the first metatarsal, going along the medial border, around the heel, and across the sole, and finish at the starting point

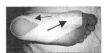

Figure 22.27 Repeat the same procedure with the fifth metatarsal

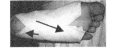

Figure 22.28 Fill the gaps with stretch tape

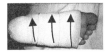

Figure 22.29 Secure edges with 3.75-cm tape, starting from the 5th metatarsal head around the heel. Put one lock over the dorsum of the foot

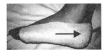

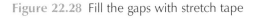

Great-toe taping

- Position: neutral.
- Indication: turf toe.

Method of application

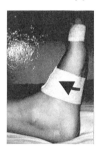

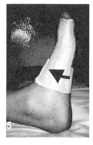

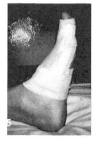

Figure 22.30
Apply one anchoring strip at the distal aspect of the great toe and another at the mid-foot

Figure 22.31
Apply 4–6 strips of tape to form a fan shape from one anchor to the other

Figure 22.32
Apply a continuing strip of 5-cm stretch tape as a spika around the great toe and mid foot

Knee support (diamond wrap)

- Position: slightly flexed.
- Indication: retropatellar pain, jumper's knee, Osgood-Schlatter disease.

Method of application

Figure 22.33
Lay 10-cm tape on the back of the knee, with gauze square in the popliteal fossa. Split both edges of tape, forming four tails. Apply tape around the patella superiorly and inferiorly, interlocking the edges

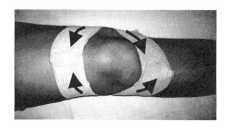

Taping for collateral ligaments of knee

- Position: slightly flexed.
- Indication: sprain of collateral ligaments.

Method of application

Figure 22.34 Cut 45 cm of stretch tape. Apply first strip of 15–20 cm below knee joint, lateral to posterior midline; direct this strip over center of medial joint line upwards, above the patella, over the anterior midline, 15–20 cm above the joint line

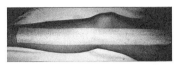

Figure 22.35 Apply second strip in a similar manner, starting anteriorly below and ending posteriorly above. Apply third strip between first two strips

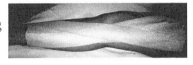

Figure 22.36 Apply anchors around lower leg, leaving 2.5 cm of earlier strips below it. Fold three supports up and continue anchor around leg to cover overlap. Fold all three supports down, rotate foot and hip outward, pull supports up till fully stretched, and apply in same direction. Now apply upper anchor in similar manner

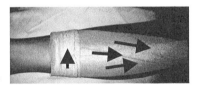

Figure 22.37 Put diamond wrap around knee joint for stabilization

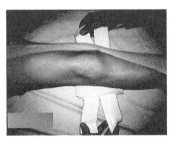

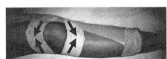

Anterior cruciate ligament taping

- Position: slightly flexed.
- Indication: sprain of anterior cruciate ligament.

Method of application

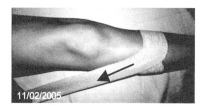 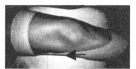

Figure 22.38 Using 7.5-cm stretch tape, begin on lateral aspect of lower leg, approximately 2.5 cm below patella. Encircle lower leg, going from lateral to medial to posterior and returning laterally. Angle tape below patella across medial joint line and spiral up to anterior portion of anchor at upper thigh

Figure 22.39 Second strip begins at anterior aspect of proximal anchor, crossing medial portion of thigh covering popliteal space, encircles lower leg, and then spirals up again to distal anchor. Repeat this step second time. Fix proximal anchor after finishing job

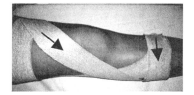

Taping for acromioclavicular (AC) joint

- Position: 30–45° abduction.
- Indication: grades I and II sprains of AC ligament.

Method of application

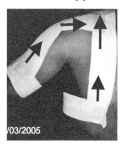 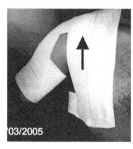 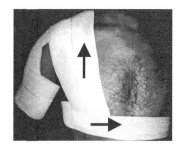

Figure 22.40 Apply anchor around upper arm and half anchor on thorax. Apply first strip along longitudinal axis of arm, over AC joint. Apply two more strips crossing AC in X shape

Figure 22.41 Apply strips starting from posterior thoracic anchor to anterior thoracic anchor under tension. Finish by covering edges

496

Elbow hyperextension taping

- Position: slightly flexed.
- Indication: elbow sprains and strains.

Method of application

Figure 22.42 Apply two anchors, proximally above belly of biceps, distally at distal one-third of forearm

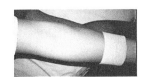

Figure 22.43 Apply five to seven strips from proximal anchor to distal anchor in hourglass fashion, under tension

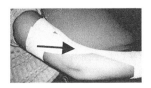

Figure 22.44 Apply second series of anchors over edges

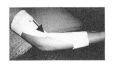

Figure 22.45 Continuous closure strip of stretch tape is applied in spiral manner from proximal to distal anchor

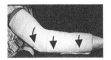

Tennis elbow: lateral epicondylitis taping

- Position: forearm pronated.
- Indication: tennis elbow (lateral epicondylitis).

Method of application

Figure 22.46 Apply three anchors, first one near elbow, second around wrist, and third around hand

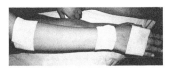

Figure 22.47 Using 3.75-cm tape, apply four strips on dorsum, from proximal to hand anchor. Cut 50-cm strip of 3-cm stretch tape; place palm of hand on center of strip. Radial strip is attached on lateral epicondyle. Ulnar strip is similarly attached on medial epicondyle. Lock strips on each anchor

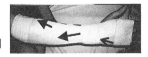

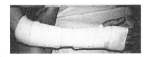

Figure 22.48 Apply fill-in strips from proximal to wrist anchors

Wrist taping

- Position: neutral.
- Indication: wrist hyperextension, hyperflexion injury.

Method of application

Figure 22.49 Apply diagonal anchor across hand and two anchors around mid forearm below muscle bulk

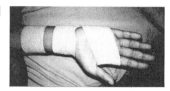

Figure 22.50 Using 2.5-cm tape, construct check rein (fan on table), overlapping each strip by half. Apply fan to anchors

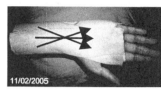

Figure 22.51 Cover anchors

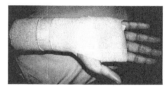

Prophylactic wrist taping

- Position: hand with palm facing up.
- Indication: prevention of injuries to wrist in sports.

Method of application

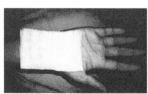 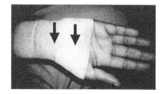

Figure 22.52 Place sponge rubber on palmar aspect of wrist; apply anchors 1, 2, and 3, starting 5 cm proximal to radial and ulnar styloid. Apply tape, so that it conforms to natural angle of hand. Overlap by repeated strips

Thumb spica taping

- Position: hand with palm down, thumb slightly flexed, and the phalanges adducted.
- Indication: thumb sprain.

Method of application

Figure 22.53 Apply anchors around wrist. Apply first of three support strips from ulnar condyle, covering dorsum of hand and surrounding thumb. Then, proceed along palmar aspect of hand to end at ulnar condyle

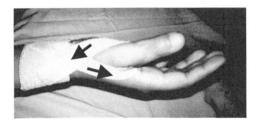

Figure 22.54 Repeat procedure three or four times. Finish by covering anchor

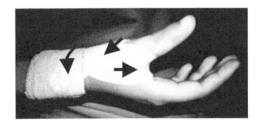

Buddy taping

- Position: finger extended in relaxed position.
- Indication: finger sprain.

Method of application

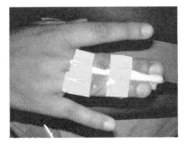

Figure 22.55 Gauze square is placed between fingers. Buddy-tape injured finger with adjacent finger around middle and proximal phalanxes

BRACES

Braces are semi-rigid orthoses used to reinforce or replace an injured or lost ligament or tendon. The purpose is to provide external support and to stabilize unstable parts. These braces include any type of neoprene sleeve and prefabricated, off-the-shelf braces.

Types of braces

Shoulder

Figure 22.56 Shoulder immobilizer (AC brace) used for grades I, II, and III ACJ dislocations

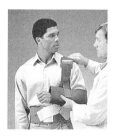

Elbow

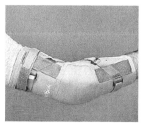

Figure 22.57
Hyperextension elbow support used for hyperextension ligament injuries, joint instability

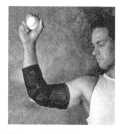

Figure 22.58
Valgus overload hinged elbow brace used to control valgus stress, ulnar collateral ligament instability

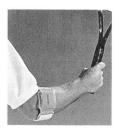

Figure 22.59
Tennis elbow band used for lateral epicondylitis

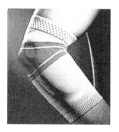

Figure 22.60
Extensor neoprene elbow sleeve used for chronic edema, medial or lateral epicondylitis, post-elbow arthroscopy, post-operative inflammatory conditions

Wrist

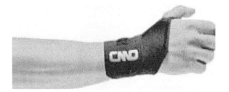 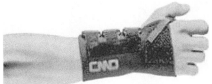

Figure 22.61
Elastic wrist support with thumb loop used for strain, sprain, and chronic weak wrist

Figure 22.62
Cock-up wrist support used for carpal tunnel syndrome, sprain, strain, post-operative rehabilitation

Thumb

Figure 22.63 Universal thumb/wrist splint used for sprains, gamekeeper injuries, collateral ligament support, and avulsion fractures

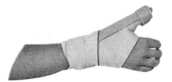

Knee

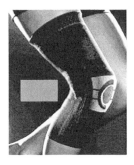 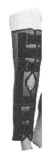

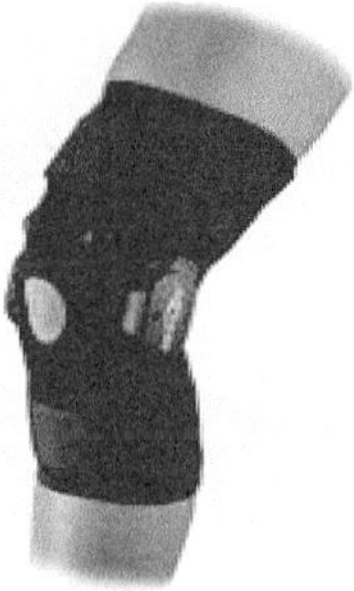

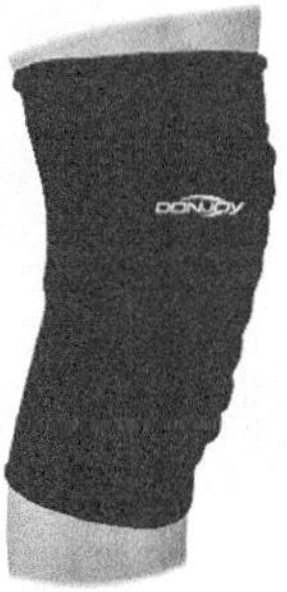

Figure 22.64
Patella stabilizers used for patellar subluxation, chondromalacia patellae, anterior knee pain, patellar instability, and to reduce chronic edema

Figure 22.65
Hinged knee braces used for collateral ligaments sprain or tear

Figure 22.66
Knee immobilizers used for immobilization following injury or surgery

Figure 22.67
Spider kneepad protector used for active sport

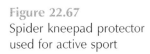
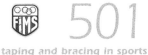

Ankle

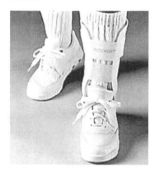

Figure 22.68
Ankle stirrups used for chronic ankle instability, sprain prevention, ligament instability

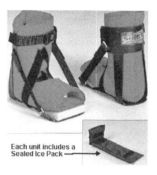

Each unit includes a
Sealed Ice Pack

Figure 22.69 Compression ankle support used for plantar fasciitis, Achilles tendinitis

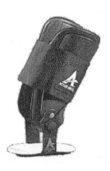

Figure 22.70 T2 active ankle support used for inversion support

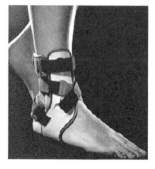

Figure 22.71 Malleiloc used for lateral ankle instability, sprain prevention, post-tibial dysfunction, post-cast, post-surgery

Back

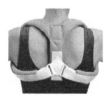

Figure 22.72
Posture corrector used for poor posture, osteoporosis

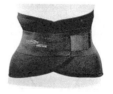

Figure 22.73
Back support used for low-back pain

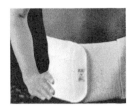

Figure 22.74
Abdominal support and binder used for weak abdominals, post-surgery, low-back pain

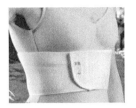

Figure 22.75
Rib support used for rib fracture

ACKNOWLEDGMENTS

We thank Ms. Mimansa Sood and Ms. Ashima Chachra, for their assistance in the preparation of this text.
Courtesy: Aircast, DonJoy, CMO, Bauerfeind, Otto Bock, Procare.

SUGGESTED READING

Alt W., Lohrer H., Gollhofer A. Functional properties of adhesive ankle taping: Neuromuscular and mechanical effects before and after exercise. *Foot Ankle Int.* 1999; 20:238–45.

Anderson D.L., Sanderson D.J., Henning E.M. The role of external nonrigid ankle bracing in limiting ankle inversion. *Clin. J. Sport Med.* 1995; 5:18–24.

Bennell K.L., Goldie P.A. The differential effects of external ankle support on postural control. *J. Orthop. Sports Phys. Ther.* 1994; 20(6):287–95.

Burks R.T., Bean B.G., et al. Analysis of athletic performance with prophylactic ankle devices. *Am. J. Sports Med.* 1991; 19:104–6.

Cordova M.L., Armstrong C.W., et al. Ground reaction forces and EMG activity with ankle bracing during inversion stress. *Med. Sci. Sports Exerc.* 1998; 30:1363–70.

Ebig M., Lephart S.M., et al. The effect of sudden inversion stress on EMG activity of the peroneal and tibialis anterior muscles in the chronically unstable ankle. *J. Orthop. Sports Phys. Ther.* 1997; 26:73–7.

Feuerbach J.W., Grabiner M.D. Effect of the aircast on unilateral postural control: Amplitude and frequency variables. *J. Orthop. Sports Phys. Ther.* 1993; 17(3):149–54.

Feuerbach J.W., Grabiner M.D., et al. Effect of an ankle orthosis and ankle ligament anesthesia on ankle joint proprioception. *Am. J. Sports Med.* 1994; 22:223–9.

Goldie P.A., Evans O.M., Bach T.M. Postural control following inversion injuries of the ankle. *Arch. Phys. Med. Rehabil.* 1994; 75(9):969–75.

Greene T.A., Hillman S.K. Comparison of support provided by a semirigid orthosis and adhesive ankle taping before, during, and after exercise. *Am. J. Sports Med.* 1990; 18:498–506.

Gross M.T., Batten A.M., et al. Comparison of DonJoy Ankle Ligament Protector and subtalar sling ankle taping in restricting foot and ankle motion before and after exercise. *J. Orthop. Sports Phys. Ther.* 1994; 19:33–41.

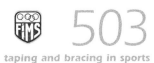

Gross M.T., Everts J.R., et al. Effect of DonJoy Ankle Ligament Protector and Aircast Sport-Stirrup orthoses on functional performance. *J. Orthop. Sports Phys. Ther.* 1994; 19:150–6.

Karlsson J., Andréasson G.O. The effect of external ankle support in chronic lateral ankle joint instability: An electromyographic study. *Am. J. Sports Med.* 1992; 20:257–61.

Löfvenberg R., Kärrholm J. The influence of an ankle orthosis on the talar and calcaneal motions in chronic lateral instability of the ankle: A stereophotogrammetric analysis. *Am. J. Sports Med.* 1993; 21:224–30.

Lohrer H., Alt W., Gollhofer A. Neuromuscular properties and functional aspects of taped ankles. *Am. J. Sports Med.* 1999; 27:69–75.

Macpherson K., Sitler M., et al. Effects of a semirigid and softshell prophylactic ankle stabilizer on selected performance tests among high school football players. *J. Orthop. Sports Phys. Ther.* 1995; 21(3):147–52.

Myburgh K.H., Vaughan C.L., Isaacs S.K. The effects of ankle guards and taping on joint motion before, during, and after a squash match. *Am. J. Sports Med.* 1984; 12:441–6.

Pienkowski D., McMorrow M., et al. The effect of ankle stabilizers on athletic performance. A randomized prospective study. *Am. J. Sports Med.* 1995; 23(6):757–62.

Quigley T.B., Cox J., Murphy J. A protective wrapping for the ankle. *JAMA* 1946; 123:924.

Rarick G.L., Bigley G., Karst R. The measurable support of the ankle joint by conventional methods of taping. *J. Bone Joint Surgery* 1962; 44A:1183.

Robbins S., Waked E., Rappel R. Ankle taping improves proprioception before and after exercise in young men. *Br. J. Sports Med.* 1995; 29:242–7.

Shapiro M.S., Kabo J.M., Mitchell P.W. Ankle sprain prophylaxis: An analysis of the stabilizing effects of braces and tape. *Am. J. Sports Med.* 1994; 22:78–82.

Tropp H., Askling C., Gillquist J. Prevention of ankle sprains. *Am. J. Sports Med.* 1985; 13:259–62.

Verbrugge J.D. The effects of semirigid Air-Stirrup bracing vs. adhesive ankle taping on motor performance. *J. Orthop. Sports Phys. Ther.* 1996; 23:320–5.

Wiley J.P., Nigg B.M. The effect of an ankle orthosis on ankle range of motion and performance. *J. Orthop. Sports Phys. Ther.* 1996; 23(6):362–9.

www.mmbrace.com

CHAPTER 23

PREVENTING SPORTS INJURIES

What the team physician needs to know

Lyle J. Micheli and Konstantinos I. Natsis

A common pronouncement on sports injuries that they are "part of the game" suggests that little can be done to prevent their incidence and severity. Recent studies have shown that this claim is totally false. By addressing risk factors associated with sports injuries, especially those seen in young athletes, both acute and overuse injuries can be reduced by 15–50%.

Needless to say, the team physician is a key player in this process.

The task of preventing acute sports injuries is relatively straightforward. Before looking at ways to prevent overuse injuries – a more complex task for the team physician – it is important to review those key areas of preventing acute injuries.

PREVENTING ACUTE SPORTS INJURIES

Pre-season fitness preparation

Athletes should participate in a directed, pre-season, physical conditioning program focusing on heart/lung endurance, strength, and flexibility. The conditioning program should also include sport-specific exercises to prevent injury – swimmers and tennis players should focus on shoulder and arm conditioning, soccer players should emphasize strength and flexibility exercises for groin and legs, and so on.

The team physician should use the off-season to help the athlete and, where appropriate, address a previous injury with an exercise program. For example, the football player who has sustained a sprained ankle the previous season should be encouraged to work on a program to build strength and flexibility in the ankle dorsiflexor and evertor muscles.

Wherever possible, teams should be encouraged to employ the services of athletic trainers or physical therapists, who can assist the team physician in instituting and monitoring pre-participation fitness programs.

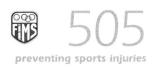

Proper warm-up and cool-down

The benefits of warming up and cooling down (sometimes called "warming down") are well established. They improve performance, prepare the athlete psychologically, create a comfort zone for the activity itself, and relieve the aches and pains of vigorous athletic activity. Most importantly, though, warm-ups and cool-downs prevent injuries from occurring.

Acute injuries are much more likely to occur when muscles, tendons, and ligaments are "tight" or "cold." Tissues that have not been warmed by increased blood flow and lengthened with gradual stretches are less pliable. Thus, they are at greater risk of being torn during the normal twists, turns, and stretches of sports. Less-pliable tissues are also more susceptible to overuse injuries.

Another important reason properly to prepare for exercise is that warm-up exercises improve coordination and minimize the risk of accidents, such as a slip, a fall, or a trip.

Furthermore, studies have shown that beginning vigorous exercise without a gradual warm-up, that is, sudden, strenuous exercise, puts athletes at risk of cardiovascular difficulties. Keep in mind also that good *preparation* will improve *performance*.

The intensity and duration of the warm-up and cool-down vary with each athlete. In order to achieve optimal elevation in body temperature and heart rate, the well-conditioned athlete probably requires a longer, more intense warm-up compared with a less-well-conditioned person.

Irrespective of the conditioning level of the athlete, every workout should include the following five stages: (1) limbering up (5 minutes); (2) stretching (5–10 minutes); (3) warm-up (5 minutes); (4) primary activity; and (5) cooling-down and cool-down stretching (10 minutes).

A team whose players experience disproportionate numbers of acute injuries such as sprains and strains may not be doing enough pre- or post-activity preparation, and, if so, the team physician should address this issue with the person responsible for this area.

Safe playing conditions

Sport injuries are less likely to occur if the athlete is using proper facilities, for example:

- playing fields free of potholes, glass, or other debris, and with padded posts;
- basketball and volleyball courts free of any debris or potentially dangerous objects (e.g., discarded sweatpants, water bottles) and without any wet spots from sweat, spillage, or roof leaks (if any occur during games or practice, they should be wiped up immediately).

Team physicians should involve themselves in inspecting the playing conditions before the sports event.

Addressing extreme temperatures

The safety of sports participation can be directly impacted by the ambient climate at the time of participation. A dramatic example of this is the Commonwealth Games of 1998, when a number of athletes were inadequately prepared for the extreme heat and humidity of the competition. Heat and cold acclimatization, as well as altitude acclimatization, are known physiological processes that can be facilitated by a proper progression in training in these environments. Both the International Federation of Sports Medicine and the American College of Sports Medicine have published position stands and recommendations on athletic participation in extreme heat, which the team physician would do well to read.

Athletes who exercise outdoors in hot and humid or cold and wet conditions can suffer a variety of ailments. Injuries due to overheating and overcooling are especially prevalent among runners. In fun runs, for instance, the most serious injuries are related to the inability to keep the body temperature from rising too high. This increase in temperature occurs when the body produces heat at a faster rate than it can disperse. In short races of 10 km (6.2 miles) or less, increased body temperature (*hyperthermia*) occurs in conjunction with the tiredness caused by the heat; fainting and dizziness can occur, even on relatively cool days. In longer races on warm days, these heat problems are common. On cool or cold days, especially when it is wet and windy, the risk to participants in running races is related to low body temperature (*hypothermia*).

Athletes may become too hot or too cold, depending on the prevailing temperature, humidity, wind conditions, and the clothing worn.

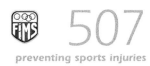

Overheating (hyperthermia)

During vigorous exercise, the amount of heat produced by the working muscles is 15–20 times what they produce at rest. This increased rate of heat production can raise the body temperature rapidly. The brain senses the rising body temperature, and thus increases the amount of blood sent to the skin and stimulates sweating. The skin is then cooled by sweat evaporation. If the cooling is inadequate, the person will overheat. Injury will occur when the person becomes too hot, that is, when body temperature goes higher than 104°F (40°C).

During long training sessions or athletic events, the amount of body fluid lost through sweat can cause athletes to lose a lot of weight. The loss of weight is directly related to how much fluid the athlete has lost, and can be up to 6–10% of total body weight. This water loss is medically known as dehydration. Severe dehydration will cause a reduction in the athlete's capacity to sweat and thereby increases the risk of getting too hot and may lead to heat stroke, heat exhaustion, and muscle cramps. Children are much more likely to get overheated or overcooled than adults and should be watched carefully during training sessions and games in hot conditions (see Chapter 9).

Dressing appropriately for the weather can reduce the risk of heat injuries. Obviously, wearing appropriate clothes to help keep the body cool will be very helpful in hot temperatures. For example, light-colored clothing made of cotton is much better than dark-colored clothing made of synthetic fibers, such as nylon.

Drinking plenty of fluids, especially cool water, reduces the risk of dehydration during long training sessions. Sometimes, the participant's body may heat up without apparent weight loss during shorter exercise sessions; athletes should therefore always be alert to the problems of heat stress. Athletes should avoid drinking liquids that contain high amounts of sugar (e.g. soft drinks) immediately before or during exercise sessions. Many sports drinks have high concentrations of glucose, which delay the absorption of water into the system. Also, the much-touted extra electrolytes of sports drinks are not necessary, because electrolyte loss from sweating is minimal in the trained athlete performing relatively short-term exercise. Most of the sugar and electrolytes can be replaced through a balanced meal after the exercise. Athletes who prefer the flavor of sports drinks should dilute them with water by half.

Athletes who frequently do vigorous exercise, especially in extremely hot temperatures, should make sure their diets contain plenty of salt, potassium, and calcium. These are the essential minerals lost through sweating. Salt tablets, however, are not suggested. They are difficult to digest, and, as a result, the salt does not get into the system where it is needed. Salt tablets may also upset the chemical and electrolyte balance of the body. Alcohol should never be used to replace lost fluids.

lyle j. micheli and konstantinos i. natsis

In hot climates, athletes should avoid exercising outdoor when the sun is strongest. It is best to exercise in the early morning or late evening. Avoid strenuous workouts when the humidity is high.

Overcooling (hypothermia)

When a person loses heat at a rate faster than that at which he/she produces it, the body can be overcooled. Even on moderately cool days, if a runner's pace becomes too slow, and/or if the weather conditions become cooler during the run, he/she may become too cold. Several deaths caused by cold conditions during fun runs, especially in the mountains, have been reported. Low body temperature is common for inexperienced marathon runners, who often run more slowly in the second half of the race: as they slow down, especially on cool, wet, or windy days, their body temperature may suddenly become too low. Early signs and symptoms of hypothermia are shivering, a false sense of well-being, and an appearance of intoxication. Shivering may stop as the body temperature drops further; excessive drowsiness and muscle weakness may then occur, accompanied by disorientation, hallucinations, and often a belligerent attitude, and finally the runner may become unconscious or die.

Injuries caused by cold temperatures are largely preventable through appropriate use of protective clothing. The appropriately clothed athlete can withstand a wide range of temperatures. In cold weather, insufficient clothing will not provide the protection necessary for a runner to keep warm, especially near the end of a race, when he/she slows down and the body produces less heat than needed for keeping warm. On a cool day, the clothing worn should consist of multiple thin layers of cotton fibers. A polypropylene fabric may be worn near to the skin and covered with an easily removed windbreaker (preferably man-made nylon). As the athlete gets warm, clothing can be removed to allow sweat to evaporate or dry. However, when the pace gets too slow for the runner to keep warm, the clothes can be put back on. In addition to being more effective in retaining body heat, multilayering allows athletes to remove layers when they get warm. When the clothing is nonconstricting, multilayering helps prevent sweat freezing on the body.

As the body loses most of its heat through the head, the importance of appropriate headgear during cold weather should not be neglected. In very cold weather, the face, nose, and ears should also be covered, as these areas are most likely to become frostbitten. During wet weather, waterproof clothing is essential.

It is also advisable to wear sweat suits while warming up during cool or cold weather. The insulation provided helps muscles, ligaments, and tendons get warmer and more flexible, which contributes to preventing both acute and overuse injuries (see Chapter 9).

Appropriate safety equipment

Protective safety equipment for many sports has been developed and recommended to help prevent and reduce the severity of injuries. The use of this equipment is usually supported by research by health professionals that identified a high risk of injury in a particular sport or recreational activity. The use of safety equipment may be advocated by the government, national medical organizations, public health professionals, safety groups, national governing bodies of sports, or sports associations to prevent different types of injury, especially catastrophic ones. It is the job of the coach and the team physician to oversee the equipment personnel in making sure athletes wear safety equipment appropriate for the sport, and that the safety equipment worn is sized correctly for the athlete.

Preventing overuse sports injuries

The risk factors of overuse injuries can be *intrinsic* or *extrinsic*. Intrinsic risk factors include previous injury, poor conditioning, muscle imbalances, anatomical abnormalities, nutritional factors, and growth (in children), whereas extrinsic risk factors are the use of improper footwear and training errors, such as an inappropriate workout structure or abrupt increases in the intensity, duration, or frequency of training.

Identifying risk factors is the key, not only to preventing sports injuries, but also to effective diagnosis, treatment, and rehabilitation. These risk factors often explain why some athletes sustain overuse injuries, while others do not. Of these factors, the ones most blamed for causing overuse sports injuries are *previous injury, poor conditioning, muscle imbalances, anatomical abnormalities*, and *training errors*.

Overuse injuries are often caused by two or more risk factors. For example, an athlete may have dramatically increased the amount of training over a relatively short period of time, while doing the training in worn-out footwear and on training surfaces that have become harder because of climatic changes such as lack of rain.

An understanding by the team physician of all the risk factors associated with overuse injuries is a crucial first step toward a comprehensive approach to injury management.

Intrinsic risk factors

Previous injury

The most reliable predictor of injury is a previous injury. Most athletes who get injured are destined to re-injure themselves. This renders injury management, especially rehabilitation, inadequate. Unless rehabilitation is done, tissues weakened by injury cannot fully regain their strength, which puts them at risk of getting damaged again.

 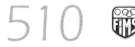

Proper rehabilitation may break the injury/re-injury cycle, but only when the program emphasizes a return to full function, not just symptom relief. The team physician must make sure injured athletes follow the rehabilitation prescription.

Poor conditioning

Unfit athletes are much more likely to get injured than those who are in shape. Studies have shown that most injuries occur early in the sports season, when athletes are less conditioned. This risk factor applies also to overuse injuries, because an unfit body is less able to cope with the repetitive stresses of a chosen activity. It is extremely important that athletes do not go from an extended period of inactivity straight into rigorous training, such as going directly into the football season after a summer off. Coaches should design off-season strength and flexibility programs for their athletes. If the program is to address weak areas that have been previously injured, the team physician should have a hand in its design.

It is also important to keep in mind that being fit for one sport does not necessarily mean that an athlete is fit for another. For example, long-distance runners may not be immediately fit for intensive swimming training, and vice versa. Thus, it is important to do exercises to condition the body and work slowly into the training when switching to different sports.

Muscle imbalances

Imbalances between adjoining muscle groups are common in athletes, and the team physician should be aware of their significance. Muscle imbalances may be caused by asymmetric muscle use that reflects the special demands of the sport.

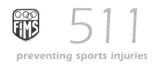

For example, ballet dancers often have excessive strength and tightness in the hip abductors and relative weakness in the adductors.

During the growth process, adolescent athletes may have muscle imbalances induced by the growth process. During adolescence, the lateral muscles in the anterior thigh have a tendency to become stronger and tighter, whereas the medial muscles are relatively weak. These muscle imbalances are commonly seen in the low back and legs.

The consequences of muscle imbalances are threefold. First, imbalances can cause stresses to the underlying tissues; second, they can pull certain parts of the anatomy out of alignment; and third, they may interfere with proper foot strike. All three can lead to overuse injuries.

- *Stresses caused by muscle imbalances*: Tight muscles can cause a variety of overuse injuries, especially in running sports. Excessive tightness in the muscles that run along the outer side of the thigh, the iliotibial band, can induce pressure on the outer side of the hip and the knee, which can cause trochanteric bursitis and iliotibial band friction syndrome, respectively. Tight muscles and tendons in the back of the lower leg (gastroc–soleus–Achilles tendon unit) can cause Achilles tendinopathy, an inflammation of the thick cord of tissue that connects the calf muscles to the back of the heel, and plantar fasciitis, an inflammation of the connective tissue underneath the foot that connects the toes to the heel (plantar fascia).
- *Alignment problems caused by muscle imbalances*: The most frequent sites of alignment problems caused by muscle imbalances are the back and knee.

Lower-back pain is common in athletes and is often caused by tightness in the muscles at the front of the hip (psoas) and behind the thigh (hamstrings) compared with the stomach muscles (abdominals) and the muscles in front of the thigh (quadriceps). Relatively weak spinal postural stabilizing muscles may also be one of the causes. Such an imbalance can cause a posture problem called "swayback" (lordosis), in which an excessive front-to-back curve in the lower spine is found. This posture problem in turn predisposes the athlete to serious overuse injuries of the lower back, such as herniated disk and spondylolysis.

Anterior knee pain is another frequent problem in athletes, especially those who have to do a lot of running during training or competition. The most common form of anterior knee pain is patellofemoral pain syndrome, which is usually caused by maltracking of the patella in the trochlea, the anterior groove of the femur. A number of factors may contribute to the imbalance of forces at the patella and result in pain, including anatomical factors and muscle imbalances. A frequent contributor to patellofemoral pain is an imbalance between the muscles on the inner and outer sides of the quadriceps, that is, the vastus medialis and vastus lateralis, respectively. The imbalance results in a tendency toward lateral tracking and posturing of the patella in its trochlear groove. Nevertheless, this imbalance can often be corrected, and pain can be relieved with early institution of appropriate exercises to strengthen the vastus medialis and stretch the vastus lateralis.

- *Foot strike problems caused by muscle imbalances*: The third problem associated with muscle imbalances is their effect on the biomechanics of running, which generally affects athletes engaged in sports that involve a lot of running.

Running causes tightness in certain areas, most often the psoas muscles in front of the hip, the hamstring muscles in the back of the thigh, and the gastroc-soleus–Achilles tendon unit in the back of the lower leg.

Athletes with this pattern of tightness tend to have a much briefer than normal foot strike when running, because their muscles are so tight that they cannot perform the optimal relaxed heel-to-toe foot strike. Their feet spend less time on the ground with each step and thus absorb more stress every time they hit the ground. Although the time differential may seem relatively minor, when one considers a runner taking 10,000 steps per hour, the consequences may be dramatic.

Anatomical abnormalities

One of the most common reasons some athletes sustain overuse injuries while others do not is that they have anatomical abnormalities that place additional stress on the surrounding structures. In daily activities, these abnormalities do not cause problems, but overuse injuries may occur when the area is subjected to repetitive stresses. The most common anatomical abnormalities of the lower extremities are flat feet, feet that pronate excessively (roll inward when running), high arches, knock-knees, bow legs, and turned-in thigh bones (femoral anteversion).

- *Flat feet/excessive pronation (pes planus)*: Some people have naturally flat feet that turn excessively inward (pronate) when they run (Figure 23.1). During normal movements of running, a certain amount of natural pronation occurs with each step an athlete takes. Excessive pronation, however, can be harmful, because it causes increased stress throughout the lower extremities, and overuse injuries may occur. The most common overuse injuries in the foot associated with flat feet and feet that excessively pronate are stress fractures and posterior tibial tendinopathy.

Flat feet and feet that excessively pronate not only cause problems in the foot, but may also affect the entire lower extremities, including the knee and hip, because both conditions cause inward rotation of the legs.

Other lower extremity problems that are believed to be partly caused by flat feet or feet that excessively pronate are compartment syndrome in the lower leg, patellofemoral pain in the knee, and trochanteric bursitis in the hip.

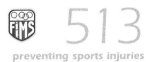

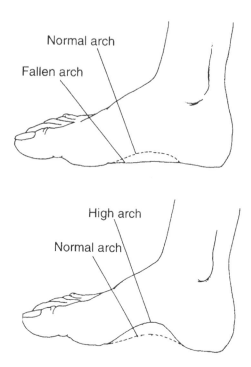

Normal arch

Fallen arch

High arch

Normal arch

Figure 23.1 Flat feet and high arches

- *High arches (pes cavus)*: High arches, or "claw foot" as this condition is sometimes known, make the feet inflexible (Figure 23.1). The rigidity of this kind of foot makes it susceptible to overuse injuries. High arches can also result in overuse injuries in the lower leg, because the inflexibility causes the force to be transmitted to the structures above. Athletes with high arches are susceptible to stress fractures in the foot, lower leg, upper thigh and pelvis, plantar fasciitis (heel spurs), and Achilles tendinopathy.

A person with high arches may also develop a "hammer toe," in which the second toe becomes buckled and cannot be straightened. A high arch causes the big toe to slide under the second toe when the athlete runs, causing the development of hammer toe.

- *Knock-knees (genu valgum)*: Knock-knees create serious problems for the knee joint. Excessive inward angling at the point where the thigh and lower leg meet (Q angle; see Figure 23.2) causes the body's weight to be borne on the inside of the knee. A Q angle greater than 10° in men and 15° in women is said to predispose that person to knee problems, if he/she participates in a sports program that involves extensive running. Knock-knee is a common cause of

lyle j. micheli and konstantinos i. natsis

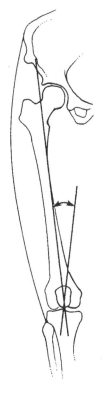

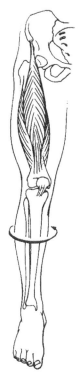

Figure 23.2 Q angle   **Figure 23.3** Femoral anteversion

patellofemoral pain syndrome and is the most common diagnosis seen in sports clinics.

- *Bow legs (genu varum)*: Bow legs are the opposite of knock-knees – they bend outward instead of angling inward. Athletes with bow legs are at greater risk for sustaining injuries on the outer side of their knees, especially iliotibial band friction syndrome. Having bowed legs creates a longer distance over which the iliotibial band (the thick swathe of tissue that runs down the side of the leg, from the hip to just below the knee) must stretch, making it tighter over the outer side of the knee joint, which is where the symptoms develop. However, it should be noted that many athletes with bow legs participate in distance running without any problems.
- *Turned-in thigh bones (femoral anteversion)*: Almost everyone has anterior rotation (anteversion) of the femoral neck with respect to the distal femur (Figure 23.3) at birth. This degree of femoral anteversion tends to decrease progressively during the growth and maturation process.

In certain cases, however, anteversion does not decrease or was initially too excessive, which makes the entire femur face inward when the athlete stands on both feet. When combined with a compensatory external tibial torsion, femoral anteversion can often increase the lateral torque at the patellofemoral groove, contributing to the onset of patellofemoral pain. Because it so often results in overuse sports injuries, the combination of femoral anteversion, genu valgum, external tibial torsion, and pes planus has been dubbed the "miserable malalignment syndrome."

■ *Unequal leg length*: Leg-length inequality is common. Having one leg longer than the other can create problems, especially in the longer leg. For example, because the iliotibial band of the longer leg must stretch over a longer distance, tissue inflammation may result where it passes over the side of the knee joint. Also, a person with unequal leg length tends to run with his/her spine curved slightly sideways, which can cause wear and tear on the concave side of the spine.

Nutritional factors

The relationship between three distinct but interrelated conditions – eating disorders, menstrual irregularities, and stress fractures – is known as the "female athlete triad." Team physicians responsible for the health of female athletes should familiarize themselves with this phenomenon.

Eating disorders are more common among female athletes than among sedentary women. Poor eating habits, combined with high activity level, can cause the fat level to drop below the level necessary for normal menstrual function. When periods stop (amenorrhea) or become irregular (oligomenorrhea), the woman loses much of the estrogen necessary for bone rebuilding, which the normal body performs on a continuous basis. This loss causes premature osteoporosis, a disease that causes the bones to become thinner and more brittle, which in turn predisposes the athlete to stress fractures. Among female athletes with menstrual irregularities, the incidence of stress fractures is almost tripled. The most common sites of stress fractures in female athletes are the back, hip, pelvis, lower leg, and foot.

The growth factor

Until quite recently, overuse injuries were seen only in adults, most often highly trained, elite athletes and "weekend warriors" – sedentary adults who do no athletic activity during the week and then play three sets of tennis on Sunday. Physicians believe that, because of this exercise pattern, too much stress is placed on aging bones, muscles, tendons, and ligaments over a short period of time, which results in overuse injuries such as tennis elbow. With the rise of rigorous, repetitive sports training regimens for children, however, it has been discovered that children are even more likely to sustain overuse syndromes.

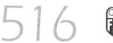

Children are more susceptible than adults to overuse injury because of growth, the fundamental feature of childhood (see Chapter 9). Growth makes children vulnerable to overuse injuries for two reasons: the presence of growth cartilage and the growth process itself. The team physician who is responsible for the sports health of young athletes must be aware of the significance of these two components of the growth factor.

- *Growth cartilage*: Growth cartilage is found at three main sites in the growing child's body: the growth plates near the ends of the long bones, the cartilage lining the joint surfaces (articular cartilage), and the points at which the major tendons attach to the bones (Figure 23.4). Growth cartilage is present until the child stops growing; it is more easily damaged by repetitive microtrauma, especially at the joint surface, than the thin, hard, and fully formed adult bone cartilage. Growth cartilage is "pre-bone," and, thus, damaging it may have serious consequences in later life.
- *The growth process*: The role of the growth process in exacerbating overuse injuries in children is less recognized than that of growth cartilage. Over the past decade, experts in pediatric sports medicine have devoted enormous amounts of time and effort to research into the growth process, unraveling the mysteries of how and why it increases the risk of overuse injuries in children. Research has identified the chief culprit – the tightness in growing muscles and tendons. Muscles and tendons do not grow at the same rate as bones; instead, they must stretch to keep up. During the adolescent growth

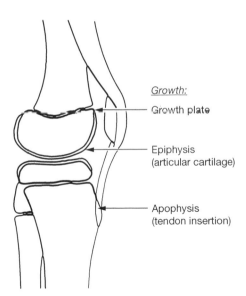

Figure 23.4 Growth cartilage is present at the growth plate, the articular cartilage, and the apophyses; each of these sites is susceptible to overuse injury

spurt, the bones in the legs grow so quickly that a 2-cm increase in height in a month is not uncommon. The muscles and tendons spanning these rapidly growing bones, however, do not elongate as quickly, and they get much tighter as a result. This tightness is particularly noticeable in muscles that cross two joints. The loss of flexibility, although temporary, increases the likelihood of overuse injuries, particularly in the knee and back.

Extrinsic risk factors

Errors in training

Training error – usually "too much too soon" – is a major cause of injury, especially overuse injury. Injuries can result when athletes suddenly increase the frequency, duration, or intensity of their workouts, where frequency refers to how often the athlete trains, duration refers to how long, and intensity refers to how hard they perform.

Intensity encompasses not only factors such as how far or fast a person jogs, or how heavy a weight he/she lifts, it refers also to less obvious aspects of the exercise regimen, such as the hardness of the training surface on which the athlete is exercising. Track athletes can be considered as having significantly increased the intensity of their workout if they have switched from running on grass or clay to road, or from flat surfaces to hills. The same applies to football players who switch from natural to artificial surfaces. Softer, however, does not always mean less stressful. For instance, running on sand stresses the Achilles tendons, which predisposes the athlete to tendinopathy in that area. Intensity can be subtle: a tennis racket that is more tightly strung provides a more intense workout for the arm. It is generally recommended that, for any athlete training exceeding 18 hours per week, careful medical monitoring should be carried out, and increases in training volume should not exceed 10% per week.

Inappropriate footwear

In sports that involve a lot of running and jumping, athletes exert forces of 3–10 times their body weight with each step on the training surface, the shoes, and the feet and legs. The fact that, the less force the limbs absorb, the lower the risk of overuse injury, explains why it is better to train on slightly softer surfaces such as clay or grass, rather than cement or asphalt, which have less "give." It also explains why shoes are the most important item in most athletes' wardrobes.

Shoes are especially important for track athletes. The right footwear makes for an enjoyable, injury-free running experience, whereas the wrong footwear can cause discomfort and ailments ranging from ankle sprains to heel spurs to knee cartilage tears. Basketball players, on the other hand, also need to wear shoes that have adequate, appropriate shock-absorption properties. Improvements in footwear technology over the past decade have, nevertheless, contributed to a decrease in the number of many footwear-related overuse injuries.

lyle j. micheli and konstantinos i. natsis

Improper workout structure

One of the most common reasons athletes get injured is because they do not prepare their bodies with a structured workout, which includes warm-up and cool-down periods, for the immediate demands of exercise.

Less-pliable tissues are more susceptible to overuse injuries. Repetitive, low-intensity stretching of inflexible tissues may cause tiny tears. Joints surrounded by tissues that are not warmed up and stretched have a restricted range of motion, which causes grinding of the cartilage against bone or other cartilage, and results in overuse injuries of the joints.

The intensity and duration of the warm-up and cool-down vary with individuals. A well-conditioned athlete probably requires a longer, more intense warm-up to achieve optimal body temperature and heart rate, compared with a less-well-conditioned person. Irrespective of the conditioning level, every athlete should complete all five stages of a workout.

A major obstacle to developing strategies for preventing injury is the lack of epidemiological data on injury rates in most sports. Without sound baseline data, the impact of measures to enhance sports safety cannot be evaluated. In 1998, the International Federation of Sports Medicine and the World Health Organization released a joint consensus statement on children and sports. One of the central themes of the document was injury prevention. This consensus statement called for a number of initiatives to be adopted by sports governing bodies, including the collection of statistics on sports injuries. This statement also called upon health professionals to take steps to improve their knowledge and understanding of the organized sports environment, as well as the risk factors associated with sports participation.

SUGGESTED READING

Fields K.B., Sykes J.C., Walker K.M., Jackson J.C. Prevention of running injuries. *Curr. Sports Med. Rep.* 2010; 9:176–82.

FIMS/WHO Ad Hoc Committee on Sports and Children. Sports and children: consensus statement on organized sports for children. *Bull. World Health Organ.* 1998; 76:445–7.

Klugl M., Shrier I., McBain K., Shultz R., Meeuwisse W.H., Garza D., Matheson G.O. The prevention of sport injury: An analysis of 12,000 published manuscripts. *Clin. J. Sport Med.* 2010; 20:407–12.

Maffulli N., Longo U.G., Spiezia F., Denaro V. Aetiology and prevention of injuries in elite young athletes. *Med. Sport Sci.* 2011; 56:187–200.

Matheson G.O., Mohtadi N.G., Safran M., Meeuwisse W.H. Sport injury prevention: Time for an intervention? *Clin. J. Sport Med.* 2010; 20:399–401.

Micheli L.J., Glassman R., Klein M. The prevention of sports injuries in children. *Clin. Sports Med.* 2000; 19:821–34.

Mountjoy M., Andersen L.B., Armstrong N., Biddle S., Boreham C., Bedenbeck H.P., Ekelund U., Engebretsen L., Hardman K., Hills A.P., Kahlmeier S., Kriemler S., Lambert E., Ljungqvist A., Matsudo V., McKay H., Micheli L., Pate R., Riddoch C., Schamasch

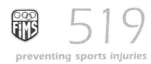

P., Sundberg C.J., Tomkinson G., van Sluijs E., van Mechelen W. International Olympic Committee consensus statement on the health and fitness of young people through physical activity and sport. *Br. J. Sports Med.* 2011; 45(11):839–48. *Erratum in: Br. J. Sports Med.* Oct. 2011; 45(13):1063.

Peterson A.R., Bernhardt D.T. The preparticipation sports evaluation. *Pediatr. Rev.* 2011; 32:e53–65.

Stojanovic M.D., Ostojic S.M. Stretching and injury prevention in football: Current perspectives. *Res. Sports Med.* 2011; 19:73–91.

Valovich McLeod T.C., Decoster L.C., Loud K.J., Micheli L.J., Parker J.T., Sandrey M.A., White C. National Athletic Trainers' Association position statement: Prevention of pediatric overuse injuries. *J. Athl. Train.* 2011; 46:206–20.

CHAPTER 24

THE PSYCHOLOGY OF SPORT INJURY AND RECOVERY

Trisha Leahy

INTRODUCTION

At any skill level, the threat of injury in sporting activities is always present. Indeed, sports injury has become a significant public health issue in many countries where sport participation is part of community life. For example, recent figures from Australia indicate that sports injuries cost approximately AUS$2 billion, with 5.2 million sports injuries incurred annually (Medibank Private, 2006). These figures appear to be relatively consistent around the world (Brewer, 2011).

In the world of high-performance sport, there is a broad consensus that individual success at the elite level is a function of the complex interplay of multiple factors acting in systemic concert. Apart from individual talent, and expert coaching to facilitate that talent, achieving and maintaining "an edge" over competitors requires a comprehensive medical, scientific, and welfare-support infrastructure to minimize risk and maximize results. Such a system requires significant funding, and, not surprisingly, governments and sponsors, as well as the athletes themselves, are heavily invested in seeing results at the highest levels in international sport. Individual livelihoods and government policies may be influenced by failure to consistently produce results. The ability to remain injury free, or recover rapidly, is central to achieving these goals and to maintaining a successful, long-term, competitive athletic career.

Medical support systems focusing on the prevention, treatment, and rehabilitation of injury are, therefore, a central part of the support infrastructure of competitive sport, particularly at the elite end of the spectrum. With current advanced procedures and technologies in the areas of sports medicine and rehabilitation, physical recovery from injury can be rapid, but, if psychological recovery has not occurred at the same pace, the risk of re-injury may be increased. The appropriate application of psychology should, therefore, be an integrated aspect of any rehabilitation program.

521

Team physicians do not need to be trained psychologists to be able to understand and apply basic principles of psychological theory to enhance the quality of care provided to injured athletes (Kolt and Andersen, 2004). In this chapter, I will attempt to present related elements of this psychological knowledge to assist team physicians to understand the psychological processes that may facilitate a speedy return to optimal performance for injured athletes. I will focus on three primary areas of discussion. In the first section, working from a theoretical backdrop grounded in a biopsychosocial model of sports injury and rehabilitation, the discussion will propose a multidisciplinary-team approach to managing injured athletes. The second section, focusing on psychosocial issues, will outline current knowledge on risk factors, prevention, and responses to sports injury. The third section will give an overview of a number of psychological interventions that team physicians can integrate into their practice, with clear guidelines for engaging effectively with injured athletes.

> With current advanced procedures and technologies in the areas of sports medicine and rehabilitation, physical recovery from injury can be rapid, but, if psychological recovery has not occurred at the same pace, the risk of re-injury may be increased. The appropriate application of psychology should, therefore, be an integrated aspect of any rehabilitation program.

A BIOPSYCHOSOCIAL APPROACH

Within behavioral medicine and the social sciences, the term biopsychosocial is used to refer to the interaction between biological, psychological, and social factors that are inextricably intertwined in the overall development of any individual. These processes are particularly involved in physical health, illness, and injury, and should always be considered in the assessment of an individual's health and in making recommendations for treatment (Brewer et al., 2002; Suls and Rothman, 2004). The biopsychosocial model fits very well within the high-performance sports system, where there has long been an explicit recognition of the complex interplay of physiological, psychological, and social factors that can influence sports performance. Indeed, many international, elite-sports support systems are underpinned by this biopsychosocial model (e.g. Australia, Hong Kong, and China), with centralized, integrated support systems targeting all aspects of medical and physiological, psychological, and social support needs. The team physician is a key player in this support structure.

In applying the biopsychosocial model to an understanding of the processes of sports injury, it can be assumed that, not only the physical characteristics of the injury itself (e.g., type, severity, chronicity, onset, etc.), but also the psychological impact of both the injury and the rehabilitation process, and the quality of the

trisha leahy

social support environment available to the injured athlete, will all interact in complex ways with the recovery process, compliance with rehabilitation regimens, and the eventual outcome (Brewer et al., 2002). Within the context of high-performance sport, team physicians and the members of the injury management team may need to be aware of the sociocultural factors that impact on the injured athlete and coach and that may facilitate or hinder appropriate help-seeking and recovery. Competitive sport at the high-performance end has often been described as a subculture with its own unique, sometimes harmful, norms (e.g., Leahy, 2010a; Sabo, 2004). For example, in some sports, the cultural norm may be one that values "mental toughness," defined as never complaining, and tolerating high levels of pain to achieve standards of excellence that are far above the norm. This has been identified as particularly prevalent in some men's sports, where definitions of masculinity become synonymous with stoic tolerance of pain and independent self-sufficiency. This has been shown to result in male athletes not seeking help in time, unless an injury is very serious (Frey et al., 2004; Sabo, 2004). In professional sports where contract renewal may depend on continued performance, athletes may be under considerable pressure to defer treatment and return to play, even before they are completely ready. Over-compliance with treatment protocols can be the risk in these cases. Conversely, the social impact of an injury requiring time off for rehabilitation, which may take place away from the team, can result in the athlete feeling alienated from, and even rejected by, team members. This can add to the distress of the injury itself, and the perceived loss of social support can lead to depressive symptoms, which may in turn interfere with recovery and compliance with the rehabilitation programs.

> The biopsychosocial model fits very well within the high-performance sports system, where there has long been an explicit recognition of the complex interplay of physiological, psychological, and social factors that can influence sports performance.

Multidisciplinary sport injury management

When understood from within the biopsychosocial framework, the process of sports injury and recovery appears as a complex, dynamic experience. It has long been recognized that a multidisciplinary, team-based approach is crucial to providing the necessary breadth and depth to service provision, allowing a broader basis for intervention decision-making and facilitating improved continuity of care across the various domains and synergism among treatments (Heil, 1993). Within this framework, recovery is viewed as a collaborative process that needs the proactive involvement of the athlete and other support people in the athlete's life. As well as the team physician, and depending on individual circumstances, the sport injury management team may include the physiotherapist, sports massage

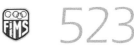

therapist, nutritionist, strength and conditioning coach, psychologist, coach, the athlete, and, in some cases, the athlete's parents/guardians and/or partners, all of whom can be recruited into supporting the athlete's recovery and adherence to the rehabilitation program (Brewer, 2011).

The obvious advantage of the multidisciplinary team approach is that all professional members of the sport injury management team bring with them different areas of expertise and clinical skills within their own discipline. Another difference, which each member of the team brings and which, some would argue, is a key variable in influencing treatment process and outcome, is each person's own personality and relational style (Kolt and Andersen, 2004). Research has identified that the quality of the working relationship between medical and allied health practitioners and the injured athlete is one of the key predictors of treatment compliance and positive outcome, regardless of the approach used (Brewer et al., 2007; Ray and Wiese-Bjornstal, 1999). Significant attention needs to be paid also to the quality of the relationships between the multidisciplinary team members and between the team as a whole and the athlete. Communication and coordination of servicing require careful monitoring, as do case management and issues of confidentiality. Shared decision-making and communication of decisions to the athlete also require collaborative negotiation. For example, it is important that the team is able to speak with a consistent voice to the athlete, so that, no matter in whom the athlete confides, the same, agreed message is provided. This is one advantage of including the athlete in the injury management team. It reduces the risk of the distressed athlete trying to manipulate the team members or play them off against one another, as s/he struggles with the ambiguity, anxiety, rigors, intensity, and frustrations of the rehabilitation process. In the third section, we will explore further the skills and competencies needed to participate as an effective member of the multidisciplinary sport injury management team.

> The quality of the working relationship between medical and allied health practitioners and the injured athlete is one of the key predictors of treatment compliance and positive outcome (Ray and Weise-Bjornstal, 1999).

A PSYCHOLOGICAL UNDERSTANDING OF SPORTS INJURY

Risk and prevention

Applying the biopsychosocial model to an understanding of sports injury risk, it is logical to expect that, although some sports injuries are clearly related to physical factors (fitness, inherent biomechanical misalignment, etc.), psychosocial elements may also be at work. A substantial body of knowledge has emerged over the past three decades focusing on the identification of the psychosocial variables associated with vulnerability or resilience to sports injury. According to what is known as the stress-injury model, individuals with a history of many stressors, who have personality characteristics that may exacerbate the stress response, and who have fewer coping resources will be more likely, when in a stressful situation, to appraise that situation as stressful and to exhibit greater physiological activation and attentional disruptions (Williams and Andersen, 1998). Consequently, such individuals are more likely to experience a more severe stress response, as a result of increased stress-reactivity. The stress-injury model proposes that it is the severity of the stress response that is the mechanism of increased injury risk.

Stemming from the stress-injury model, a number of primary prevention measures become immediately obvious and are commonly an important component of psychology work with high-level athletic individuals and teams (Johnson, 2007). For example, at the premier sports institutes around the world, primary prevention not only includes regular medical and musculoskeletal screening, and physiological and biochemical monitoring of adaptation to training, but it also includes a comprehensive program targeting psychological skills training. These include stress-management skills, such as appropriate cognitive appraisals and rational, positive self-talk, relaxation and visualization with biofeedback training, skills to enhance self-confidence, relationship and communication skills, conflict-management skills, eating-disorder prevention programs, etc.

Primary prevention also includes working with coaching and support staff to ensure that the athletes' environment is one that provides social support and that values and rewards proactive help-seeking behaviors, particularly in terms of early warning signs of injury. Each member of the multidisciplinary sport injury team has a significant role to play in this primary prevention work. Consistent coaching messages that advocate proactive recovery after training and that position help-seeking as a key component of the athletes' training and monitoring responsibilities need to be reinforced by the support staff. In my experience with working with elite athletes who left it too late to report a niggling discomfort, it was often the case that the athletes felt that reporting such discomfort would be perceived as weakness, as not being "mentally tough." For example, an elite male athlete described it to me as follows:

> I tried to ignore the pain and I just hoped it would go away or something, or else that it would, you know, that a more obvious symptom could be seen, rather than just me complaining about pain. The coach and the psychologist were always going on about being "mentally tough" and I just knew it would affect my selection if I started bringing it up too early, 'cause they would just see me as a whinger and not tough enough. So I tried to wait it out, but then look what happened [sighs], now I am completely out of action until I don't know when.

The team physician is also in a key position to monitor the maintenance of a safe sporting environment for athletes. This is particularly relevant for youth teams, as young people in many of our societies are relatively powerless compared with adults and can be vulnerable to exploitation. I am using the word "safety" here to refer to both psychologically and physically healthy environments. Lack of psychological safety can occur where the sporting environment is marked by abusive, threatening, or humiliating coaching styles. This not only significantly increases the immediate stress on athletes, but has also been found to be associated with long-term psychological harm (Leahy et al., 2008). Lack of physical safety can occur where extreme physical activities are used as a punishment for errors or failure to perform. Sexual abuse of young athletes has also been documented in many countries, with some research reporting long-term post-traumatic stress symptomatology (Leahy, 2010b; 2011; Leahy et al., 2008).

Team physicians, because of their close involvement with the team, are often the first point of contact for athletes, and, therefore, they need to be aware of the potential for these forms of injury, and the relevant social policy and procedures for reporting and referring. By providing well-timed advice, guidance, and other interventions, team physicians can also use their position within the multi-disciplinary support team to contribute effectively to the prevention of these forms of injury and to advocate for appropriate child and youth protection policies within the sports system.

Impact of sports injury

It is important for team physicians to understand the potentially profoundly disorganizing dynamics related to the impact of sports injury on athletes for whom both career and identity may be deeply enmeshed with athletic skills and abilities. Applying the framework of the biopsychosocial paradigm, we can conceptualize the stresses of injury impacting across the domains of physical, psychological, and social well-being. For example, the stress of the physical pain of the injury at the time of occurrence may soon be replaced by the physical and sometimes painful demands of treatment and rehabilitation. There may be significant psychological trauma where the events leading to the injury are themselves traumatic. For example, an athlete who previously worked with me was seriously injured while attending an overseas event, when a bridge, on which a large number of athletes were standing, collapsed, causing death and severe injury. This athlete barely escaped with his life. An athlete who has experienced this level of trauma may need a more in-depth and focused psychotherapeutic intervention to fully recover psychologically from the various implications of this type of traumatic injury experience.

Other psychological challenges brought about by sports injury may include possible threats to future performance, goals, and athletic identity. An athlete poignantly describes her gradual realization that successive injuries were preventing her from realizing her sporting goals, which were closely bound up with her identity:

> I used to be, like even when it was tough, I used to really enjoy training and loved competing [long pause]. My dream had been to go to the Olympics, and I was giving up my dream, and so many people associated me as an athlete [pause], but [long pause, weeping] I knew in my heart, I had known for a long while that it was happening [pause], like you know, my sport has been the defining thing for me as a person.

Athletes may experience a loss of key social roles and self-concept, and move from being, as one athlete explained to me, "the team captain who controls everything and who always works harder to push everyone along, and on whom everyone depends for support to being completely dependent [on the sports medicine team] and useless to anyone [on the sports team]."

Psychological theories of the aftermath of sport injury

A number of conceptual models have been proposed to explain the process of sport injury and rehabilitation and provide a frame of reference for understanding psychological responses to sport injury. Most physicians will be familiar with the work of Kübler-Ross (1969) who, based on her work with terminally ill patients, describes a series of stages that patients typically face: disbelief, denial, isolation, anger, bargaining, depression, acceptance, and, finally, resignation. Kübler-Ross's model was initially adapted to the context of sport injury, with researchers proposing that injured athletes' psychological responses suggest a sequence of stages of denial, bargaining, and depression, before final acceptance. However, empirical support for the proposition that there is a typical, stage-based set of responses to athletic injury has not been strong (Brewer, 2001; Wiese-Bjornstal, 2004). Nevertheless, the advantage of the Kübler-Ross model is that it provides a non-anthologizing framework for describing the dynamic, transformational experience of grief and loss that can characterize an individual's experience of serious sport injury.

Recent conceptualizations of psychosocial responses to sport injury represent an integration of stage models of grief and loss into frameworks that recognize that the complex interaction of characteristics of the individual (especially cognitive appraisals of the event), the injury itself (e.g., severity), and the social or situational context within which it occurs, results in considerable variability in individual responses (Wiese-Bjornstal, 2004).

What we do know from the empirical literature is that sport injury can be a significant source of stress, and that emotional reactions appear to be related to rehabilitation outcomes (Brewer et al., 2002; Podlog and Eklund, 2007). There is general consensus that the majority of emotional distress experienced by injured athletes does not usually reach clinical levels. Nevertheless, a significant minority of injured athletes, between 5 and 24% in some epidemiological studies, will manifest clinically significant psychological symptomatology (Brewer, Linder, et al., 1995; Brewer, Petitpas et al., 1995; Leddy, Lambert, and Ogles, 1994). However, those not reaching clinical cut-off scores on diagnostic tests may also be experiencing significant distress, and the presence of sub-clinical levels of psychological distress should be monitored by the team psychologist.

Stages of the injury process

What, then, might the team physician and the members of the sport injury management team expect to see as part of the injury presentation and process? Let's take a step-by-step look at the injury process to demonstrate the possible range of psychosocial factors that may be manifested in the injured athlete's presentation. Petitpas and Danish (1995) propose a three-stage process to consider in treatment planning: the crisis phase, the rehabilitation phase, and the recovery target date.

The crisis period, immediately post-injury, is the time when we can expect the maximum emotional upheaval, including shock, denial, fear, and anxiety. At this stage, denial can be adaptive and need not necessarily be challenged by the sport injury team. Denial can indicate some level of peritraumatic dissociation, a form of numbing or disconnection from the immediate traumatic pain and shock. This type of dissociation is a very useful initial coping strategy, as it prevents the full extent of the injury and pain from overwhelming the athlete, facilitates emergency medical aid, and gives the athlete time come to a realization of what has happened. For example, an athlete who had a life-threatening mountaineering accident recalls that the first thought that came to his mind when he regained consciousness at the bottom of a cliff, with his "legs and feet pointing at odd angles," was the fact that he still had a few days to recover and so could still make his planned skiing holiday the following week. This protective denial allowed him to be able to cope with the protracted and difficult rescue attempts.

Key tasks during the early part of the crisis stage are to establish a rapport by validating the athlete's feelings and helping the athlete to feel understood. The athlete's anxiety needs to be alleviated, and the athlete needs to be assisted in moving toward realistic expectations regarding recovery and to adaptive coping. This is particularly important, as the athlete may need to be involved in treatment decisions regarding surgery. Active coping, or what Heil (1993) calls determined coping, requires the athlete to be able to move from an emotionally reactive frame of mind, to rational, calculated decision-making. Denial could very well hinder the process at this point.

Where surgery is needed, a surge in anticipatory anxiety may replace the reactive anxiety of the injury. At this stage, it is not uncommon to encounter another form of denial, manifested through statements expressing that, after surgery, everything will be perfect, and the athlete will be able quickly to return to play. This may not be realistic, and the athlete may need to be appropriately helped to understand the impact and possible immediate and long-term outcomes of surgery. If the denial is not empathically addressed, then, in the early post-operative period, which may involve significant pain and physical restriction and, perhaps, complications, high levels of anxiety, feelings of being betrayed by the treatment team, and a breakdown in trust and therefore the therapeutic alliance may occur, leaving the athlete feeling isolated and helpless and potentially leading to a depressive episode.

The rehabilitation phase follows the crisis phase (Petitpas and Danish, 1995). Early on in this phase, it is important to help the athlete to focus on productive activity organized around appropriate, short-term rehabilitation goals. As the rehabilitation phase progresses, we would expect that the athlete may be feeling a sense of self-efficacy and increasing confidence as s/he successfully completes the rehabilitation tasks. Risks during this phase may come from treatment setbacks, as well as the day-to-day drudgery of rehabilitation. Motivation may decrease, resulting in anger and irritability with treatment providers and questioning of the team's competence and of the effectiveness of the program. If treatment providers fail to recognize these signs as indicators of distress, and react defensively or in a punishing manner to these perceived criticisms (see the section below on transference and counter-transference), then the athlete will feel alienated from those who should be helping. This can contribute to depression. What is essential at this point for the recovering athlete is continued and consistent support, encouragement, and coping skills to successfully negotiate the ups and downs of the rehabilitation path. Members of the sport injury management team may also need to support each other during this phase and provide supportive debriefing for front-line team members. This will ensure that every one is in the best emotional shape when dealing directly with the athlete.

The third phase proposed by Petipas and Danish (1995) is what they call the recovery target date. During this phase, also referred to as the specificity period (Steadman, 1993), the athlete needs to test the injured body part in his/her specific sport conditions. At this stage, ongoing success in rehabilitation should have successfully reduced any depression, and increased fitness should improve energy levels and sense of well-being. However, there may be a resurgence in anxiety, significant fears of re-injury, and worries about loss of skills when returning to play. With appropriate psychological preparation, and with ongoing support from the sport injury management team, these fears may soon be alleviated with a planned, successive, goal-directed return to play. It might be important during this phase to remind the coach, teammates, parents/guardians, and partners to also provide support and help to strengthen the athlete's confidence. Where return to play is not possible, and there is permanent impairment, then helping the athlete accept this loss may require significant psychological intervention and social support.

PSYCHOLOGICALLY BASED INTERVENTIONS

The goals of a psychologically based sport injury management program are to contribute to rehabilitation and, ultimately, recovery and successful return to sport performance, by facilitating emotional and psychological equilibrium and growth, mobilizing and strengthening existing coping resources, and ensuring that psychological readiness for return to play complements physical readiness. Important elements in psychologically based interventions with high-performing athletes, which non-psychology professionals can successfully implement, build on skills already well known to the athlete. High-performance athletes are generally experienced in psychological skills applied to sporting performance, such as goal setting, task-orientation focus, visualization, relaxation, and positive self-talk. The key to optimizing an athlete's active cooperation and adherence to the program is to set up the recovery as a performance task, with phased rehabilitation tasks conceptualized as the periodized training program. Once we move into the terminology of performance, we are speaking a language the athlete understands and we are explicitly validating the athletes' identity as an elite performer, rather than as an injured or ill person, which may have counterproductive connotations and associated role behaviors in the athlete's culture.

The fundamental components of an effective, psychologically based sport injury management program should incorporate an educational approach, where knowledge and skills are shared with the athlete. Additionally, a task-oriented, goal-setting approach, where sequential steps lead to successful completion of rehabilitation tasks, will facilitate active coping and adherence to the program. An approach that optimizes the benefits of appropriate social support to effect and maintains motivation is as important as the application of basic mental skills such as relaxation and visualization. Finally, no matter what psychological strategies are applied, practitioners must be able to use basic counseling skills to engage effectively with the injured athlete in delivering the program. These psychological strategies will only be effective within the context of a high-quality working alliance with the injured athlete.

Education

The primary goal of education is to help athletes gain a clear and accurate insight into the structure of the injury itself and the rehabilitation mechanisms and recovery processes. This will result in optimizing adherence by engaging the athlete as an active, motivated collaborator. It will aid in reducing worries, fears, and related mood disturbances, which, in some studies, have been found to correlate negatively with adherence (e.g., Brewer, 2011). As well as detailed knowledge of the anatomy of the injured part and the effects of the injury, athletes also need to be able clearly to differentiate the discomfort due to rehabilitation from pain that may indicate a problem.

It is never safe to assume that, just because the individual is engaged in sport, s/he therefore has in-depth knowledge of his/her own anatomy! An educational approach to sport injury management encourages a view of rehabilitation as a learning process, a set of skills to be learned and performed well to achieve a desired outcome. Again, this is the fundamental basis of sports training and is a familiar conceptualization for athletes.

Goal setting

Originating from the action-oriented behavior therapies, and widely used in high-performance sport, goal setting is defined very precisely. Effective goals are specific, measurable, time-based, and challenging but achievable, and outcome goals are very tightly linked to process goals. Athletes use goals every day as part of training and preparation for competition. A number of recent studies have lent empirical evidence to the long-advocated importance of goal setting in the injury rehabilitation process (e.g., Evans and Hardy, 2002).

In addition to setting goals to structure the rehabilitation process as a task-oriented set of skills to be mastered, identification of possible barriers to goal attainment can also provide useful information to attenuate the lack of adherence or apparent decrements in motivation. Fear of re-injury, concerns about pain, and lack of understanding of the task are often factors that underlie compliance problems. Another useful function of goal setting can be applied to the use of medications and modalities, including wearing of braces etc. Goals for coping with the routine drudgery of rehabilitation and attendant negative emotions (e.g., boredom, impatience, frustration, etc.), pain management, and adherence to activity proscriptions are also commonly set up. Goals of this nature, involving psychological coping skills, may be usefully set up and monitored as a collaborative activity between the athlete, the team physician, the physiotherapist, and the psychologist, thus affirming the importance of the activities, but, at the same time, acknowledging the challenges therein.

Social support

Sport injury rehabilitation is essentially a social process with, not just the sport injury management team, but also the athlete's teammates, family, and friends forming a support network. Social support is understood as a multidimensional construct consisting of listening support, emotional support, emotional challenge, task appreciation, task challenge, reality confirmation, and material and personal assistance (Richman et al., 1993). It has been applied in research on athletes and recently in the sport injury research area. All of the significant people in the athlete's life can potentially contribute to a perception of support, or lack thereof. Research findings with injured athletes reveal that friends, family members, and significant others appear to be more frequently nominated as providers of emotional support. On the other hand, medical practitioners and coaches are more frequently nominated as providers of technical and informational support (e.g., Johnston and Carroll, 1998).

PSYCHOLOGICALLY BASED SPORTS INJURY MANAGEMENT STRATEGIES

- Education.
- Goal setting.
- Social support.
- Relaxation and visualization.
- Therapeutic working alliance with injured athlete:
    - Empathic engagement
    - Transference and countertransference.

Research has shown that positive social support for rehabilitation is generally correlated with better adherence and outcome (Brewer, Linder, et al., 1995; Udry, 1997). To be effective, social support must be perceived as supportive by the recipient. All members of the sport injury management team must be proactive in asking the athlete what his/her support needs are. Assumptions are frequently incorrect and can lead to the injured athlete feeling unsupported. Indeed, injured athletes have reported family members and teammates as being more supportive than coaches and medical professionals (Udry et al., 1997).

What psychologists also recognize is that social support systems can sometimes fail significantly when they are most needed. This can happen where the support providers are themselves overwhelmed with anxiety or fear about the situation. For example, individuals in the sport injury management team may be struggling with heavy caseloads. Family and friends may avoid talking about the injury because they assume this is the best way to avoid upsetting the injured athlete. Coaches and teammates may miscalculate their attempts to reassure the athlete and unwittingly cause increased stress, by what the athlete perceives as pressure to return to play too quickly and challenges to the validity of their impairment or pain. Compassion fatigue, or burnout, can lead to a withdrawal of support and, in some cases, to the athlete being blamed for not recovering quickly enough in rehabilitation programs that extend over long periods of time.

The team physician is in a key position to be able to assess, advise, and plan, with the other sport injury team members, corollary interventions with key support providers to ensure the athlete's support needs are being met throughout the rehabilitation process. For example, help and information can be provided to coaches, family, and friends on how to cope with the various stages of the rehabilitation process, and how to support the athletes through the challenges of each stage.

Relaxation and visualization

Stemming from the cognitive-behavioral school of therapy and frequently used in stress-management protocols, relaxation, and visualization (or mental rehearsal) are skills routinely used by elite athletes. Relaxation and visualization can be applied to performance enhancement, recovery from training, preparation for competitions, learning or refining new skills, etc. The use of these mental skills neatly converges with the needs of a rehabilitation program set up as a performance task. The team physician, in conjunction with the coach and the psychologist, can be instrumental in encouraging the athlete to continue using these skills to maintain mental readiness for performance and to apply them to the challenges of rehabilitation. For example, while undergoing painful treatment protocols, or to cope with post-surgical pain, the athlete can control autonomic arousal by engaging in muscle relaxation and diaphragmatic breathing. Visualizing peaceful, relaxing scenes can also help to alleviate the discomfort of painful treatments and control anxiety. Athletes can mentally rehearse particularly challenging rehabilitation tasks prior to appointments, as they do for competition, focusing on mastery, successful execution, and positive self-talk.

Research on this aspect of rehabilitation and recovery supports the use of these basic mental skills (e.g., Cupal, 1998; Ross and Berger, 1996; Theodorakis et al., 1997), even though the exact mechanisms are not well understood. Proponents of the biopsychosocial framework suggest that these strategies have direct and indirect effects (mediated by biological factors) on rehabilitation outcome. In other words, these mental skills may contribute to attitude or behavioral changes (e.g., positive mood, better adherence) and physiological responses (e.g., blood circulation) that contribute to recovery outcomes (Brewer et al., 2002).

All members of the sport injury management team who are themselves competent in using relaxation and visualization can effectively teach and apply these basic skills in their practice with injured athletes.

533

Engaging effectively with the injured athlete

As mentioned earlier, there is considerable evidence that the quality of the working relationship between the practitioner and the injured athlete is one of the key predictors of treatment compliance and positive outcome (Ray and Weise-Bjornstal, 1999). All members of the sports injury management team – and particularly the team physician, who may be the case manager – need to be able to establish and maintain a therapeutic working alliance with the injured athlete. By "therapeutic alliance," I mean a relationship that is defined as existing solely to help another person. In other words, it is a one-way relationship, with one person's recovery needs (the athlete's) as the focus. One of the key elements in this process is the provision of a safe, respectful, nonjudgmental environment, where the athlete feels understood, validated, and listened to and is free to express distress and difficulties. What are the elements of this quality relationship and how can they be maximized? In this section, I will describe some basic counseling skills that are fundamental to effective engagement in a therapeutic alliance with injured athletes.

Empathy

Empathy is the term we use to describe a way of communicating that involves listening to, understanding, and communicating that understanding to, another person. Implicit in the concept of empathy is the ethic of care, a genuine wish to engage with the other person's perspective, and an acknowledgment that accurate understanding is crucial to effective care-giving. Lack of appropriate empathic engagement with injured athletes is perhaps one of the reasons that athletes in the social support research mentioned earlier did not perceive medical practitioners to be particularly supportive (Udry et al., 1997).

Empathic engagement starts with active listening. Active listening requires giving your full attention to the athlete, adopting an open, relaxed posture (and not taking phone calls or finishing off previous case notes!). Communication techniques such as open questions – "How are you feeling today?" – allow the opportunity for an open-ended answer. Closed questions – "Are you feeling better today?" – requiring only "Yes" or "No" answers, close down dialogue options, as do multiple-choice questions – "Is your leg feeling better or worse today?".

Another useful technique to show that you are interested in clearly understanding an athlete's communication is to paraphrase it. Paraphrasing can contain three components:

1. an introductory stem such as, "It sounds like what you are saying is . . .";
2. the basic idea, with any key words used by the athlete;
3. a perception check for accuracy, such as, "Is that correct?" or "Have I understood you correctly?".

For example, an athlete who is entering the specificity stage of the rehabilitation in preparation for return to play, tells you,

> You know, I really can't wait to get back out there on the track, it has been so hard not being able to train properly. But I am a bit worried I will not be as fast as I was before.

What is the key issue being expressed by the athlete? Paraphrasing the core content of the message might look like this: "It sounds like you are having conflicting feelings about getting back out on the track and are not sure what it will be like. have I understood you correctly?" These communication skills are not ones that we usually use in our daily lives. You will find that they require focused practice before they become natural and automatic. Without appropriate practice, they will sound forced and inauthentic. Try adding them into your daily conversations and experiment with different ways of expression that most suit your personality. There are other common phrases that we use in normal, daily conversation that, in the context of a therapeutic working alliance, can harm rather than support the injured athlete. Table 24.1 provides some examples of these, with suggestions for helpful, therapeutic alternatives. Training yourself not to automatically fall back on these "stock" phrases will take some time!

Table 24.1 Dos and don'ts of therapeutic conversations

Do not say	Why not?	Do say
I know how you feel	You can never really know how someone else feels. Even if you have gone through exactly the same experience, your individual experience may differ in significant ways	I am sorry this has happened to you
You shouldn't feel that way	This is a direct invalidation of someone's lived emotional experience	I can see that you are very upset about this
Put it behind you and move on	There is no pre-set timetable for people to overcome and move on from distressing experiences. Implying that there is will make the person feel like a failure. This will add unnecessary and harmful feelings of shame or guilt to the emotional distress of the injury itself	It is very challenging, and it may take some time before you feel better
It could have been worse	This statement is invalidating, as it implies that the person's distress is somehow unreasonable. Considering hypothetically worse scenarios or comparing with other's distress does not alleviate personal pain. Additionally, this might very well be the worst thing that has happened in this athlete's life	I am sorry this has happened to you. It must be very challenging for you. Let's work together and see how we can get the best outcome possible

Remember that providing medical interventions grounded in an empathic working alliance does not require the team physician to resolve psychological issues and emotional distress. Resolving these issues requires a deeper level of psychotherapeutic work that is the psychologist's area of expertise. However, the very simple process of being empathic and actively listening to the injured athlete will, in itself, be sufficient to provide a safe, containing space for the athlete to feel supported, which, as mentioned previously, is one of the factors correlated with adherence and positive rehabilitation outcome.

Transference and countertransference

Central to an effective, empathic, working alliance between the sport injury management team and the injured athlete is an awareness of, and ability to deal with, two key relational processes. These processes, called transference and countertransference, invariably arise in the context of helping relationships. They are prime catalysts in the failure of empathy and the impairment or even destruction of the therapeutic working alliance. To express it very simply, in any relational dyad, and particularly in care-giving relationships, transference is the label we assign to the process where the client transfers his/her feelings about something, or someone, on to the treatment provider. For example, as the frontline team physician, genuinely concerned and caring about the injured athlete who has presented in your office, you may be confronted with an extremely frustrated and angry athlete, whose anger may be projected on to you personally, and on to your profession. Countertransference, in this case, would arise if you were to respond to the personalized, transferred anger (by being defensive and getting angry) rather than to the real issue (the athlete's frustration and fear about the injury). The countertransferential response of defensive anger and withdrawal from empathic, authentic engagement with the athlete is a relational error that will impede the establishment and maintenance of a good treatment alliance and will result in the athlete remaining isolated in his/her distress and feeling unsupported. An appropriate response in this situation might be, "It sounds like you are really upset and worried about this injury. I am sorry this has happened, and it's quite normal to be upset at this point." With this short response, you have shown that you are an empathic listener, you have placed the athlete's needs (rather than your own) at the forefront of the interaction, and you have correctly identified and normalized the core issue for the injured athlete – the initial distress s/he is experiencing. A follow-up comment, such as, "Let's work together to see how we can best deal with this injury and work out a plan for recovery," then invites the athlete to participate as an active member of the treatment team.

Transference and countertransference can work on a number of levels to impede or assist the working alliance of the multidisciplinary team. For example, I was involved in a multidisciplinary team helping a young, elite athlete who was self-injuring. The team physician found himself responding in a very strict and punishing way to the young athlete: "You must stop this. If you don't stop this behavior, you will be thrown out of the team." Of course, this response exacerbated the athlete's

trisha leahy

distress even further, leading to more incidents of self-injury as a way of coping with the tension. What the team physician came to realize was that, as the father of a daughter of the same age as the athlete, he found himself being extremely anxious and worried, even panicked, about her well-being. The more he identified with the athlete as a daughter, the more he felt completely responsible for "curing" her. This sense of responsibility, coupled with the fact that treating self-harming behaviors was outside his domain of expertise, increased his anxiety. So, he fell back on another set of competencies that he did have – his parenting skills. When the athlete did not respond by ceasing the self-harming behavior, he began to act in the role of a strict father. Once he realized the impact of his countertransferential responses, he was able to understand and positively modify his responses to the athlete and effectively support the psychological aspects of the treatment.

A common countertransferential dynamic that occurs in helping relationships within the health professions arises where the athlete, who may have suffered great pain and anxiety at the time of the injury, is now, owing to your caring, compassionate, and effective treatment, free from pain and well on the way to full recovery. For this athlete, you are a hero. You have saved his/her career. You have been kind and have listened and understood, and the athlete has never before experienced such a positive relationship experience. You find that the athlete praises you and tells you that you are the only member of the sport injury management team who has truly understood him/her, and you are the best sports physician in the world! Of course, this is gratifying, and it is important to acknowledge your own good work. Where a countertransferential response might be evident is where you find yourself beginning to believe you really are the best in the world, and that you have no need of input from the other injury team members. In fact, their input is just not relevant, as they do not understand the athlete and the injury like you do. Before long, you are independently giving all kinds of advice to the athlete, without reference to the multidisciplinary team members. You have a sense of omnipotence – you can do no wrong! The dangers of this slippery countertransferential slope are obvious.

Not so obvious is the situation where you have been providing the best care that you can, having consulted with colleagues and the injury management team, but, after a few weeks with less than expected recovery progress, you find yourself in a consultation with the athlete and realize that you are feeling unsure, overwhelmed, and helpless about the case. There may be a countertransferential dynamic at work here, stemming from the athlete's transferred feelings about the recovery process. By recognizing these feelings as coming from the athlete, you are in a good position to address them helpfully. Remember that, as the team physician, your task is not to try to resolve these feelings for the athlete; rather, your task is to name, acknowledge, and normalize these feelings for him/her. Generally, once people experience that their concerns have been acknowledged and affirmed, they can get on with active coping. If they feel they are not being heard, or are being invalidated (e.g., by being told, "You shouldn't feel that way"),

Table 24.2 Understanding yourself in the countertransferential process

Exercise 1	• Reflect on a case that you have worked on, which you found particularly challenging in terms of relational issues with the client.
	• List the behaviors of the client that you found challenging.
	• How did you feel when the client displayed those behaviors?
	• What did you think when the client displayed those behaviors?
	• Identify the transferential or countertransferential dynamics that were in operation for you by reflecting on possible reasons why particular behaviors result in particular responses from you.
Exercise 2	• Divide a sheet of paper into two columns. In the first column, write the name of the client that you usually look forward to meeting, and list the behaviors that you really appreciate under that person's name.
	• In a parallel column, write the name of a client that you usually dislike meeting, and list the behaviors that challenge you under that person's name.
	• Ask yourself what characteristics, experiences, assumptions, and beliefs about the world and about relationships are you bringing into the practitioner–client interaction that are influencing your responses.

the feelings may escalate into depression and a real sense of hopelessness that will impede recovery and compliance.

The dynamics of transference and countertransference will occur during all stages of the recovery and rehabilitation process. The responsibility rests with us, the professionals, to monitor ourselves, and to seek help where our own "blindspots" may hinder our ability effectively to engage with our clients. For example, are you comfortable when people express pain and distress differently to you? How about anger? Harmful countertransferential errors with vulnerable, distressed individuals occur where the helper defensively withdraws from the client because of discomfort with the client's emotional expression (Leahy et al., 2003). Explore your own possible countertransferential "triggerpoints" in the exercises provided in Table 24.2.

Self-care for the team physician

For the team physician, working within the organized, competitive sport arena, opportunities for working with teams at club, regional, and national levels are more and more common. Increasingly, sports teams are requesting team physicians, as well as other sports science and allied health professionals, to work as part of the designated support team. This may involve working with a team of athletes on an ongoing basis over a number of years. To successfully perform this role, all members of the support team are required to have an in-depth knowledge of the sport and the individual athletes and, ultimately, be present at their important

trisha leahy

events, up to and including the Olympics. The demands on the team physician can be considerable, and the stress and expectations can be exhausting.

To continue to function effectively, team physicians, like all care professionals, need to carefully monitor their own health and well-being. In the environment of high-level sport, the team physician may have a very public role and may be viewed as a role model in terms of health behaviors and lifestyle. However, we also know that front-line health-care professionals are a high-risk group for stress and burnout. If you find yourself having difficulty sleeping or eating, feeling irritable, anxious, or even not feeling much of anything at all, and not enjoying the activities that used to give you pleasure, then you may be in need of a recovery break. Using colleagues to debrief and get supportive feedback after difficult cases or client interactions is a technique commonly used by psychologists and other mental-health professionals to maintain a sense of balance. In the long term, prevention in the form of a balanced, healthy lifestyle, with adequate rest, recreation, and social support, is crucial.

CONCLUSION

In this chapter, I have attempted to outline the elements of a biopsychosocial approach to understanding sport injury, with a focus on the psychosocial aspects. Managing injury is a part of the game that athletes must learn to play well in order to maintain a long and successful career in sport. Team physicians may be in the unique position of being able to spend considerable time with injured athletes relative to physicians in private or hospital clinics. They can play a crucial role in the effective functioning of the multidisciplinary sport injury management team in optimizing the recovery environment. To this end, the fundamentals of psychosocial theory and knowledge can be effectively incorporated into the team physician's repertoire of clinical skills.

SUGGESTED READING

Brewer, B., 2001. Psychology of sport injury rehabilitation. In: *Handbook of Sport Psychology*. 2nd ed. New York: John Wiley & Sons, pp. 787–809.

Brewer, B., 2011. Adherence to sport injury rehabilitation. In: *Routledge Handbook of Applied Sport Psychology*. London: Routledge, pp. 233–41.

Brewer, B., Andersen, M., and Van Raalte, J., 2002. Psychological aspects of sport injury: Toward a biopsychosocial approach. In: D. Mostofsky and D. Zaichkowsky, eds. *Medical and Psychological Aspects of Sport and Exercise*. Morgantown, WV: Fitness Information Technology, pp. 41–54.

Brewer, B., Linder, D., and Phelps, C., 1995. Situational correlates of emotional adjustment to athletic injury. *Clinical Journal of Sports Medicine*, Volume 5, pp. 241–5.

Brewer, B., Petitpas, A., Van Raalte, J., Sklar, J.H., and Ditmar, T.D., 1995. Prevalence of psychological distress among patients at a physical therapy clinic specializing in sports medicine. *Sports Medicine, Training, and Rehabilitation*, Volume 6, pp. 138–45.

Brewer, B., Van Raalte, J., and Petitpas, A., 2007. Patient–practitioner interactions in sport injury rehabilitation. In: D. Pargman, ed. *Psychological Bases of Sport Injuries*. Morgantown, WV: Fitness Information Techology, pp. 79–94.

Cupal, D., 1998. Psychological intervention in sport injury prevention and rehabilitation. *Journal of Applied Sport Psychology*, Volume 10, pp. 103–23.

Evans, L., and Hardy, L., 2002. Injury rehabilitation: A goal setting intervention study. *Research Quarterly in Exercise and Sport*, Volume 73, pp. 310–19.

Frey, J., Preston, F., and Bernhard, B., 2004. Risk and injury: A comparison of football and rodeo subcultures. In: K. Young, ed. *Sporting Bodies, Damaged Selves: Sociological Studies of Sports-Related Injury*. Oxford: Elsevier, pp. 59–80.

Heil, J., 1993. A psychologist's view of the personal challenge of injury. In: J. Heil, ed. *Psychology of Sport Injury*. Champaign, IL: Human Kinetics, pp. 33–48.

Johnson, U., 2007. Psychosocial antecedents in sport injury prevention. In: D. Pargman, ed. *Psychological Bases of Sport Injuries*. 3rd ed. Morgantown, WV: Fitness Information Techology, pp. 39–52.

Johnston, L. and Carroll, D., 1998. The provision of social support to injured athletes: A qualitative analysis. *Journal of Sport Rehabilitation*, Volume 7, pp. 267–84.

Kolt, G. and Andersen, M., 2004. Using psychology in the physical and manual therapies. In: G. Kolt and M. Andersen, eds. *Psychology in the Physical and Manual Therapies*. London: Churchill Livingstone, pp. 3–8.

Kübler-Ross, E., 1969. *On Death and Dying*. New York: Macmillan.

Leahy, T., 2010a. Safeguarding child athletes from abuse in elite sport: The role of the sport psychologist. In: D. Gilbourne and M. Andersen, eds. *Critical Essays in Applied Sport Psychology*. Champaign, IL: Human Kinetics, pp. 251–66.

Leahy, T., 2010b. Sexual abuse in sport: Implications for the sport psychology profession. In: T. Ryba, R. Scinke, and G. Tenenbaum, eds. *The Cultural Turn in Sport Psychology*. Morgantown, WV: Fitness Information Techology, pp. 315–34.

Leahy, T., 2011. Working with adult athlete survivors of sexual abuse. In: S. Hanrahan and M. Andersen, eds. *Routledge Handbook of Applied Sport Psychology*. London: Routledge, pp. 303–12.

Leahy, T., Pretty, G., and Tenenbaum, G., 2003. Childhood sexual abuse narratives in clinically and non-clinically distress adult survivors. *Professional Psychology, Research and Practice*, Volume 34, pp. 657–65.

Leahy, T., Pretty, G., and Tenenbaum, G., 2008. A contextualized investigation of traumatic correlates of childhood sexual abuse in Australian athletes. *International Journal of Sport and Exercise Psychology*, Volume 4, pp. 366–84.

Leddy, M., Lambert, M., and Ogles, B., 1994. Psychological consequences of athletic injury among high-level competitors. *Research Quarterly for Exercise and Sport*, Volume 65, pp. 347–54.

Medibank, private, 2006. Author.

Petitpas, A. and Danish, S., 1995. Caring for injured athletes. In: S. Murphy, ed. *Sport Psychology Interventions*. Champaign, IL: Human Kinetics, pp. 255–81.

Podlog, L. and Eklund, R., 2007. Psychological considerations of the return to sport following injury. In: D. Pargman, ed. *Psychological Bases of Sport Injuries*. 3rd ed. Morgantown, WV: Fitness Information Techology, pp. 109–30.

Ray, R. and Wiese-Bjornstal, D. eds., 1999. *Counseling in Sports Medicine*. Champaign, IL: Human Kinetics.

Richman, J., Rosenfeld, L., and Hardy, C., 1993. The social support survey: A validation study of a clinical measure of the social support process. *Research on Social Work Practice*, Volume 3, pp. 288–311.

Ross, M.J., and Berger, R.S. 1996. Effects of stress inoculation training on athletes' post surgical pain and rehabilitation after orthopedic injury. *Journal of Consulting and Clinical Psychology*, Volume 64, 406–10.

Sabo, D., 2004. The politics of sports injury: Hierarchy, power and the pain principle. In: K. Young, ed. *Sporting Bodies, Damaged Selves: Sociological Studies of Sports-Related Injury*. Oxford: Elsevier, pp. 59–80.

Steadman, J., 1993. A physician's approach to the psychology of injury. In: J. Heil, ed. *Psychology of Sport Injury*. Champaign, IL: Human Kinetics, pp. 25–32.

Suls, J. and Rothman, A., 2004. Evolution of the biopsychosocial model: Prospects and challenges for health psychology. *Health Psychology*, Volume 23, pp. 119–25.

Theodorakis, Y., Beneca, A., Malliou, P., and Goudas, M. 1997. Examining psychological factors during injury rehabilitation. *Journal of Sport Rehabilitation*, Volume 6, pp. 355–63.

Udry, E., 1997. Coping and social support among injured athletes following surgery. *Journal of Sport and Exercise Psychology*, Volume 19, pp. 71–90.

Udry, E., Gould, D., Bridges, D., and Tuffey, S., 1997. People helping people? Examining the social ties of athletes coping with burnout and injury stress. *Journal of Sport and Exercise Psychology*, Volume 19, pp. 368–95.

Wiese-Bjornstal, D., 2004. Psychological responses to injury and illness. In: *Psychology in the Physical and Manual Therapies*. London: Churchill Livingstone, pp. 21–38.

Williams, J. and Andersen, M., 1998. Psychosocial antecedents of sports injury: Review and critique of the stress and injury model. *Journal of Applied Sport Psychology*, 10: pp. 5–25.

CHAPTER 25

REHABILITATION IN SPORTS MEDICINE

Sheila A. Dugan and Walter R. Frontera

INTRODUCTION

Perhaps when the team physician thinks about rehabilitation, he or she may not automatically consider its application to initial injury management. Rehabilitation begins at the time of injury and continues beyond the time the athlete returns to competition. What is done at fieldside may be more relevant to the athlete's recovery of musculoskeletal health than at any other time. We will discuss briefly the basic principles, phases, and techniques of rehabilitation. While they will be introduced individually, one must remember that rehabilitation occurs on a continuum, with much overlap. For example, there is no sharp cutoff between acute and subacute management techniques. The team physician must regularly re-evaluate the athlete's status and progress him or her appropriately. Comprehensive management uses multiple approaches. Additional approaches can be added or deleted, based on the athlete's response.

Our review summarizes the different modalities, medications, and therapy techniques and the rationale for their use in the rehabilitation of sports injuries. The team physician chooses which modality to use, based on the specific injury and feasibility. Athletes require a rehabilitation approach that is based on physiologic principles, is directed by the individual's response, and goes beyond resolution of the acute injury to prevent repeat injury. It is important to note that the quality of the scientific evidence that supports the use of modalities and techniques in rehabilitation is variable.

The following are principles to guide sports rehabilitation: minimize damage/inflammation/pain at the site of injury; promote healing; maintain/increase range of motion (ROM); prevent atrophy/increase strength; maintain/increase endurance; facilitate functional recovery; and avoid maladaptive compensatory movement patterns.

542 FiMS

Pathophysiology of injury and repair

Knowledge of the pathophysiology of tissue injury and the healing process is important in planning for treatment. The healing process involves three stages: the inflammatory stage; the fibroblastic-repair stage; and the maturation–remodeling stage. Understanding the chemical and physiological events can help the practitioner to select rehabilitation interventions that maximize restorative events and minimize maladaptive responses. One must identify the tissues injured and the extent of the injuries. Previous chapters of this book review diagnosis and management of injury by anatomic location. Injury classification guides the rehabilitation process. For instance, a fracture of the radius requires different management than a soft-tissue injury of the forearm such as wrist extensor tendinitis.

THE STAGES OF INJURY

The inflammatory stage

The inflammatory response lasts for 2–4 days. It presents clinically as increased warmth, redness, swelling, and tenderness. The initial trauma to the tissue or primary injury is followed by secondary injury resulting from hypoxia and enzymatic activity. At the time of injury, a cascade of events is set in motion. After a 5–10-minute period of vasoconstriction, a locally mediated influx of cells presents at the injury site. Chemical mediators, such as histamine from mast cells, increase membrane permeability and vasodilatation. Phagocytic cells and leukocytes invade the area. Waste products are broken down and removed via local and vascular effects. At the site of vessel injury, platelets adhere to the exposed collagen fibers, starting clot formation. Fibrin clot formation ensues via the cascade stimulated by thromboplastin. Eventually, a walling-off effect facilitates the healing process. Clot formation begins about 12 hours post-injury and is complete within 48 hours.

Initial rehabilitation techniques focus on minimizing the inflammatory response. This is done to prevent further loss of function and to decrease pain. The influx of inflammatory mediators is necessary to keep up with the metabolic demands and remove waste products. This prepares for the fibroblastic-repair stage of healing. However, the resulting inflammation and tenderness can cause impairments in strength, joint ROM, endurance, and tissue mobility. If left unchecked, these impairments can become a significant problem for the athlete. An exuberant inflammatory response can also compress tissues adjoining the injury, widening the extent of the injury.

Let us consider the example of a soccer player with knee swelling. Swelling in the tibiofemoral and patellofemoral joint space can mechanically limit joint ROM. Inhibition of quadriceps contraction in the setting of knee effusion occurs via central mechanisms. If the effusion persists untreated, significant impairment in knee strength results. Pain can lead to muscle spasm and disuse. These impairments cause a disability in gait and sport-specific movement patterns. A rehabilitation approach that limits the knee effusion, increases tibiofemoral and patellofemoral ROM, and improves quadriceps strength is the most effective.

The fibroplastic-repair stage

The fibroplastic-repair stage begins during the inflammatory response and continues for the next 4–6 weeks. It starts by scar filling in the injury defect. The fibrin clot is replaced with granulation tissue made up of collagen and fibroblasts. Critical nutrients are delivered via new capillaries. The collagen fibers are randomly laid down in an extracellular matrix of proteins and ground substance produced by the fibroblasts. The tensile strength of the scar is based on the collagen deposition.

Let's consider a complete rupture of the Achilles tendon, treated non-surgically, in a tennis player. Application of a cast will control inflammation and enhance scar formation. After about 3 weeks, a firm, strong, non-vascular scar exists. After 3 weeks of complete immobilization, the tendon should be ready for a controlled remobilization process. Impairments minimally include decreased soft-tissue mobility, loss of foot and ankle ROM, decreased strength of the foot and ankle muscles, and limited ankle proprioception. Disabilities in position changes, gait, and sport-specific movement patterns are to be expected. The rehabilitation process must address all of these issues.

The maturation–remodeling stage

The maturation–remodeling stage begins as the tensile strength of the scar tissue increases, and fibroblast activity declines. During this stage, stress on the collagen fibers causes them to realign in parallel with the forces applied, via Wolff's law. It may take months to years to normalize the strength of the tissue. Controlled mobilization at this time maximizes the reorientation of healing fibers, ultimately resulting in improved tensile strength and function. Pain can guide the rate of progression of stress on the remodeling tissue. Whereas pain may be significant during the inflammatory response, it will typically subside during the repair and remodeling stages. Any exacerbation of pain in this stage indicates that the rehabilitation program is too stressful on the tissue for the level of maturation attained.

Let's consider an overhead-throwing athlete with a partial tear of the supraspinatus tendon. In the maturation–remodeling stage, rehabilitation will shift to activity that will apply strain to the tendon along lines of tensile force parallel to the movements he will use in throwing. This can be achieved initially with bilateral activities such as overhead toss with an exercise ball. This limits the degrees of freedom at the glenohumeral joint and the workload. A progression could include the same activity with a medicine ball or done unilaterally. Ongoing impairments in soft-tissue mobility, glenohumeral and scapulothoracic ROM, scapular and upper extremity musculature strength, and shoulder proprioception must be addressed.

Sport-specific training is necessary for neuromuscular re-education, in addition to tissue remodeling.

MEDICATIONS IN SPORTS MEDICINE

A comprehensive discussion of the medications used in sports medicine is beyond the scope of this chapter. Pharmacologic agents are used to minimize inflammation and provide analgesia. This allows the athlete to get on with the rehabilitation program. The use of medications to limit inflammation, control pain, and limit muscle spasm is appropriate. There are multiple agents that are routinely used with injured athletes. These include the following categories: analgesics; NSAIDs; and muscle relaxants. The use of corticosteroids in the setting of athletic injury is controversial and will not be addressed.

Analgesics

Pure analgesic agents are used to decrease pain to allow participation in an active rehabilitation program as early as feasible. Centrally acting agents in the opioid group are used for a short course for severe pain. However, narcotics are banned by the International Olympic Committee. Acetaminophen is a peripheral analgesic without anti-inflammatory action. Because it does not interfere with prostaglandin synthesis, prostaglandin-related toxicities such as gastric ulceration do not occur. For patients in whom NSAID use is contraindicated, acetaminophen can be substituted.

Aspirin in low doses has an analgesic and anti-pyretic effect. In higher doses, it demonstrates significant gastrointestinal side effects. It also impairs platelet aggregation and can increase the bleeding associated with the initial injury.

Non-steroidal anti-inflammatory agents

NSAIDS are the most frequently prescribed medication in the setting of sports medicine. They directly affect the inflammatory cascade by blocking the conversion of arachidonic acid to prostaglandin by inhibiting the action of cyclooxygenase. The main side effect, causing morbidity and mortality, is gastric ulceration. There is some theoretical concern that NSAID use may slow or delay healing by interfering with the inflammatory response, but clinical studies with humans have not proved this. Newer NSAIDs and enteric-coated aspirin cause fewer gastro-intestinal side effects. A more selective group of NSAIDs has been developed, COX 2 inhibitors, which block only a subset of cyclooxygenase enzymes. Although they demonstrated a more limited gastrointestinal side-effect profile, some studies have

545

demonstrated a significant cardiovascular thrombogenic potential with particular COX 2 inhibitors. Efficacy between different NSAIDs is user-dependent and involves many factors.

Muscle relaxants

Muscle relaxants are frequently prescribed in addition to an analgesic agent or NSAIDs. In the short run, reduction in muscle spasm is in keeping with other goals of the acute rehabilitation period. Sedation is the major side effect that may limit patient tolerance; they may be helpful acutely to improve sleep.

MODALITIES

The team physician can order many different physical modalities to treat athletes. Refer to Table 25.1 for an overview of modalities. The guiding principle for their use should be minimization of injury and time away from sport. They are helpful in managing pain and edema and promoting healing. A thorough understanding of the indications, contraindications, and expected physiological response ensures appropriate utilization. They are an adjunct to care and do not provide a cure. They do not replace active exercise and are used to promote activity. This philosophy should be conveyed to the coach and the athlete being treated. Coaches and athletes can be instructed in the proper use of modalities; some modalities require direct setting up and monitoring by the physical therapist or athletic trainer.

Modalities can be grouped in the following way: cold, heat, electricity, and traction. Hydrotherapy can be used for both cold (cryotherapy) or heat transfer. Aquatherapy is a hybrid agent and will be discussed after the section on exercise. An athlete can exercise in water while benefiting from the modality.

Cold modalities

Superficial cold
Cold therapy, or cryotherapy, is a very helpful modality in the sports medicine practice. There are multiple applications of cryotherapy. Ice massage involves using an ice cube or lolly to apply ice directly to the inflamed tissue with gentle stroking, for 5–10 minutes. It combines the effects of cooling with massage. Crushed ice can be placed in a plastic bag to make an ice pack. Commercially available gel or a silicon cold pack cooled in a freezer to –12°C can be applied. Packs are applied for 10–30 minutes at a time, while tolerance is monitored. A compressive bandage may enhance the effect. Immersion in cold water provides circumferential cooling of a limb via convection, with a water temperature of 15°C. Cryotherapy–compression units combine cold therapy and pneumatic compression. A cuff is used for 10–30 minutes, through which cold water circulates while static or serial pneumatic compression is applied.

Table 25.1 Modalities used in sports medicine

Modality	Physiologic effects	Indications for use	Contraindications
Superficial cold	Slow nerve conduction ↓ blood flow due to cutaneous vasoconstriction ↑ firing muscle spindle and GTO ↓ collagenase activity and ↓ collagen distensibility	Analgesia, ↓ pain ↓ swelling ↓ muscle spasm Anesthetic skin	Raynaud's phenomenon Cryoglobulinemia Cold allergy (cold based urticaria) PVD/aortic insufficiency
Superficial heat	Sedation and general relaxation ↑ blood flow via vasodilatation ↑ collagenase activity	↓ pain ↑ tendon distensibility and ↓ joint stiffness ↑ metabolism and tissue temperature	Impaired sensation Bleeding diasthesis Directly over fetus, gonads Malignancy Impaired circulation Acute inflammation
Deep heat	Same as superficial heat	Same as superficial heat	Near brain, eyes, heart, gravid uterus Near spine laminectomy site Skeletal immaturity/growth plate Methyl methacrylate High-density polyethlylene Near pacemaker
Electrotherapy	Promote muscle relaxation ↑ local blood flow Stimulate muscle contraction Drive ions into skin	↓ pain and ↓ muscle spasm Promote tissue healing ↓ disuse atrophy ↓ edema	Proximity to cardiac sinus, eyes, fetus Pacemakers Anesthetic skin Area with metal
Traction	Distract cervical vertebral facet joints Stimulate joint mechanoreceptors Elongate and improve blood flow to paraspinal muscles Decrease intradiscal pressure	Improve healing by nutrition of articular cartilage ↓ pain ↓ muscle guarding Improve alignment	Acute inflammation Lesion compromising spinal stability, for example: neoplasm, spondylolisthesis, spinal infection, rheumatoid arthritis

Notes: GTO = Golgi tendon organ; PVD = peripheral vascular disease

rehabilitation in sports medicine

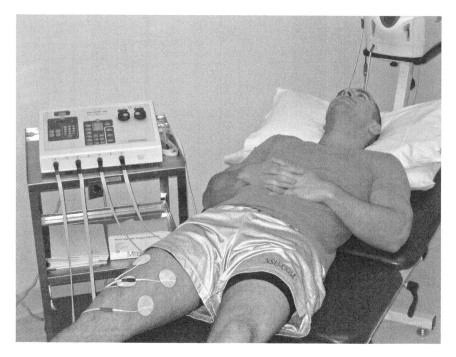

Figure 25.1 Interferential current: Electrotherapy modality requiring direct set-up and supervision

Source: Sol M. Abreu Sosa, MD

Heat modalities

Superficial heat

Superficial agents penetrate less than 2 cm. Maximal tissue temperatures are in skin and subcutaneous fat. Hydrocollator pads are an example of superficial conductive heat transfer. They are made of silicone oxide in a canvas cover and are immersed in water at 77°C. They are applied with a layer of towels and maintain heat for about 30 minutes. Electric heating pads and paraffin are two other examples of superficial heating via conduction.

Whirlpool-bath immersion is an example of a superficial heating modality that transfers energy via convection. The water temperature is based on the extent of the body immersed. For a distal limb, up to 45°C is tolerated. For immersion to the waist, up to 41°C is tolerated. Maintaining a water temperature below 38°C is appropriate with immersion of most of the body, or in a patient with cardiac precautions. Detergent or iodine can be added to the whirlpool for wound care. Fluidotherapy is another convective superficial heating agent. Like a whirlpool, it allows active range of motion but provides protection from skin contamination.

Cornhusks are circulated by warm air in an enclosed container, with the extremity in an isolated sheath.

Deep heat

Deep-heating agents penetrate deeper than 2 cm. Maximal temperatures are beneath the subcutaneous tissue, with conversion to heat at the bone–muscle interface. There is a smaller margin between a therapeutic temperature range and a temperature for potential thermal injury. The thermal pain threshold is 45°C, and the therapeutic goal temperature is 40°C.

Ultrasound is an example of a deep-heating agent. Molecular vibration is converted to heat, which penetrates 6–8 cm. Dosage is expressed as intensity. The usual therapeutic intensity range is 0.5–3.0 W/cm^2. Ultrasound can be delivered via continuous or pulsed output, and it is typically applied with a stroking technique. Non-thermal effects such as cavitation, media motion, and standing waves must be considered. Ultrasound waves can be used to deliver biologically active molecules into tissue via phonophoresis. Short-wave diathermy is another deep-heating modality, where electromagnetic energy is converted to thermal energy. Its use is limited by its significant side effects, including interference with pace-makers and focal heating of metal.

Electrical modalities

Electrotherapy has been used for centuries. Muscle and nerve respond differently to electrical stimulation. The team physician can take advantage of this and use different therapeutic electricity techniques. Depending on the goal of therapy, an agent is chosen. There are many types to choose between, with either alternating current (AC) or direct current (DC). The parameters, such as waveform, amplitude, and duration, can be manipulated. Transcutaneous electrical nerve stimulation (TENS) is used to treat painful conditions, with either local or segmental elec-trode placement, depending on the underlying condition. High-voltage galvanic stimulation (HVGS) transmits higher voltage, with higher peaks than traditional TENS. This allows for deeper tissue penetration. Neuromuscular electrical stimulators (NMESs) are used to maintain strength, limit atrophy, and re-educate injured muscles. Interferential current is used to increase blood flow in the region of intersecting waveforms and can be applied in conjunction with electrical muscle stimulation, with a massage effect. Neuroprobe can be used over motor points or trigger points, as well as acupuncture points. It produces anesthesia via hyper-stimulation.

Percutaneous electrical nerve stimulation (PENS) is applied via acupuncture needles. Iontophoresis involves driving biologically active agents through the skin to treat conditions in the soft tissues. Laser (light amplification by stimulated emission of radiation) therapy comes in two types, high powered versus low powered or cold. Gallium arsenide (GaAs) and helium neon (HeNe) are two types of cold laser that are used for the treatment of localized injury in superficial tissue.

Traction

Manual traction treats painful conditions of the spine. Pain reduction most likely occurs owing to relaxation of soft tissues overlying the spine. To achieve distraction of the vertebral bodies or facet joints, a mechanical apparatus with weights is necessary. Mechanical distraction may occur in the cervical spine if the weight is sufficient to overcome the weight of the head. The usefulness of mechanical traction in sports medicine is limited. Mechanical traction is contraindicated if any spinal instability, infection, or tumor is present.

ORTHOTICS IN SPORTS

An orthosis, or brace, is an external device that is applied to a body part to provide reduction of pain, support or stability, limited ROM, improvement in function, prevention of deformity, and kinesthetic reminder, among other things. Orthotics can be divided into two major categories: corrective or accommodative. Corrective devices are meant to improve the position of the limb segment, either by stretching a contracture or correcting the alignment of skeletal structure. Accommodative devices are meant to provide additional support to an already deformed tissue, to prevent further deformity, and ultimately to provide function. Orthoses can be further subdivided into static or dynamic. The use of orthotics during sport rehabilitation or injuries needs to be discussed in detail with a sports physician in order to choose the most suitable device.

Athletic taping is a technique used to stabilize muscles and joints to prevent injury. Athletic tape can also be used to help minimize additional damage to existing injuries, particularly on the hands, feet, and wrists, where many athletes are most vulnerable. Kinesio Taping® is an alternative taping technique. Unlike traditional athletic tape, Kinesio Tape® is elastic, and it can be stretched to 140% of its original length before being applied to the skin. Once applied, it provides a constant pulling (shear) force to the skin. It is of note that the fabric of this specialized tape is air permeable and water resistant and can be worn repeatedly for days. Kinesio Tape® is currently being used to treat a variety of orthopedic and neuromuscular conditions, immediately following injury and during the rehabilitation process. Proposed treatment mechanisms may include: (1) correcting muscle function by strengthening weakened muscles; (2) improving circulation of blood and lymph; (3) decreasing pain through neurological suppression; and (4) repositioning subluxed joints by relieving abnormal muscle tension. However, despite the increased use of Kinesio Tape® for the management and/or prevention of sports injuries, further research is required to validate its effect and efficacy.

STAGES OF REHABILITATION AND MANAGEMENT PRINCIPLES

In general, rehabilitation follows a logical sequence. Pain and edema must be controlled initially. Modalities, medications, and some form of immobilization may be necessary. Massage, manual therapy, and acupuncture are useful to reduce pain and promote activity. Flexibility and ROM can be addressed once pain decreases. Once mobility is restored, strengthening can be achieved in the appropriate range, with closed- and open-chain kinetics. Endurance training is added to the strengthening regiment. Finally, function and sport-specific activities are integrated. This necessitates neuromuscular re-education, balance, proprioception, and agility training. We will review this progression in order.

ACUTE STAGE (FIRST 48–72 HOURS)

Rehabilitation in this stage is focused on limiting the inflammatory response. The letters RICE summarize the methods used to control inflammation and pain: rest, ice, compression, and elevation.

- *Rest*: Continued unlimited movement of the injured area will cause increased bleeding and swelling. Depending on the extent of the injury, partial or relative rest through to complete rest with immobilization may be appropriate. The team physician faces the dilemma of balancing the protective effects of immobilization with its negative physiologic results.
- *Ice*: The inflammatory response is brought about by vasodilatation and tissue exudates, including white blood cells, breakdown products of damaged cells, and various chemical mediators. Ice decreases local metabolism and oxygen

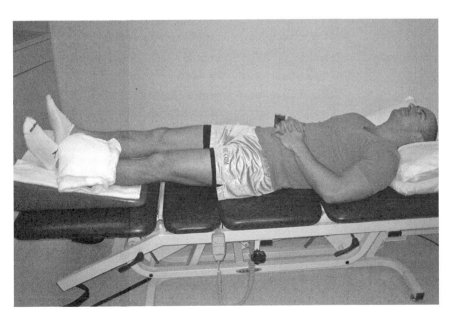

Figure 25.2 RICE treatment: Rest, ice, compression, and elevation
Source: Sol M. Abreu Sosa, MD

demand. A recent study showed that ice reduced the secondary injury that occurs after musculoskeletal trauma by retarding the hypoxia and enzymatic cascade. Ice controls pain and local muscle guarding. It is most effective minimizing the effects of inflammation when used with compression.

▪ *Compression*: Compression with a firm material can reduce bleeding and swelling at the site of injury. Pain should not be increased with the dressing; if application of compression causes pain, it may be too tight. It should be applied with the greatest pressure distal to the injury site and with declining pressure proximally.

▪ *Elevation*: Elevation decreases blood flow to, and increases venous and lymph return from, the injured body part. For lower-limb injuries, the injured part should be positioned above the level of the pelvis. For upper-limb injuries, the injured part should be positioned above the level of the heart.

Table 25.2 Acute rehabilitation stage

Intervention	Example	Indication
Modality	Superficial cold	Decrease pain, decrease swelling
	Interferential current	Facilitate participate in active rehabilitation program
Medication	Analgesics	Decrease pain, decrease swelling
	NSAIDs	Decrease muscle spasm
	Muscle relaxants	Facilitate active exercise
Immobilization	Air cast	Relative rest for injured joint/limb
	Walking boot	Protect from further injury
	Fiberglass cast	Reduce swelling
		Allow overall mobility
Massage	Effleurage	Reduce swelling
		Decrease pain
Manual therapy	Joint mobilization	Restore physiological movement
Acupuncture	Tendinomuscular meridian acupuncture	Decrease pain
Exercise	Static strengthening (isometrics)	Reduce atrophy and weakness
	Gentle static stretching	Limit loss of range of motion
Aquatherapy	Walking in pool	Maintain general cardiovascular endurance
		Limit weight-bearing of affected lower extremity

Medications and modalities, especially cryotherapy and electrotherapy, are important tools during this stage. Maintenance of general flexibility, strength, and conditioning should be ongoing. For example, a runner with a tibial stress fracture can cross-train with swimming instead of running. Cross-training is also beneficial because of the cross-over effect. Owing to neural adaptation, flexibility and strength training with the contralateral uninjured limb has been shown to be beneficial to the injured limb. Other components of the acute management of injury include immobilization, massage, manual therapy, and acupuncture. See Table 25.2 for the elements of rehabilitation in the acute stage.

Rehabilitation techniques

Immobilization

Often, in the acute stage of injury management, immobilization is necessary to prevent continuation of the inflammatory cascade, allow healing, or prohibit loading in particular planes while allowing other planes of movement. Complete immobilization is needed in the setting of a bony injury, especially an acute fracture. In a more subacute stage, it may be indicated, as with some stress fractures. Plaster casting has traditionally been used most for complete immobilization. Fiberglass casting also provides immobilization with a more lightweight and waterproof material. Alternative agents such as rigid braces, air splints, thermoplastic orthotics, and taping provide less-rigid stabilization but allow for easier wear, observation of the area, and hygiene and are appropriate for protected mobilization. The team physician monitors healing and can progress the athlete from partial to complete mobilization when appropriate. Prolonged immobilization can cause side effects, including muscle atrophy and weakness, loss of ROM, and degenerative changes in articular cartilage.

Manual techniques

Manual therapy

The application of manual-therapy techniques to restore normal joint, soft-tissue, and neural mobility is imperative to normalize the biomechanics of the musculoskeletal system. Manual therapy is done in conjunction with the re-education of muscle function. Joint mobilization is used to treat deficiencies in the accessory or physiological movements of a joint. It is graded in intensity and provides passive movement in the available ROM only. Joint manipulation includes movement through the barrier of available ROM. This is done via thrusting or high-velocity translation of one component of a joint, while the other component is fixed. Contraindications to joint mobilization and manipulation include: local malignancy; local bony infection or fracture; spinal cord or caudaequina compression; rheumatoid arthritis at C1–C2; vertebral artery insufficiency; spondylolisthesis; prepubertal children with open growth plates; and joint instability.

Massage

Massage involves direct physical action on an injured or painful area. It may decrease pain and facilitate healing by reducing muscle spasm, aiding in removal of chemical substances, promoting efficient scar formation, or breaking down abnormal scar tissue. It should be used to facilitate active exercise whenever possible. Various techniques are used, including stroking or effleurage; kneading or petrissage; tapping or tapotement; and deep pressure or cross-friction. Cross-friction is contraindicated in the acute stage, owing to increased local blood flow and tissue reactivity.

Acupuncture

Acupuncture has been used for many centuries for the control of pain. It continues to have a role in the acute treatment of athletic injuries. Although its mechanism of action is not fully understood, its effects are related to stimulation of endorphins, the autonomic nervous system, or pain control mechanisms at the local, meridian, or segmental level. It can be used in a variety of settings. It is safe in the hands of a trained professional. It has few contraindications.

SUBACUTE OR RECOVERY STAGE (FROM 3 DAYS TO WEEKS)

The focus during this stage of rehabilitation is restoration of joint and soft-tissue flexibility, strength endurance, and proprioception. These are the building blocks for normal movement and sport-specific activity. After initial focus on inflammation control, protected mobilization begins. The focus shifts from resolution of clinical signs and symptoms to restoration of function. The athlete must be closely monitored in regard to his or her response to the treatment, and any resumption of the inflammatory response signifies a need to reduce the level of rehabilitation activities. A gradated progression in force generation and degrees of freedom is necessary. Any setbacks can delay this phase of rehabilitation. It is generally the longest stage. Ongoing medications, modalities, and therapy technique use is constantly re-evaluated and minimized. Exercise prescription is the main feature of this stage of rehabilitation. A summary of interventions used in the recovery stage of rehabilitation is found in Table 25.3.

The exercise prescription

The team physician must identify deficits in flexibility, strength, and endurance. The exercise prescription is based on addressing these deficits. The components of the prescription are: type of exercise; frequency; duration; and intensity. See Table 25.4 for an overview.

Stretching

Athletes use stretching techniques to increase ROM and prevent injuries. In the setting of an injury, stretching decreases pain and reduces loss of ROM and

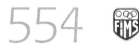

554

Table 25.3 Recovery rehabilitation stage

Intervention	Example	Indication
Exercise	Contract–relax stretching	Improve flexibility
	Closed kinetic chain exercise	Improve limb strength and co-contraction
	Open kinetic chain exercise	Improve strength
	Medicine ball	Prepare for sport-specific activity
	Exercise ball	Improve trunk strength
Aquatherapy	Flutter kick with kick board	Improve strength and conditioning
Modality	Superficial and deep heating	Facilitate stretching
	Superficial cold	Decrease post-exercise swelling
Medication	Analgesics	Reduce exercise related pain and swelling
	NSAIDs	
Immobilization	Taping	Improve kinesthetic sense
	Neoprene sleeve	
Massage	Cross-friction	Promote efficient scar formation
Manual therapy	Joint mobilization and/or manipulation	Restore physiological movement

Table 25.4 The exercise prescription

Element	Definition
Type of exercise	Specific activity the athlete will engage in
Frequency	Number of times per week
Duration	For strength training: – number of repetitions per set *and* – number of sets per session For endurance training: – total number of minutes
Intensity	For strength training: – % of repetition, maximum For endurance training: – % VO_2, or – % maximum heart rate

rehabilitation in sports medicine

flexibility. Vigorous stretching may be contraindicated with an acute muscle or myotendinous injury. Passive stretching is when another individual applies a stretch to a relaxed extremity; it must be done gently and slowly to avoid eliciting the stretch reflex. The stretch reflex is a protective reflex that prohibits injury to the muscle or joint after a rapid stretch. Heating modalities to increase the viscoelastic nature of collagen, used prior to stretching, can improve the results. Prolonged static stretching is a commonly used technique by athletes. With hands-on assistance or after instruction in correct positioning, the stretch should be held at the end of the available ROM for 30–60 seconds. Recognizing and utilizing physiologic responses can maximize the results. For example, reciprocal inhibition involves static stretching with contraction of the antagonist muscle group. The athlete moves the joint to the end of the available ROM and then isometrically contracts the antagonist muscle group for 30 seconds. This reduces the tendency to elicit the stretch reflex in the muscle being stretched. One type of proprioceptive neuromuscular facilitation (PNF) technique involves static stretching with contraction of the agonist muscle group. The athlete moves the joint to the end of the available ROM and then isometrically contracts the muscle group being stretched. The isometric contraction may increase the flexibility by relaxing the muscle via the golgi tendon organ or via stretching the connective tissue about the joint. Studies with athletes demonstrate the efficacy of this type of stretching. Flexibility can be addressed in post-surgical patients using a continuous passive machine (CPM) when active ROM is contraindicated or too painful. It minimizes joint stiffness and encourages nourishment of articular cartilage. The CPM encourages alignment of healing fibers via Wolff's law.

Strengthening

Strength is the maximal force that can be generated by a muscle at a specific velocity. Throughout the rehabilitation stages, an athlete should continue with his/her usual resistance training programs, with the exception of the injured extremity or region.

In the injured limb, static strengthening with isometric muscle contraction can be done during the acute stage and beyond, as, in some instances, limited joint stress but continued strengthening may be appropriate. For example, exercises such as straight leg raises can be done in the setting of a ligamentous knee injury. Dynamic strengthening can begin once the athlete tolerates static strengthening. Closed-kinetic-chain (CKC) exercises are introduced first (see Figure 25.3). The distal component of the extremity is fixed, thereby limiting the degrees of freedom of the extremity and joint forces. Once through the phase of protected mobilization, open-kinetic-chain (OKC) exercises can be prescribed (see Figure 25.4). The distal component of the limb is free, increasing the degrees of freedom of movement and increasing joint forces. The transition from CKC to OKC is particularly important in the upper extremity, which functions primarily in an open-kinetic-chain manner.

sheila a. dugan and walter r. frontera

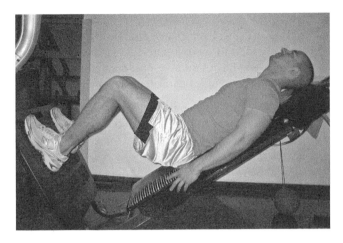

Figure 25.3 Closed-kinetic-chain exercise: Distal lower extremity is fixed
Source: Sol M. Abreu Sosa, MD

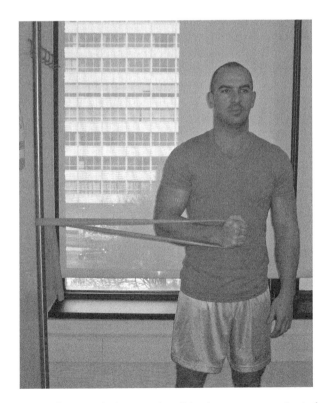

Figure 25.4 Open-kinetic-chain exercise: Distal upper extremity is free
Source: Sol M. Abreu Sosa, MD

The specific adaptation to imposed demand (SAID) principle requires that a muscle must be worked at a level higher than it is accustomed in order to increase strength. The workload can be varied to meet a particular goal. For example, exercising with a lower resistance and higher number of repetition builds endurance. Low-repetition, high-resistance workouts build strength.

Trunk (core) stabilization strengthening exercises are an important part of the rehabilitation process. When you consider the kinetic chain and the transmission of forces from the distal extremity to the proximal extremity to the trunk, it is key to maintain or increase core stability. The core is defined anatomically by the diaphragm superiorly, pelvic floor inferiorly, abdominals anteriorly and lumbar extensors posteriorly. Core-strengthening programs incorporate specific exercises, some that isolate and others that combine the muscular activation of the core. The muscles most frequently targeted include the transversus abdominis, multi-fidus, lumbar paraspinals, gluteus maximus and medius, and the pelvic-floor musculature.

Eccentric exercise (plyometrics)

Eccentric exercise uses the viscoelastic properties of muscle to increase force production. An eccentric action is applied to the muscle just prior to a concentric action (see Figure 25.5). This loads the sarcomeres and connective tissue. This type of contraction sequence is utilized in sport-specific activities. For example, basketball players will pre-load their calf muscles prior to jumping to rebound. Plyometric activities can be progressed by adding height to jumping surfaces or increasing the speed of the activity.

Power

One important aspect of an athlete's therapeutic exercise prescription, besides restoration and/or increase of ROM and increase of strengthening, is power training. Power is defined as the rate at which work is performed, or, in other words, the ability to move a weight, either an object or a human body, over a distance in relation to time. The ability to generate power is necessary in most sports. Power training is a form of strength training, where the main goal is to decrease the amount of time it takes you to apply a given force, or to increase the amount of force that can be generated in a given amount of time.

Kettlebells have been used for strength training, dynamic flexibility, and power training. The unique shape of the kettlebell allows an individual to develop power by performing the swinging exercise. During kettlebell training, an athlete undergoes a short, initial phase of concentric action, followed by momentum generated by the initial phase, and ending with a deceleration phase governed by eccentric muscle action. Power may be developed by swinging the kettlebell at a faster rate or by increasing the weight of the kettlebell.

sheila a. dugan and walter r. frontera

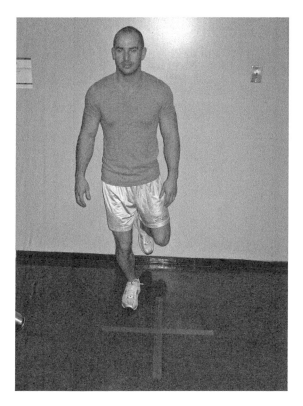

Figure 25.5 Plyometric exercise: Eccentric gastrocnemius–soleus action prior to concentric action

Source: Sol M. Abreu Sosa, MD

Endurance

Even with a brief injury time frame, significant deconditioning occurs. The muscles at the site of injury and muscles proximal and distal to the site are affected. Cross-training, or ongoing endurance training utilizing a different exercise type, should begin immediately. Aquatherapy, including water jogging or swimming, an upper body exerciser (UBE), or one-legged exercycle can be used in the setting of a lower-extremity injury. For upper-extremity injuries, walking, running, or exercycle can continue, if tolerated.

As recovery continues, high-repetition, low-resistance strength training programs can target involved muscles. Taping or bracing provides protected mobility. As recovery continues, conditioning deficits must be addressed prior to safe return to sport. A structured, stepwise progression of training time and activity level should be set and followed.

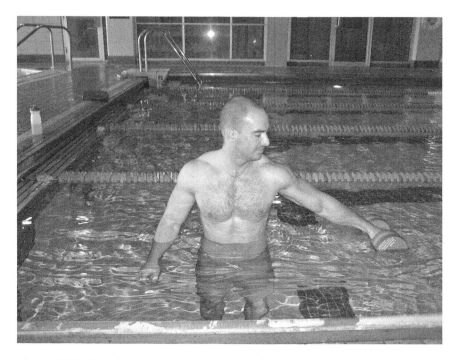

Figure 25.6 Aquatherapy: Using properties of water to facilitate exercise
Source: Sol M. Abreu Sosa, MD

Aquatherapy

Aquatherapy is a hybrid technique used in rehabilitation. As reviewed previously, whirlpools can be used for heating or cooling modalities. More importantly, the injured athlete can take advantage of the properties of the water to exercise (Figure 25.6). Exercise in water facilitates movement, prevents muscle atrophy, and limits loss of ROM. The aquatic environment can also be used generally for cross-training and earlier and more aggressive rehabilitation of sports injuries. Buoyancy supports body weight and can allow active exercise, even when reduced weight-bearing through an injured extremity is necessary. Hydrostatic pressure can reduce edema and aid in removal of cellular waste products. The viscosity of the water can add to the athlete's proprioceptive joint sense. It allows progression of resistance proportional to the effort exerted, flotation device applied, and direction of movement. Control of water temperature can be helpful for pain management. There are significant effects on the cardiac and pulmonary systems with immersion in water, and this should be taken into account.

FUNCTIONAL STAGE (FROM WEEKS TO MONTHS)

The focus of this stage of rehabilitation includes improved neuromuscular control, sport-specific and multiplane activity, and cessation of maladaptive behaviors that could lead to a future injury. The athlete completes this stage when he or she can meet the return-to-play criteria. Therapeutic-modality and medication use is only needed intermittently, related to exacerbation. An exercise program including flexibility, strengthening, and proprioception is well established. Progression of sport-specific activity allows for successful return to play. The focus on correct technique will prevent future injury.

See Table 25.5 for a review of interventions in this phase.

Table 25.5 Functional rehabilitation stage

Intervention	Example	Indication
Exercise	Balance beam	Improve balance
	Minitrampoline	Increase proprioception
	Figure-8 drills	Improve agility and foot placement
	Jump training	Improve tensile strength of muscle–tendon unit and ligaments
	Overhead throwing	Regain sport-specific neuromuscular control
	Exercise-ball program	Maintain proximal stability and alignment
		Prevent future injury

Functional retraining

The athlete must go beyond the improvement in flexibility, strength, and conditioning and practice sport-specific activity prior to returning to play. Forces of gravity, momentum, and ground reaction in multiple planes of motion dictate sports-related function. Functional or sport-specific retraining includes kinetic-chain, balance, proprioception, and agility drills. The athlete must be closely supervised during this critical period and progressed appropriately.

Kinetic chain

The team physician must evaluate the entire kinetic chain of movement. Biomechanical deficits in joints outside the injured limb can lead to re-injury. In fact, this may have led to the current injury. For example, a baseball pitcher transmits forces from the lower limbs, via the trunk, to augment force production in the upper limb. Therefore, identifying and treating flexibility and strength deficits in the lower limbs and trunk are an important part of the rehabilitation process. Motion analysis using videotaping can also be helpful in reinforcing correct movement patterns once biomechanical deficits have been addressed. Lower-extremity weight-bearing exercise must be done in the frontal, sagittal, and transverse planes, training both concentric and eccentric lower-extremity musculature in a functional way. Eccentric contractions are crucial in slowing or decelerating segments of the body that have acquired kinetic energy, such as the lower limbs in running. Let's consider an athlete with an ACL injury. The goal of rehabilitation is to provide exercise training that simulates sports-related activities. This expands his/her biomechanical and neurophysiological repertoire so that he/she is prepared to return to the field of play with enhanced performance and reduced re-injury rate.

Balance and proprioception

Balance is a dynamic component of sports performance. Early dynamic balance activities such as wobble-board training are followed by activity at varying speeds and intensities (Figure 25.7). Simulation of sport-specific movement patterns can help identify functional balance deficits. Proprioceptive deficits result from injury, depending on the tissue injured and the length of immobilization. Injuries to the anterior talofibular ligament (ATFL) or ACL can impair sensory feedback from the ankle or knee. Unilateral stance or step-ups and -downs allow co-contraction about

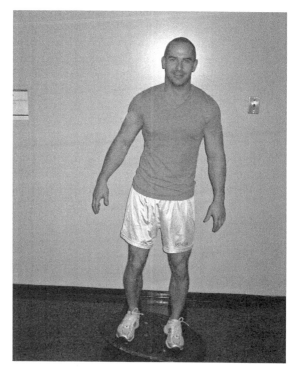

Figure 25.7 Wobble board: Retraining balance and proprioception
Source: Sol M. Abreu Sosa, MD

562

the lower-extremity joints, increasing the joint position sense. Upper-extremity proprioception and co-contraction can be enhanced with closed-chain weight-bearing activities over an exercise ball.

Agility drills

Agility drills are incorporated prior to returning to play. Tasks such as figure-8 or star drills require cutting and pivoting, causing rotational and translation moments in many planes at the joints. Hand–eye coordination and appropriate foot placement are required. This improves the neuromuscular control of the athlete. The athlete should perform sport-specific agility drills on the surface of play and with the correct sporting equipment prior to returning to competition.

CONCLUSION

The purpose of our chapter is to acquaint the reader with rehabilitation in sports medicine. We have covered the stages of injury and repair. We have discussed the use of medications, physical modalities, and therapy techniques. We have defined the three stages of sports rehabilitation, the acute, recovery, and functional stages, and reviewed the management of each. We hope this review provides a practical framework from which the team physician can prescribe treatment. This treatment should be based on physiologic principles. The ultimate goal of rehabilitation is the safe, expedient return of the athlete to the field of play. The team physician should focus on treatments that limit the inflammatory response and promote healing, to provide functional recovery as early as possible. By identifying and treating biomechanical deficits, the team physician can also strive to prevent future injuries in the athlete. Rehabilitation truly does begin at the time of injury and continues beyond the time of return to play.

ACKNOWLEDGMENTS

Photographs courtesy of Sol M. Abreu Sosa, MD, Chief Resident, Physical Medicine and Rehabilitation, Rush University Medical Center, with thanks to demonstrator model James B. Spendley, DO.

SUGGESTED READING

Acute Pain Management Guideline Panel, 1992. Acute pain management: Operative medical procedures and trauma. Clinical practice guidelines. *AHCPR Pub No. 92–00332*, February.
Akuthota, V. and Nadler, S., 2004. Core strengthening. *Arch. Phys. Med. Rehabil.*, Volume 85, pp. 886–92.
Almekinders, L., 1993. Anti-inflammatory treatment of muscular injury in sports. *Sports Med.*, Volume 15, pp. 139–45.
Bruckner, P. and Khan, K., 1993. *Clinical Sports Medicine*. Sydney, Austrailia: McGraw-Hill.

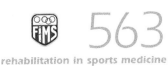

Brummit, J., En Gilpin, H., Brunette, M., and Meira, E., 2010. Incorporating kettlebells into a lower extremity sports rehabilitation program. *North American Journal of Sports Physical Therapy*, Volume Dec 5(4), pp. 257–65.

Chandler, T. and Kibler, W., 1992. The role of muscular strength in injury prevention. In: P. Renström, ed. *The Encylopedia of Sports Medicine, Sports Injuries, Basic Prevention and Care*. Oxford: Blackwell Scientific Publications, pp. 252–61.

Childs, J. and Irrgang, J., 2003. The language of exercise and rehabilitation. In: J. DeLee, D. Drez, and M. Miller, eds. *DeLee & Drez's Orthopaedic Sports Medicine: Principles and Practice*. 2nd ed. Philadelphia: WB Saunders, pp. 319–35.

Corrigan, B. and Maitland, G., 1994. *Musculoskeletal & Sports Injuries*. Oxford: Butterworth-Heinemann.

Cucurullo, S., 2008. *Physical Medicine and Rehabilitation Board Review*. 2nd ed. New York: Demos Medical.

DeLisa, J., 2010. *Physical Medicine and Rehabilitation: Principles and Practice*. 5th ed. Philadelphia: Lippincott, Williams & Wilkins.

Dreyfuss, P. and Stratton, S., 1993. The low-energy laser, electro-acuscope, and neuroprobe. *Phys. Sports Med.*, Volume 21(8), pp. 47–57.

Dugan, S., 2005. Sports-related knee injuries in female athletes: What gives?. *Am. J. Phys. Med. Rehabil.*, Volume 84, pp. 122–30.

Fleck, S. and Falkel, J., 1986. Value of resistance training for the reduction of sports injuries. *Sports Med.*, Volume 3, pp. 61–8.

Gann, N., 1991. Ultrasound: Current concepts. *Clin. Manage.*, Volume 11(4), pp. 64–9.

Gersh, M., 1992. *Electrotherapy in Rehabilitation*. Philadelphia: FA Davis.

Greenman, P., 1996. *Principles of Manual Medicine*. 2nd ed. Baltimore: Williams and Wilkens.

Halseth, T. et al., 2004. The effects of Keniso taping on proprioception at ankle. *Journal of Sports Science and Medicine*, Volume 3, pp. 1–7.

Harrison, R. and Bulstrode, S., 1987. Percentage weight-bearing during partial immersion in the hydrotherapy pool. *Physiother. Pract.*, Volume 3, pp. 60–3.

Jay, K. et al., 2011. Kettlebell training for musculoskeletal and cardiovascular health: A randomized controlled trial. *Scandinavian Journal of Work, Environment and Health*, 37(May), pp. 196–203.

Kaltenborn, F., 1975. *Manual Therapy of the Extremity Joints*. Oslo: Bokhandel.

Kaplan, R., 2005. Current status of nonsteroidal anti-inflammatory drugs in physiatry: Balancing the risks and benefits in pain management. *Am. J. Phys. Med. Rehabil.*, Volume 84, pp. 885–94.

Kibler, W., Herring, S., and Press, J. eds., 1998. *Functional Rehabilitation of Sports and Musculoskeletal Injuries*. Gaithersburg, MD: Aspen Publications.

Kraemer, W., Duncan, N. et al., 1998. Resistance training and elite athletes: Adaptations and program considerations. *J. Orthop. Sports Phys. Ther.*, Volume 28, pp. 110–17.

Leadbetter, W., 1994. Soft tissue injuries. In: F. Fu and D. Stone, eds. *Sports Injuries – Mechanisms, Prevention and Treatment*. Baltimore: Williams and Wilkins, pp. 733–80.

Lephart, S. and Henry, T., 1995. Functional rehabilitation for the upper and lower extremity. *Orthop. Clin. North Am.*, Volume 26, pp. 572–9.

Magee, D., 2008. *Orthopedic Physical Assessment*. 5th ed. St. Louis, MO: Saunders Elsiever.

Maitland, G., 1986. *Vertebral Manipulation*. 5th ed. London: Butterworths.

Merrick, M., Rankin, J., et al., 1999. A preliminary examination of cryotherapy and secondary injury in skeletal muscle. *Med. Sci. Sports Exerc.*, Volume 31, pp. 1516–21.

Prentice, W., 1994. *Rehabilitation Techniques in Sports Medicine*. 2nd ed. St. Louis, MO: Mosby.

Richardson, C., Jull, G., Hodges, P., et al., 1999. *Therapeutic Exercise for Spinal Segmental Stabilitation in Low Back Pain: Scientific Basis and Clinical Approach*. Edinburgh: Churchill Livingstone.

Ryan, E. and Stone, J., 1991. Specific approaches to rehabilitation of athletic injury. In: W. Grana and A. Kalenak, eds. *Clinical Sports Medicine*. Philadelphia: WB Saunders Company, pp. 255–63.

Sharkey, B., 1991. Training for sport. In: R. Cantu and L. Michelli, eds. *ACSM's Guidelines for the Team Physician*. Philadelphia: Lea & Febiger, pp. 34–47.

Shellock, F. and Prentice, W., 1985. Warming up and stretching for improved physical performance and prevention of sports-related injuries. *Sports Med.*, Volume 2, pp. 267–78.

Standen, R., 1997. Rehabilitation and physiotherapy of the elite athlete. In: E. Sherry and D. Bokor, eds. *Sports Medicine Problems and Practical Management*. London: Greenwich Medical Media, pp. 309–17.

Thacker, S., Gilchrist, J., Stroup, D., et al., 2004. The impact of stretching on sports injury risk: A systematic review of the literature. *Med. Sci. Sports Exerc.*, Volume 36, pp. 371–8.

Thein, J. and Brody, L., 1998. Aquatic-based rehabilitation and training for the elite athlete. *J. Orthop. Sports Phys. Ther.*, Volume 27, pp. 332–41.

Tippet, S. and Voight, M., 1995. *Functional Progressions for Sports Rehabilitation*. Champaign, IL: Human Kinetics.

Vleeming, A., Pool-Goudzwaard, A., Stoeckart, R., et al., 1995. The posterior layer of the thoracolumbar fascia: Its function in load transfer from spine to legs. *Spine*, Volume 2, pp. 753–8.

Young, J. and Press, J., 1994. The physiologic basis of sports rehabilitation. *Phys. Med. Rehabil. Clin. North Am.*, Volume 5, pp. 9–36.

INDEX

index

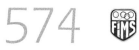

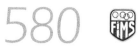

584